Current Research in Herbal Medicine

Current Research in Herbal Medicine

Edited by Cameron James

STATES
ACADEMIC PRESS
www.statesacademicpress.com

States Academic Press,
109 South 5th Street,
Brooklyn, NY 11249, USA

Visit us on the World Wide Web at:
www.statesacademicpress.com

ISBN: 978-1-63989-136-8

Cataloging-in-Publication Data

Current research in herbal medicine / edited by Cameron James.
p. cm.
Includes bibliographical references and index.
ISBN 978-1-63989-136-8
1. Herbs--Therapeutic use. 2. Pharmacognosy. 3. Herbal abortifacients.
4. Herbal contraceptives. I. James, Cameron.

RM666.H33 C87 2022
615.321--dc23

Table of Contents

Preface

A plant or a part of a plant which is utilized for its therapeutic properties is termed as an herb. The branch of complementary medicine which makes use of biologically active natural products for the treatment and management of various diseases is termed as herbal medicine. It can also be used to boost health and immunity. Along with parts of plants, it can also encompass minerals, shells and fungal products. One of the fundamental aspects of herbal medicine is the usage of unrefined plant and animal extracts, with minimal processing. It is believed within this field that less processing makes the products safer and more effective. Such selected concepts that redefine herbal medicine have been presented in this book. There has been rapid progress in this field and its applications are finding their way across multiple industries. Those in search of information to further their knowledge will be greatly assisted by this book.

The information contained in this book is the result of intensive hard work done by researchers in this field. All due efforts have been made to make this book serve as a complete guiding source for students and researchers. The topics in this book have been comprehensively explained to help readers understand the growing trends in the field.

I would like to thank the entire group of writers who made sincere efforts in this book and my family who supported me in my efforts of working on this book. I take this opportunity to thank all those who have been a guiding force throughout my life.

Editor

1

Quality Control by Immunoaffinity Concentration using Monoclonal Antibody

Takuhiro Uto and Nguyen Huu Tung
Nagasaki International University
Japan

1. Introduction

The rapid and sensitive methods for separation and quantification of bioactive compounds are essential for quality control of the traditional Chinese medicine (TCM) and crude extracts. However, it seems that the current systems in use are not necessarily optimum approaches. For example, various methods for separation and quantification of glycyrrhizin (GC), the main active constituent in licorice (*Glycyrrhiza* spp.), have been used such as gas chromatography, high performance liquid chromatography (HPLC), and micellar trokinetic chromatography (Ong, 2002; Lay et al., 2004; Tan et al., 2002). Commercial purification of GC typically progressed through several steps, including crystallization, column chromatography, and liquid partitioning. However, these methods are far from satisfactory analytical purpose in terms of high sensitivity, reproducibility, large amounts of extraction solvents and time-consuming factors.

Owning to the rapid development of the molecular biosciences and their biotechnological applications, immunoassays using monoclonal antibodies (MAbs) against target molecules such as proteins, drugs and low-molecular-weight bioactive compounds have become one of the important tools by taking advantage of their specificity. Immunoassay by MAbs is used in a wide variety of analysis such as receptor binding assays, enzyme assays, and quantitative and qualitative analytical techniques both *in vivo* and *in vitro* studies.

Immunoaffinity purification is a highly specific technique that has the potential to be used for the one-step isolation of a target molecule from many complex mixtures like a cellular lysate. Immunoaffinity columns are conjugated with MAbs and work by specifically binding and removing the target molecules. Several immunoaffinity columns like a protein G affinity column for MAbs expressed by hybridoma and a metal chelate affinity column for single chain variable fragment (Fv) proteins expressed by *E. coli* have been commonly used for the purification of peptides and proteins. Application of an immunoaffinity column may decrease the amount of solvent used and the number of purification steps, shorten analysis time, and simplify sample analysis compared to traditional cleanup techniques. Although immunoaffinity purification against higher molecule analyte such as peptides and proteins are widely used in the research and commercial ways, there are too few cases of immunoaffinity purification targeting a small molecule compound. Fortunately, in our ongoing studies of naturally occurring bioactive compounds we have prepared many kinds of MAbs against terpenoids (Sakata et al., 1994; Xuan et al., 1999; Lu et al., 2003), alkaloids (Shoyama et al., 1996; Kim et al. 2004), plant saponins (Tanaka et al., 1999; Fukuda et al.,

2000b; Zhu et al., 2004; Shan et al., 2001; Ishiyama et al., 1996), and phenolics (Morinaga et al., 2000; Morinaga et al., 2001; Tanaka et al., 1996; Loungratana et al., 2004), and set up the enzyme-linked immunosorbent assay (ELISA) for quality control of the TCM. Furthermore, we have been establishing several affinity column with MAb against a kind of terpenoid, forskolin (Yanagihara et al., 1996), solasodine glycosides (Putalun et al., 1999), ginsenosides Rb1 (Fukuda et al., 2000c), and GC (Xu et al., 2007).

In this chapter, we introduce the new strategy to isolate and concentrate the target bioactive compounds from the crude extract by immunoaffinity column using individual MAb. We succeeded one-step purification of target compounds by MAb-conjugated immunoaffinity column, which leads to the knock-out (KO) extract which contains all components except an antigen molecule. The KO extract will be useful for the pharmacological investigation to reveal real effects of bioactive compound in the crude extract and the interaction between the target compound and other compounds.

2. One step concentration by immunoaffinity column conjugated with anti-ginsenoside Rb1 MAb

Ginseng, the crude drug of *Panax ginseng* root, has been used as a therapeutic herbal medicine in Asian countries and one of the most important components in TCM for thousands of years. The pharmacological and biological activities of ginseng have been reported to have anti-aging, anti-cancer, anti-inflammation, anti-diabetics, anti-stress, maintenance of homeostasis, and to affect on central nervous system and immune function (Gillis et al., 1997). Ginsenosides are believed to account for the pharmacological activities of ginseng. It is well known that the concentrations of ginsenosides vary in the ginseng root or the root extracts depending on the method of extraction, subsequent treatment, or even the season of its collection (Kitagawa et al., 1989; Tanaka et al., 1989). Recently, the individual ginsenosides in ginseng are purified by preparative HPLC. However, the repeated purification is required and may result in the decrease of the final yield. Therefore, the developed approaches for quality control are required in the field of TCM.

Ginsenosides are normally fractioned into two groups based on the types of aglycone, namely the protopanaxadiol group and the protopanaxatriol group. Within more than 30 different ginsenosides, ginsenoside Rb1 (G-Rb1), one of the protopanaxadiols, is considered the most important active factor (Washida & Kitanaka, 2003). G-Rb1 has various biological activities, including facilitating acquisition and retrieval of memory (Mook-Jung et al., 2001), scavenging free radicals (Lim et al., 1997), inhibition of calcium over-influx into neurons (Liu & Zhang, 1995), and preserving the structural integrity of the neurons (Jiang & Qian, 1995).

To control the quality of ginseng, the preparation of anti-G-Rb1 MAb, set up of ELISA, and a new immunostaining method named Eastern blotting were reported (Tanaka et al., 1999; Fukuda et al., 2000a). Herein, we describe an immunoaffinity column procedure for G-Rb1 and its application in single step isolation from crude extract of ginseng root.

2.1 Preparation of immunoaffinity column against G-Rb1

Purified anti-G-Rb1 MAb (10 mg) in diluted Affi-Gel Hz coupling buffer was dialyzed against the coupling buffer two times. The dialyzed anti-G-Rb1 MAb was treated by $NaIO_4$ to give dialdehyde group in sugar moiety which was coupled to Affi-Gel Hz hydrazide gel. The immunoaffinity gel was packed into plastic mini-column (Figure 1).

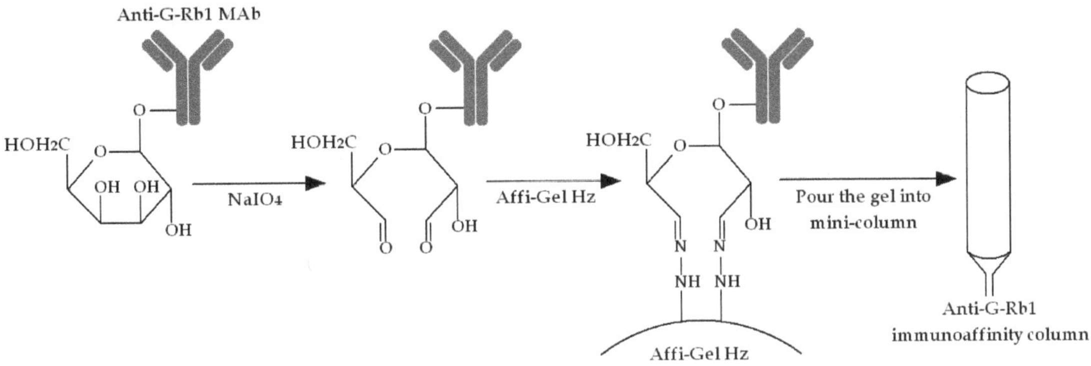

Fig. 1. Scheme of preparation of anti-G-Rb1 immunoaffinity column

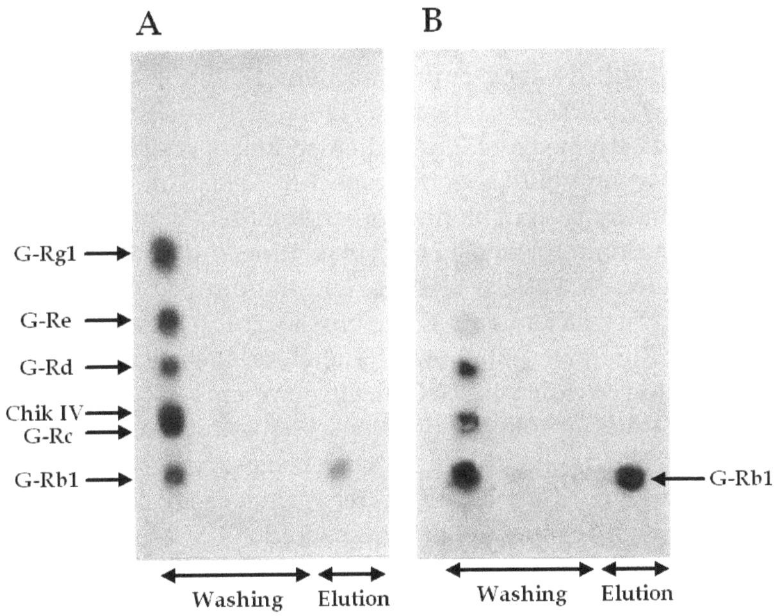

Fig. 2. TLC (A) and Eastern blotting (B) profiles for a standardized ginsenosides mixture. The TLC plate and Eastern blotting membrane were stained by H_2SO_4 and incubated with anti-G-Rb1 MAb, respectively

2.2 Optimal buffer systems for separation of G-Rb1

Firstly, to examine the optimal conditions of adsorption and elution, 400 μg of G-Rb1 was dissolved in phosphate buffer (PB) and loaded on anti-G-Rb1 affinity column. After washing with washing buffer (20 mM PB containing 0.5 M NaCl), various buffer solutions for elution were loaded on the column, and then the recovery efficiency was determined by ELISA. The G-Rb1 concentration was slightly increased by eluting with a 20 mM PB containing 0.5 M KSCN and 10 % MeOH. When the 20 mM PB was changed to 100 mM AcOH buffer (pH 4), the elution ability reached the optimal level. Since 20 % MeOH could elute G-Rb1 efficiently, higher MeOH concentration of over 20 % was ineffective. Thus, 100 mM AcOH buffer containing 0.5 M KSCN and 20 % MeOH could be used as an elution buffer in subsequent immunoaffinity chromatography.

2.3 One step purification of G-Rb1 from a standardized ginsenosides mixture by anti-G-Rb1 immunoaffinity column

To confirm the concentration of G-Rb1 by anti-G-Rb1 affinity column, a ginsenoside mixture containing 100 μg each of ginsenoside Rg1, Re, Rd, Rc, and chikusetsusaponin IV (chik IV; an oleanane-type saponin) were loaded on the column. Figure 2 shows the TLC and Eastern blotting profiles of ginsenosides and chik IV in washing and elution buffers flowed from the affinity column. When the column was washed with washing buffer (20 mM PB containing 0.5 M NaCl), ginsenoside Rg1, Re, Rd, Rc, chik IV, and overcharged G-Rb1 were detected. After these compounds were completely washed out by washing buffer, the G-Rb1 bound to anti-G-Rb1 MAb was eluted by elution buffer (100 mM AcOH buffer containing 0.5 M KSCN and 20 % MeOH).

2.4 One step purification of G-Rb1 from crude extract of P. ginseng roots by anti-G-Rb1 immunoaffinity column

A crude extract of *P. ginseng* roots (3.8 mg) was loaded onto anti-G-Rb1 immunoaffinity column. After washing with washing buffer (fractions 1-20), the column was eluted with elution buffer (fractions 21-40). As shown in Figure 3, the G-Rb1 concentration in the collected fractions was determined by ELISA. After loading of crude extract, overcharged G-Rb1 was detected in washing buffer of fractions 1-8. G-Rc, Rd, Re, and Rg1 were also detected in these fractions by Eastern blotting procedure (data not shown). A sharp peak of G-Rb1 was observed around fractions 21-24 of elution buffer. However, these eluted fractions were investigated by Eastern blotting, and the purified G-Rb1 in these fractions was still contaminated by a small amount of malonyl-G-Rb1, which having almost the same cross-reactivity with G-Rb1 (data not shown). Therefore, the mixture was treated with a mild alkaline solution (0.1 % KOH in MeOH) at room temperature to give pure G-Rb1. Overcharged G-Rb1 in washing solution (fractions 1-8) was repeatedly loaded and finally isolated in pure form. The anti-G-Rb1 MAb was stable during all procedures, and the immunoaffinity column showed almost no decrease in capacity (20 μg of G-Rb1/ml gel) after repeated use more than 10 times under same conditions.

After washing the column, each fraction of washing and elution were deionized and the solvent was lyophilized. Figure 4 demonstrated that TLC profile of the purification steps. Lane 1 and 2 were spotted the standard of ginsenosides (G-Rd, G-Rc, G-Rb1, G-Rg1, and G-Re). Lane A, B, and C were the crude extract, the washing fraction, and the eluted fraction, respectively. In the crude extract (lane A), all spots of ginsenosides were clearly detected. Interestingly, the washing fraction (lane B) contained all of the ginsenosides in the crude extract except G-Rb1. Furthermore, the spot of G-Rb1 was detected in the eluted fractions (lane C). These data strongly indicated that G-Rb1 molecule in the ginseng extract can be eliminated by an anti-G-Rb1 immunoaffinity column and the washing fractions was knock-out only by the antigen molecule, G-Rb1. Thus, we named the washing fractions a knock-out (KO) extract (Wang & Shoyama, 2006; Tanaka et al., 2007).

Since we succeeded the preparation of MAbs having a wide cross-reactivity like anti-solamargine MAb (Ishiyama et al., 1996), anti-saikosaponin a (Zhu et al., 2004) and ginsenoside-Re (Morinaga et al., 2006), the related total saponins can be removed by an immunoaffinity column conjugated with MAb in the case of solasodine glycosides, as reported previously (Putalun et al., 1999). The newly developed KO extract may be useful for the determination of real pharmacologically active principle in the TCMs.

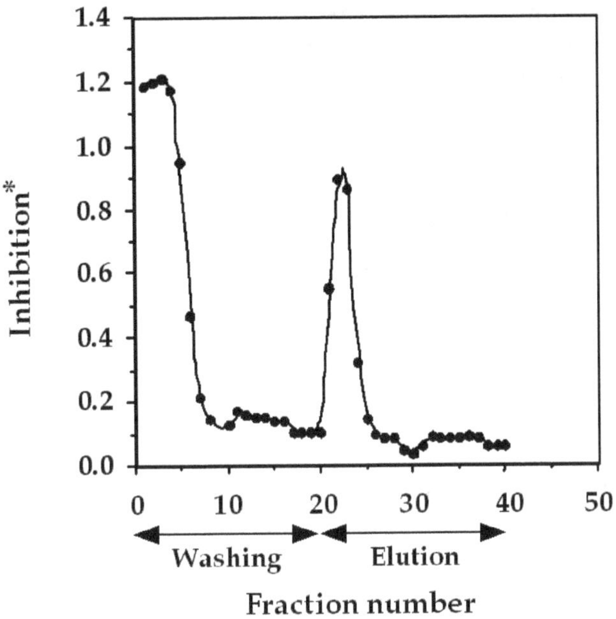

Fig. 3. Elution profile of *P. ginseng* crude extract by anti-G-Rb1 immunoaffinity column. G-Rb1 of each fraction was monitoring by ELISA using anti-G-Rb1 MAb. The volume of individual fraction was 2 mL. *Inhibition = $(A_0\text{-}A)/A_0$;A_0 is the absorbance in the absence of the test compounds. A is the absence in the presence the test compounds (Fukuda et al., 2000c)

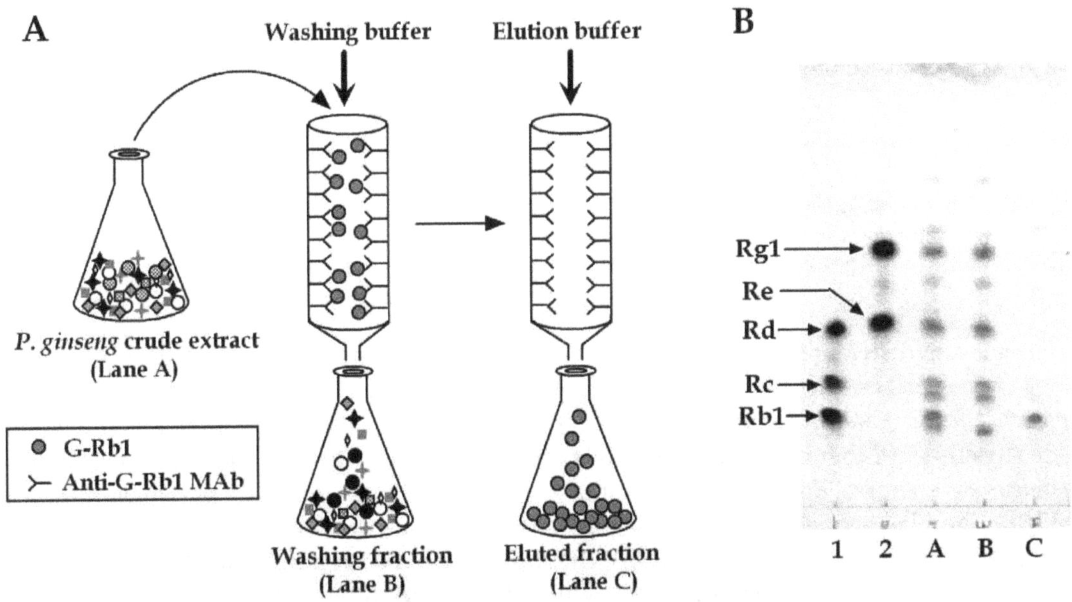

Fig. 4. Scheme of the preparation of G-Rb1 KO extract from *P. ginseng* crude extract using anti-G-Rb1 immunoaffinity column (A) and TLC profile of the separated fractions by the column (B). Lane 1 and 2 indicate the standard of ginsenosides (G-Rd, G-Rc, G-Rb1, G-Rg1, and G-Re). Lane A, B, and C were the crude extract, the washing fraction, and the eluted fraction, respectively (Fukuda et al., 2000c)

2.5 Isolation and determination of ginsenosides by anti-G-Rb1 immunoaffinity column

The anti-G-Rb1 immunoaffinity column could separate G-Rb1 from the crude extract of *P. ginseng*. In this case, malonyl-G-Rb1 was also eluted by elution buffer together with G-Rb1, because that this anti-G-Rb1 MAb has the cross-reactivity with malonyl-G-Rb1. Therefore, the pre-treatment of *P. ginseng* extract with a mild alkaline solution was needed to convert into pure G-Rb1.

Table 1 indicates the G-Rb1 concentration in several ginseng roots determined by ELISA by anti-G-Rb1 MAb and HPLC after pre-treatment under mildly alkaline condition. The fibrous ginseng made from the active growing part of *P. ginseng* showed the highest G-Rb1 concentration. White ginseng was prepared from *P. ginseng* simply by drying. The concentration of G-Rb1 was higher than that red ginseng, but lower compared with the other samples except Japanese ginseng. Red ginseng is prepared by steaming and drying the root of *P. ginseng*. Eastern blotting analysis indicated that the red ginseng contained few of malonyl-G-Rb1, which is a distinctive feature of it (data not shown). These data suggests that the steaming step for the preparation of red ginseng decreases the concentration of G-Rb1 by conversion into C-20 hydroxy free ginsenosides (Kitagawa et al., 1983). Among these tested samples, the lowest concentration of G-Rb1 was detected in Japanese ginseng (*P. japonicus*). Interestingly, the G-Rb1 concentration of *P. japonicus* was not correlated between ELISA and HPLC.

Sample	G-Rb1 content (μg/mg dry wt.)	
	ELISA	HPLc
White ginseng (*P. ginseng*)	5.49 ± 0.75	4.96 ± 0.05
Red ginseng	3.57 ± 0.62	3.93 ± 0.34
Fibrous ginseng	64.44 ± 3.64	69.75 ± 1.45
San-chi ginseng (*P. notoginseng*)	47.08 ± 3.34	42.39 ± 1.39
American ginseng (*P. quinquefolium*)	48.51 ± 1.79	47.96 ± 1.04
Japanese ginseng (*P. japonicus*)	1.37 ± 0.34	0.63 ± 0.06

Table 1. G-Rb1 content of various ginseng samples after pre-treatment with mildly alkaline condition

P. japonicus is distributed in Japan and China and it is morphologically different from the other *Panax* species. The phytochemical profiles indicated that no G-Rbl was detected in *P. japonicus*, and isolated oleanane-type saponins named as chikusetsusaponins and elucidated their structures (Yahara et al., 1977). Morita et al. examined the varieties of saponins in *P. japonicus* by chemical analysis (Morita et al., 1985). From these results, the concentration of G-Rb1 might be trace level in *P. japonicus*. However, as shown in Table 1, G-Rb1 was detected by ELISA in *P. japonicus* crude extract pre-treated with a mild alkaline solution and found higher concentrations compared with HPLC and previous reports (Morita et al., 1985). This data suggest that anti-G-Rb1 MAb using ELISA has the cross-reactivity with some unknown compounds.

To investigate the unknown compounds bound to anti-G-Rb1 MAb, the crude extract of *P. japonicus* was concentrated by immunoaffinity column using anti-G-Rb1 MAb. The crude root extract was loaded on the column and washed with the washing buffer, followed by the elution buffer as indicated in Figure 4. Figure 5 shows the H_2SO_4 staining (A) and the Eastern blotting (B) profiles of the two fractions separated by the immunoaffinity column. Fractions eluted with the washing buffer (lane A-D) showed many spots, including ginsenosides and chikusetsusaponins, similar to the original extract of *P. japonicus*. After washing, the column was eluted by elution buffer (lane E), and then one spot was detected. Interestingly, Eastern blotting indicated two different spots on lane A (the washing fraction containing the overcharged compounds) and one spot on each lane B and E. These compounds bound with anti-G-Rb1 MAb have a dammarane saponin having protopanaxadiol as a framework.

Compound 1 detected in the washing fraction had an Rf value close to that of G-Rd, indicating that this compound has three sugar moieties in a molecule. Considering the previous study compound 1 is chikusetsusaponin III (chik III) has three sugars, one xylose and two glcoses in a molecule (Morita et al., 1985) (Figure 6). Finally, this compound was identified as chik III in a direct comparison with authentic sample. These data indicated that the specificity of anti-G-Rb1 MAb against chik III of immunoaffinity column is higher than that of Eastern blotting because the antigen (chik III) conjugated with carrier protein via sugar chain to fix on the membrane in case of Eastern blotting, so the structure of chik III was changed.

Another unknown spot, compound 2 appeared in fraction A of the overcharged washing fraction and fraction E of the eluted fraction. G-Rb1 was not detected by Eastern blotting although it was determined by TLC as indicated in Figure 5. It can be suggested that compound 2 has a similar molecular structure and cross-reactivity with G-Rb1, and seems to be related ginseng saponin having protopanaxadiol as an aglycone. Moreover, compound 2 is more polar than G-Rb1, indicating that it possess 5 sugar moiety compared with G-Rb1. Although compound 2 was treated with a mild alkaline solution, no change occurred. From these evidences compound 2 might be chikusetsusaponin III-20-*O*-gentiobiose (chikusetsusaponin VI; Figure 6) having 5 sugars in a molecule in good agreement with the R_f value previously reported (Kohda et al., 1991) and we confirmed that compound 2 is chik VI by the direct comparison with authentic sample (Fukuda et al., 2000a).

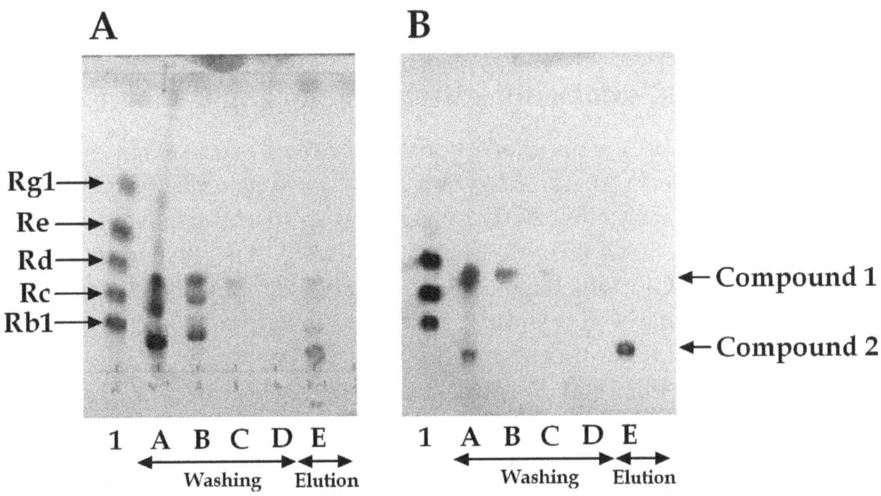

Fig. 5. TLC (A) and Eastern blotting (B) profiles of the separated fractions from *P. japonicus* crude extract by the anti-G-Rb1 immunoaffinity column. Lane 1 indicates the standard of ginsenosides (G-Rd, G-Rc, G-Rb1, G-Rg1, and G-Re). Lane A-D and Lane E were the washing fractions and the eluted fraction, respectively (Fukuda et al., 2000a)

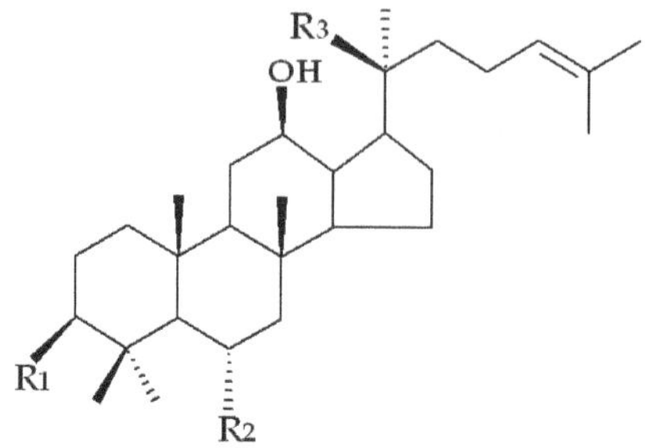

Compound	R1	R2	R3
G-Rb1	-O-Glc-^{2}Glc	-H	-O-Glc-^{6}Glc
Chik III	-O-Glc-^{6}Xyl ^{2}\ Glc	-H	-OH
Chik VI	-O-Glc-^{6}Xyl ^{2}\ Glc	-H	-O-Glc-^{6}Glc

Fig. 6. Chemical structures of G-Rb1 and chikusetsusaponins purified from *P. japonicus* by the anti-G-Rb1 immunoaffinity column

Taken together, *P. japonicus* root contains no G-Rb1 as previously reported (Yahara et al., 1977). However, the immunoaffinity column conjugated with anti-G-Rb1 MAb could concentrate some unknown structurally resemble compounds having cross-reactivity against anti-G-Rb1 MAb. Thus, this purification system will be applied to survey new compounds related to target compound of MAb. In a previous report, a immunoaffinity purification against solasodine glycosides purified all solasodine glycosides by one-step purification. In this case, all solasodine glycoside have almost same cross-reactivity against anti-solamargine MAb (Ishiyama et al., 1996).

3. Preparation of GC-knock out extract and its application for in vitro assay

Licorice (*Glycyrrhiza* spp.) is another important crude drug used in over 70 % of TCMs. It mainly consists of dried roots and stolons of *Glycyrrhizae uralensis, G. inflate* and *G. glabra.* Licorice is prescribed with other herbal medicines as an anti-tussive, an expectorant, and an anti-inflammatory agent (Asl & Hosseinzadeh, 2008). The pharmacological properties of licorice depend upon GC, which is considered to be its main active constituent (Figure 7). It has been reported that GC exhibits numerous pharmacological effects such as anti-inflammation, anti-ulcer, anti-cancer, and anti-viral activities (Asl et al., 2008; Wang & Nixon, 2001; Doll & Hill, 1962; Pompei et al., 1979). Clinically, GC has been used to treat patients with chronic hepatitis (Schalm et al., 1999; Coon & Ernst, 2004). Moreover, GC is used in food additives and cosmetics as a well-known natural sweetener (Kim & Kinghorn, 2002). The quality standardization of licorice is usually based on its GC content. Recently, the utilization volume of licorice is rapidly increasing, while the availability of wild licorice has declined to curb overexploitation of the natural resources (Yamamoto et al., 2003; Hayashi et al., 2003). For the promotion of effective cultivation of licorice as an additional and stable herbal resource, the rapid and easy measurement methods of the GC content are required. Previously, we established anti-GC MAb and a fast and sensitive assay system using the MAb for the screening of GC concentration in large numbers of samples (Tanaka & Shoyama, 1998; Shan et al., 2001), the sensitive detection of GC by surface plasmon resonance-based immunosensor (Sakai et al., 2004), and the rapid detection by immunochromatographic assay (Putalun et al., 2005). The purpose of our recent studies is to purify and quantify GC from licorice crude extract by anti-GC-MAB immunoaffinity chromatography to expand the possibilities for pharmacological research and other applications.

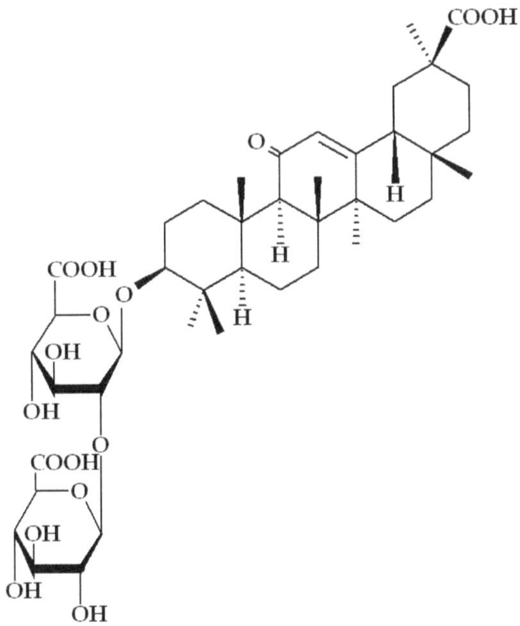

Fig. 7. Chemical structure of GC

3.1 Preparation of GC-KO extract by anti-GC immunoaffinity column

Previously, we have reported the preparation of anti-GC MAb, and its cross-reactivity of the anti-GC MAb against glycyrrhetic acid-3-*O*-glucuronide and glycyrrhetic acid were 0.585 % and 1.865 %, respectively, compared with GC (Tanaka & Shoyama, 1998; Shan et al., 2001). The other related compounds such as deoxycholic acid, ursolic acid, and oleanolic acid, were all less than 0.005 %. The purified 60 mg of the anti-GC MAb was coupled to 25 ml of an Affi-Gel Hz gel and used to prepare the immunoaffinity column.

Twelve milligrams of licorice crude extract containing 1275.0 μg of GC was dissolved in loading buffer (5 % MeOH), and then applied on the anti-GC-MAb immunoaffinity column. The column was washed with washing buffer (5 % MeOH) and then eluted with elution buffer (20 mM phosphate buffer containing 30 % MeOH). After separation, each fraction was deionized and the solvent was lyophilized. Table 2 indicates the GC concentration of washing and eluted fractions determined by ELISA. The washing and eluted fractions contain and 3.50 μg and 1269.26 μg of GC, respectively. These data indicate that the anti-GC column could eliminate 99.55 % of the loading GC. Thus, we named this washing fraction "GC-knock out (GC-KO) extract". The capacity of the anti-GC immunoaffinity column was effective to capture GC compared with the immunoaffinity columns for forskolin and solasodine glycosides (Yanagihara et al., 1996; Putalun et al., 1999). This result may also infer that when the GC concentration is trace level or cannot be analyzed by even ELISA, this anti-GC immunoaffinity column can concentrate GC to the detectable level. The combination of the established anti-GC-MAb immunoaffinity column and ELISA provided a reliable and very high sensitive analysis for GC in different extracts of various medicinal herbs or other drugs.

	GC content (μg)	GC content rate (% of loading GC)
Loading sample	**1275.0** (12 mg licorice extract)	**100**
Washing fraction	**3.50**	**0.27**
Eluted fraction	**1269.26**	**99.55**

Table 2. GC content of the loading licorice extract and the separated fractions by anti-GC immunoaffinity column

To investigate the profiles of GC-KO extract, we performed the TLC analysis and Eastern blotting. As shown in Figure 8A, several spots of GC and other compounds were detected in licorice extract (lane 2). However, although all other spots were clearly detected, the spot of GC was completely disappeared in GC-KO extract (lane 3). Furthermore, Eastern blotting by anti-GC MAb indicated that GC was detected in licorice extract (lane 2), but the spot of GC was disappeared in GC-KO extract (lane 3) (Figure 8B). Taken together, these data suggest that GC was specifically eliminated from licorice extract by anti-GC MAb immunoaffinity column.

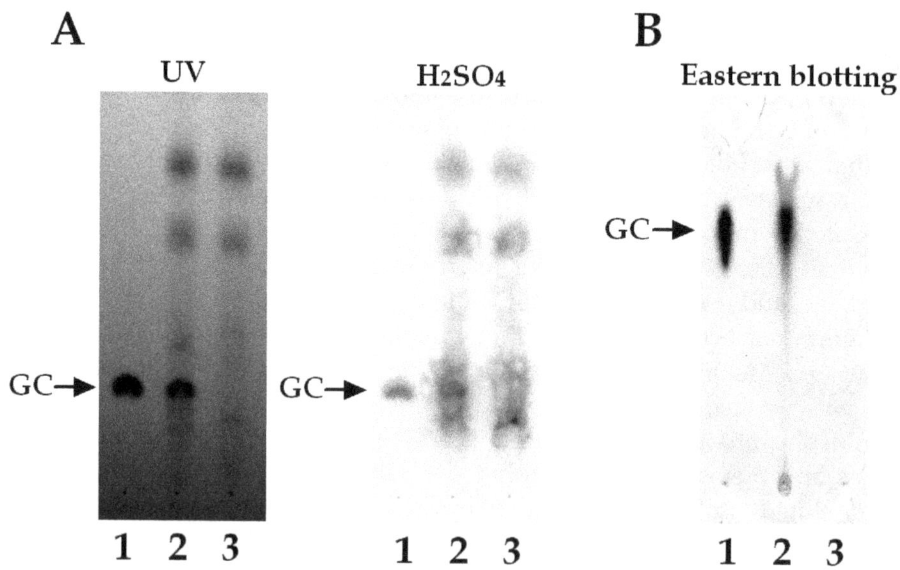

Fig. 8. TLC profiles (A) and Eastern blotting by anti-GC MAb (B) of licorice extract and GC-KO extract. Lane 1; GC strandard, Lane 2; licorice extract, Lane 3; GC-KO extract

3.2 The application of GC-KO extract prepared by anti-GC immunoaffinity column to in vitro assay

Inflammation leads to the up-regulation of a series of enzymes and signaling mediators in the affected tissue and cells. Nitric oxide (NO) is a highly reactive free radical involved in multiple physiological functions, such as vasodilatation, neurotransmission and inflammation (Moncada et al., 1991). During inflammatory process, a large amount of NO is produced by inducible nitric oxide synthase (iNOS) by inflammatory cytokines and/or bacterial lipopolysaccharide (LPS) in various cell types including macrophages (Nathan & Xie, 1994). Overproduced NO synthesized by iNOS triggers the pathogenesis of septic shock and organ destruction in certain inflammatory and autoimmune diseases (Naseem et al., 2005; Guzik et al., 2003; Abramson et al., 2001). Therefore, inhibiting NO production by blocking iNOS expression may be useful strategy to treat a variety of inflammatory diseases.

Initially, we examined whether licorice crude extract suppress NO release in LPS-treated mouse RAW264 macrophages. LPS evoked a dramatic increase of NO production, and this induction was blocked by treatment of licorice extract dose dependently (12.5-100 μg/mL) (data not shown). Next, we performed Western blot analyses and RT-PCR to investigate the effect of licorice extract on iNOS protein and mRNA expressions. LPS markedly up-regulated iNOS protein and mRNA level, and pretreatment of licorice extract reduced these up-regulations in the same concentration range as was used for NO production (data not shown). At 100 μg/mL of licorice extract, iNOS protein and mRNA were completely suppressed. ELISA by using anti-GC MAb demonstrated that 100 μg of licorice extract contains 10.6 ± 0.618 μg of GC. To examine whether GC alone can reduce NO production and iNOS expression, we pretreated the cells with GC around 10.6 μg/ml before exposure to LPS. However, GC did not exert any significant influence on LPS-induced NO production and iNOS protein expression (data not shown).

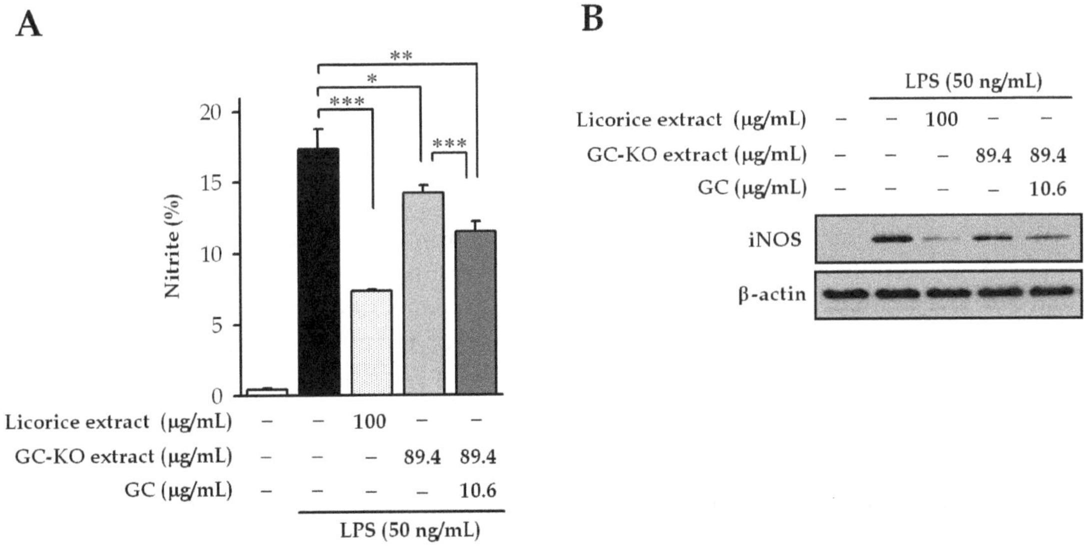

Fig. 9. Effect of licorice extract, GC-KO extract, and the co-treatment of GC-KO extract and GC on NO production (A) and iNOS protein expression (B) in LPS-treated RAW264 cells. Each bar represents the means ± S.D. from four separate experiments. *P<0.05, **P<0.01, *P<0.001 compared with LPS alone

To further elucidate the effect of GC on NO inhibition by licorice extract, we used GC-KO extract prepared by anti-GC immunoaffinity column. According to data of ELISA, 100 μg of licorice extract contains 10.6 μg of GC and 89.4 μg of the other compounds. Thus, the cells were treated with licorice extract (100 μg/mL), GC-KO extract (89.4 μg/mL), or combination of GC-KO extract (89.4 μg/mL) and GC (10.6 μg/mL). As shown in Figure 9A, although treatment of licorice extract lead to an inhibition of NO production as compared to LPS treatment [inhibition ratio (IR) = 57.7%], the inhibitory effect of GC-KO extract was decreased compared with licorice extract (IR = 17.8 %). Interestingly, the combination of GC-KO extract and GC significantly improved the inhibitory ability (IR = 33.5 %). Furthermore, we performed Western blotting to determine whether the combinational effect of GC-KO extract and GC was related to iNOS expression (Figure 9B). Inhibitory activity of iNOS expression by licorice extract was reduced in treatment of GC-KO extract. The addition of GC to GC-KO extract improved the inhibition. These data suggest that GC alone cannot suppress iNOS expression, but combinational inhibition of iNOS expression may occur when GC coexists with the other constituents contained in licorice extract.

In conclusion, this study demonstrate that KO extract prepared by anti-natural compound specific MAb-conjugated immunoaffinity column is a useful approach for determination of potential function of natural compound on *in vitro* and in *vivo* assays.

4. Conclusion

We describe the new strategy of one-step purification of target compounds from crude extract by anti-natural compound MAb-conjugated immunoaffinity column. The combination of the immunoaffinity column and ELISA by using MAb provided a reliable and high sensitivity analysis for target compound in various crude extracts and TCMs. Furthermore, by the use of the cross-reactivity of MAb, the affinity column can identify new unknown compounds related to target compound of MAb and determine their structures. Finally, we demonstrate that KO extract, which contains all components of crude extract except an antigen molecule, may be useful approach to determine the potential function of one principal compound on the crude extract or TCM by *in vitro* and *in vivo* assays.

5. Acknowledgment

We thank Prof. Yukihiro Shoyama and Dr. Osamu Morinaga (Nagasaki International Univ.) for useful suggestions in this work. This work was supported by a Grant in Aid from the Japan Society for the Promotion of Science (JSPS) Asian CORE Program, the Ministry of Education, Culture, Sports, Science and Technology of Japan, and grants from the Asahi Beer Science Promoting Foundation and Takeda Science Foundation.

6. References

Abramson, S.B.; Amin, A.R.; Clancy, R.M. & Attur, M. (2001) The role of nitric oxide in tissue destruction. *Best Pract. Res. Clin. Rheumatol.*, 15(5) 831-845

Asl, M.N. & Hosseinzadeh, H. (2008) Review of pharmacological effects of Glycyrrhiza sp. and its bioactive compounds. *Phytother. Res.*, 22(6) 709-724

Coon, J.T. & Ernst, E. (2004) Complementary and alternative therapies in the treatment of chronic hepatitis C: a systematic review. *J. Hepatol.*, 40(3) 491-500

Doll, R. & Hill, I.D. (1962) Triterpenoid liquorice compound in gastric and duodenal ulcer. *Lancet*, 2(7266) 1166-1167

Fukuda, N.; Tanaka, H. & Shoyama, Y. (2000a) Applications of ELISA, western blotting and immunoaffinity concentration for survey of ginsenosides in crude drugs of Panax species and traditional Chinese herbal medicines. *Analyst*, 125(8) 1425-1429

Fukuda, N.; Tanaka, H. & Shoyama, Y. (2000b) Formation of monoclonal antibody against a major ginseng component, ginsenoside Rg1 and its characterization. Monoclonal antibody for a ginseng saponin. *Cytotechnology*, 34(3) 197-204

Fukuda, N.; Tanaka, H. & Shoyama, H. (2000c) Isolation of the pharmacologically active saponin ginsenoside Rb1 from ginseng by immunoaffinity column chromatography. *J. Nat. Prod.*, 63(2) 283-285

Gillis, C.N. (1997) Panax ginseng pharmacology: a nitric oxide link? *Biochem. Pharmacol.*, 54(1) 1-8

Guzik, T.J.; Korbut, R. & Adamek-Guzik, T. (2003) Nitric oxide and superoxide in inflammation and immune regulation. *J. Physiol. Pharmacol.*, 54(4) 469-487

Hayashi, H.; Hattori, S. ; Inoue, K.; Khodzhimatov, O.; Ashurmetov, O.; Ito, M. & Honda, G. (2003) Field survey of *Glycyrrhiza* plants in Central Asia (3). Chemical characterization of *G. glabra* collected in Uzbekistan. *Chem. Pharm. Bull.*, 51(11) 1338-1340

Ishiyama, M.; Shoyama, Y.; Murakami, H. & Shinohara, H. (1996) Production of monoclonal antibodies and development of an ELISA for solamargine. *Cytotechnology*, 18(3) 153-158

Jiang, K.Y. & Qian, Z.N. (1995) Effects of Panax notoginseng saponins on posthypoxic cell damage of neurons *in vitro*. *Zhongguo Yao Li Xue Bao*, 16(5) 399–402

Kim, J.S.; Tanaka, H. & Shoyama, Y. (2004) Immunoquantitative analysis for berberine and its related compounds using monoclonal antibodies in herbal medicines. *Analyst*, 129(1) 87-91

Kim, N.C. & Kinghorn, A.D. (2002) Highly sweet compounds of plant origin. *Arch. Pharm. Res.*, 25(6) 725-746

Kitagawa, I.; Taniyama, T.; Yoshikawa, M.; Ikenishi, Y. & Nakagawa, Y. (1989) Chemical studies on crude drug processing. IV. Chemical structures of malonyl-ginsenosides Rb1, Rb2, Re and Rd isolated from the root of Panax Ginseng C.A. Meyer. *Chem. Pharm. Bull.*, 37(11) 2961–2970

Kitagawa, I.; Yoshikawa, M.; Yoshihara, M.; Hayashi, T. & Taniyama, T. (1983) Chemical studies of crude drugs (1). Constituents of Ginseng radix rubra. *Yakugaku Zassh*, 103(6) 612-622

Kohda, H.; Tanaka, S.; Yamaoka, Y. & Ohhara, Y. (1991) Saponins from Amaranthus hypochondriacus. *Chem. Pharm. Bull.*, 39(10) 2609-2612

Lay, H.L.; Chen, C.C. & Chiang, S.T. (2004) Simultaneous analysis of nine components in" Byi-Liang-Tang" preparation by high performance liquid chromatography. *J. Food Drug Anal.*, 12(2) 115-119

Lim, J.H.; Wen, T.C.; Matsuda, S.; Tanaka, J.; Maeda, N.; Peng, H.; Aburaya, J.; Ishihara, K. & Sakanaka, M. (1997) Protection of ischemic hippocampal neurons by ginsenoside Rb1, a main ingredient of ginseng root. *Neurosci. Res.*, 28(3) 191–200

Liu, M. & Zhang, J. (1995) Effects of ginsenoside Rb1 and Rg1 on synaptosomal free calcium level, ATPase and calmodulin in rat hippocampus. *Chin. Med. J. (Engl.),* 108(7) 544-547

Loungratana, P.; Tanaka, H.; & Shoyama, Y. (2004) Production of monoclonal antibody against ginkgolic acids in Ginkgo biloba Linn. *Am. J. Chin. Med.,* 32(2) 33-48

Lu, Z.; Morinaga, O.; Tanaka, H. & Shoyama, Y. (2003) A quantitative ELISA using monoclonal antibody to survey paeoniflorin and albiflorin in crude drugs and traditional Chinese herbal medicines. *Biol. Pharm. Bull.,* 26(6) 862-866

Moncada, S.; Palmer, R.M. & Higgs, E.A. (1991) Nitric oxide: physiology, pathophysiology, and pharmacology. *Pharmacol. Rev.,* 43(2) 109-142

Mook-Jung, I.; Hong, H.S.; Boo, J.H.; Lee, K.H.; Yun, S.H.; Cheong, M.Y.; Joo, I.; Huh, K. & Jung, M.W. (2001) Ginsenoside Rb1 and Rg1 improve spatial learning and increase hippocampal synaptophysin level in mice. *J. Neurosci. Res.,* 63(6) 509-515

Morinaga, O.; Nakajima, S.; Tanaka, H. & Shoyama, Y. (2001) Production of monoclonal antibodies against a major purgative component, sennoside B, their characterization and use in ELISA. *Analyst,* 126(8) 1372-1376

Morinaga, O.; Tanaka, H. & Shoyama, Y. (2000) Production of monoclonal antibody against a major purgative component, sennoside A, its characterization and ELISA. *Analyst,* 125(8) 1109-1113

Morinaga, O.; Tanaka, H. & Shoyama, Y. (2006) Detection and quantification of ginsenoside Re in ginseng samples by a chromatographic immunostaining method using monoclonal antibody against ginsenoside Re. *J. Chromatography B,* 830(1) 100-104

Morita, T.; Tanaka, O. & Kohda, H. (1985) Saponin composition of rhizomes of *Panax japonicus* collected in South Kyushu, Japan, and its significance in oriental traditional medicine. *Chem. Pharm. Bull.,* 33(9) 3852-3858

Nathan, C. & Xie, Q.W. (1994) Regulation of biosynthesis of nitric oxide. *J. Biol. Chem.,* 269(19) 13725-13728

Naseem, K.M. (2005) The role of nitric oxide in cardiovascular diseases. *Mol. Aspects Med.,* 26(1-2) 33-65

Ong, E.S. (2002) Chemical assay of glycyrrhizin in medicinal plants by pressurized liquid extraction (PLE) with capillary zone electrophoresis (CZE). *J. Sep. Sci.,* 25(13) 825-831

Pompei, R.; Flore, O.; Marccialis, M.A.; Pani, A. & Loddo, B. (1979) Glycyrrhizic acid inhibits virus growth and inactivates virus particles. *Nature,* 281(5733) 689-690

Putalun, W.; Tanaka, H. & Yukihiro, S. (1999) Rapid separation of solasodine glycosides by an immunoaffinity column using anti-solamargine monoclonal antibody. *Cytotechnology,* 31(1-2) 151-156

Putalun, W.; Tanaka, H. & Shoyama, Y. (2005) Rapid detection of glycyrrhizin by immunochromatographic assay. *Phytochem. Anal.,* 16(5) 370-374

Sakai, T.; Shinahara, K.; Torimaru, A.; Tanaka, H.; Shoyama, Y. & Matsumoto, K. (2004) Sensitive detection of glycyrrhizin and evaluation of the affinity constants by a surface plasmon resonance-based immunosensor. *Anal. Sci.,* 20(2) 279-283

Sakata, R.; Shoyama, Y. & Murakami, H. (1994) Production of monoclonal antibodies and enzyme immunoassay for typical adenylate cyclase activator, Forskolin. *Cytotechnology,* 16(2) 101-108

Schalm, S.W.; Brouwer, J.T.; Bekkering, F.C. & van Rossum, T.G. (1999) New treatment strategies in non-responder patients with chronic hepatitis C. *J. Hepatol.*, 31(Suppl.1) 1184-1188

Shan, S.J.; Tanaka, H. & Shoyama, Y. (2001) Enzyme-linked immunosorbent assay for glycyrrhizin using anti-glycyrrhizin monoclonal antibody and an eastern blotting technique for glucuronides of glycyrrhetic acid. *Anal. Chem.*, 73(24) 5784-5790

Shoyama, Y.; Fukada, T. & Murakami, H. (1996) Production of monoclonal antibodies and ELISA for thebaine and codeine. *Cytotechnology,* 19(1) 55-61

Tan, T.W.; Huo, Q. & Ling, Q. (2002) Purification of glycyrrhizin from glycyrrhiza uralensis fisch with ethanol/phosphate aqueous two phase system. *Biochem. Lett.*, 24(17) 1417-1420

Tanaka, H.; Fukuda, N. & Shoyama, Y. (1999) Formation of monoclonal antibody against a major ginseng component, ginsenoside Rb1 and its characterization. *Cytotechnology,* 29(1) 115-120

Tanaka, H.; Fukuda, N. & Shoyama, Y. (2007) Eastern blotting and immunoaffinity concentration using monoclonal antibody for ginseng saponins in the field of traditional chinese medicines. *J. Agric. Food Chem.*, 55(10) 3783-3787

Tanaka, H.; Goto, Y. & Shoyama, Y. (1996) Monoclonal antibody based enzyme immunoassay for marihuana (cannabinoid) compounds. *Immunoassay,* 17(4) 321-342

Tanaka, H. & Shoyama, Y. (1998) Formation of a monoclonal antibody against glycyrrhizin and development of an ELISA. *Biol. Pharm. Bull.,* 21(12) 1391-1393

Tanaka, O. (1989) Saponin-composition of Panax species. In recent advances in ginseng studies. Shibata, S.; Ohtsuka, Y. & Saito, H., (Eds.), 43-47, Hirokawa Publishing, Tokyo, Japan

Wang, C.A. & Shoyama, Y. (2006). Herbal medicine: identification, analysis, and evaluation strategies, In: *Textbook of complementary and alternative medicine, second edition,* C.S. Yuan; E.J. Bieber & B.A. Bauer, (Ed.), 51-70, Informa Healthcare, ISBN 1-84214-297-6, London, UK

Wang, Z.Y. & Nixon, D.W. (2001) Licorice and cancer. *Nutr. Cancer,* 39(1) 1-11

Washida, D. & Kitanaka, S. (2003) Determination of polyacetylenes and ginsenosides in Panax species using high performance liquid chromatography. *Chem. Pharm. Bull.,* 51(11) 1314–1317

Xu, J.; Tanaka, H. & Shoyama, Y. (2007) One-step immunochromatographic separation and ELISA quantification of glycyrrhizin from traditional Chinese medicines. *J. Chromatog. B,* 850(1-2) 53-58

Xuan, L.; Tanaka, H. ; Xu, Y. & Shoyama, Y. (1999) Preparation of monoclonal antibody against crocin and its characterization. *Cytotechnology,* 29(1) 65-70

Yahara, S.; Kasai, R. & Tanaka, O. (1977) New dammarane type saponins of leaves of *Panax japonicus* C.A. Meyer. (1). Chikusetsusaponins L_5, L_{9a} and L_{10}. *Chem. Pharm. Bull.,* 25(8) 2041-2047

Yamamoto, Y.; Majima, T.; Saiki, I. & Tani, T. (2003) Pharmaceutical evaluation of *Glycyrrhiza uralensis* roots cultivated in eastern Nei-Meng-Gu of China. *Biol. Pharm. Bull.,* 26(8) 1144-1149

Yanagihara, H.; Sakata, R.; Minami, H.; Shoyama, Y. & Murakami, H. (1996) Immunoaffinity column chromatography against forskolin using an anti-forskolin monoclonal antibody and its application. *Anal. Chim. Acta,* 335(1-2) 63-70

Zhu, S.; Shimokawa, S.; Tanaka, H. & Shoyama, Y. (2004) Development of an assay system for saikosaponin a using anti-saikosaponin a monoclonal antibodies. *Biol. Pharm. Bull.,* 27(1) 66-71

2

Procedures of Food Quality Control: Analysis Methods, Sampling and Sample Pretreatment

Nancy Ornelas-Soto[1],
Oracio Barbosa-García[1] and Pedro L. Lopez-de-Alba[2]
[1]*Centro de Investigaciones en Óptica, León, Gto.*
[2]*Departamento de Química. Universidad de Guanajuato. Gto.*
México

1. Introduction

The development of new methods that might or might not involve sophisticated techniques for the quality control of food products continues increasing according to consumer requirement of food safety and authenticity issues. The production of fakes is a worldwide problem that includes food products. Some examples can be found on olive oils, honeys and alcoholic beverages such as table wines and spirits (Contreras et al., 2010; Gallardo et al, 2009; Marcos et al., 2002; Zhang et al., 2001; Zhu et al., 2010). Therefore, food authentication concerns both authorities and food processors to avoid the unfair competition from counterfeiters who exploited the economic advantage by producing and selling fake food products.

Food companies have adopted different strategies to improve the positioning of their brands on the market. These strategies not only include the food quality control based on the identification and reduction of forbidden compounds but also on monitoring the key compounds that enhance the food value. In this chapter a practical review of methods for quality control on compounds and on the confirmation of food authenticity is presented. Non-destructive testing sample methodologies that have found new applications in the field of quality assurance are discussed in terms of their potential use in food industry. Thus, the use of spectroscopic techniques with chemometric analysis for the classification of food samples based on quality attributes is also discussed in this chapter.

The optimization of the analytical methods is based on the selection of fundamental working conditions (sampling, pretreatment, selectivity, linearity, range determination, sensitivity, limit of detection, precision and accuracy, etc.) according to which the suitability of a selected method might be evaluated. One of the most important steps in the analytical method for compound determination in biological matrices is the sample pretreatment. The purpose of a pretreatment is to release analytes from compounds and phases as well as to remove components which have adverse impacts on the analytical signal.

On the other hand, before any analytic treatment it is necessary to take into account some preliminary procedures that involve statistic analysis (Cochran, 1977; Hinkelmann &

Kempthorne, 1994). When making surveys within different research fields, the access to the entire population of items/subjects/individuals/samples is almost impossible and expensive and thus, sampling techniques come into play. Industry and business make use of sampling techniques to increase the efficiency of their internal operations. In particular, for industry sampling techniques are important tools for quality control to ensure that final items are ready for marketing. In particular, for food processing decisions regarding any change on the quality control to accept or reject lots would be well grounded if the selected data from the population is done with the appropriate sampling technique. In this way you can be confident that your decision about acceptance or rejection of lots is right. That is, sampling procedures are focused on the selection of a subset of sample observations within a population attempted to yield some knowledge about the entire population of concern. Sample observations bring out data values of some measurable properties of the subject. Therefore, the cost of collecting data about a population by gathering information from a subset instead of the entire population is reduced. In addition to this, making use of the appropriate sampling technique the data can be collected and summarized more quickly since the data set is smaller and the accuracy and quality of the data can be improved. Therefore, this chapter starts with the sampling procedures followed by the most common analytic methods focused on food quality control.

2. Sampling procedures

If the population regarding any survey is almost impossible to reach and expensive to try every single sample, then how large should the subset of samples be to ensure that the results obtained from it would be generalized? A single answer to this question is not possible. However, it is clear that the larger the sample size the more closely your sample data will match that from the entire population. For sampling procedures one counts with the *probability sampling* and *non-probability sampling* procedures.

The *probability sampling procedure* refers to a given population where one is able to identify distinct samples; each possible sample has some known probability of selection and thus, one can select, and identify, any sample through a random process. That is, each sample within the population has its own probability to be randomly selected. In contrast, the *non-probability sampling procedure* refers to the case when the sample to be selected is part of the population that is readily accessible or it might occur that the population consists of volunteers or that the samples were haphazardly selected. In any case, for this procedure some samples have no chance of selection and information about the relationship between samples and the entire population is very limited. For the non-probability sampling no known probability is assigned to the samples of the population and it will almost certainly contain sampling biases.

When the sample is selected on a random basis 3 main types of random sampling techniques can be identified, i.e., the *simple random sampling, stratified random sampling* and *systematic sampling*.

For the *simple random sampling* method, any sample from the population has an equal chance of being drawn, that is, every sample has the same probability of being selected. If the selected sample is removed from the population for subsequent draws, then the method is random sampling without replacement. However, if the selected sample is not removed from the population in such way that for any new draw the population remains fixed to the original, then the simple random sampling is without replacement.

The *stratified random sampling* method is based on the fact that sometimes the entire population might embrace certain number of distinct samples which would be divided into subpopulations. If this is the case, these subpopulations are called strata and the sum of them is the total population. For stratified random sampling each stratum is sampled independently and each individual in the subpopulation is randomly selected, i.e., a simple random sample is taken in each stratum. For this method, each subpopulation can be considered as independent and thus each stratum is a population in its own and one is able to get inferences from each of them.

When the population can be ordered in some scheme and the samples are drawn at regular intervals through that ordered list, then the sampling method is called *systematic sampling*. For this method and to start the sampling is convenient to select the first sample randomly and then drawn the next samples at regular fixed intervals till the end of the list. That is, the first element to draw should be selected randomly instead of selecting the first of the list. Notice that for this method the complete list defines a stratum and each regular interval defines a stratum that contains the fixed number of elements defined by the interval. Thus, the difference between this method and the stratified is that the former is defined by regular strata and each individual occurs at the same relative position within the stratum. On the other hand, for the later the strata might not be regular and the individuals are selected randomly in each stratum.

2.1 Normal distribution

By doing a survey with the appropriate sampling method one ends up with a collection of data that represents the measurement of one or more properties of the chosen samples from the given population. To make predictions based on statistical inference it is convenient to make use of the probability functions. The *normal distribution* is a continuous probability function and it is considered one of the most important in the field of statistics. This probability distribution is used in different fields such as statistics, natural sciences, medical sciences, business and social sciences. Some of its advantages come from the fact that the random variables get around a single mean value and a large number of results can be derived in explicit form. The normal distribution is also called Gaussian distribution and because its plot is a curved flaring shape, it is recognized as a bell curve.

Therefore, the simplest case for a normal distribution is

$$F(x)=\left(\frac{1}{\sqrt{2\pi}}\right)e^{\left(-\frac{1}{2}\right)x^2} \tag{1}$$

where x is the random variable. This expression corresponds to the so called *standard normal distribution*. The shape of this expression is a "bell curve" where the coefficient $(1/\sqrt{2\pi})$ ensures that the total area under the curve is equal to one; meanwhile the coefficient ½ in the exponent makes the width of the bell curve also equal to one. If μ is the mean value and σ^2 the variance of a population, the above equation can be expressed in a more general form as

$$F(x)=\left(\frac{1}{\sqrt{2\pi\sigma^2}}\right)e^{\left(-\frac{1}{2\sigma^2}\right)(x-\mu)^2} \tag{2}$$

The parameter μ localizes the peak of the bell curve while the root square of σ^2 is the standard deviation, σ, which defines the width of the distribution. This expression is called *probability density function* and is represented in Figs. 1 and 2. In Fig. 1 the mean value μ and variance σ^2 have different values to see how the shape of f(x) changes; notice that by making $\mu=0$ and $\sigma^2=1$ one obtains the standard normal distribution. μ and σ^2 are two important parameters in sampling, probability theory and statistics. Most of the time μ is referred as the mean of a set of values and corresponds to the arithmetic mean, that is,

$$\mu = \left(\frac{1}{N}\right)\sum_i x_i \tag{3}$$

where N is the total number of values $\{x_i\}$. In statistics μ is the expected value of a random variable and when sampling a statistical population the used term for mean is the sample mean.

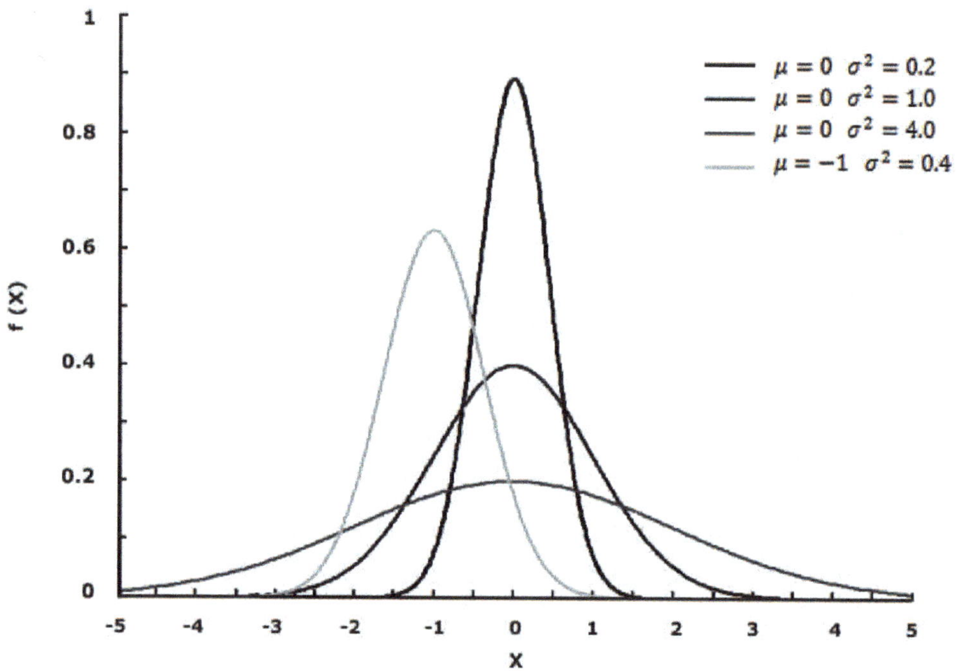

Fig. 1. The normal probability density function with different μ and σ^2 values

The variance measures how far a set of samples are spread out from each other and it is defined as,

$$\sigma^2 = \left(\frac{1}{N}\right)\sum_i (x_i - \mu)^2 \tag{4}$$

For a discrete distribution P(X) with N possible values of x_i, the variance is

$$\sigma^2 = \sum_i P(x_i)(x_i - \mu)^2 \tag{5}$$

and for a continuous distribution,

$$\sigma^2 = \int P(x)(x-\mu)^2 dx \tag{6}$$

If variance tells us how far a set of samples are spread out from each other, the root square of the variance tell us how far samples lie from μ, i.e., it describes the spread of the data around the mean, see Fig.2. In this figure the values of $2|\sigma_1|$, $2|\sigma_2|$, $2|\sigma_3|$ and $2|\sigma_4|$ are 68.2, 95.4, 99.6 and 99.8 %, respectively, of the unit area under f(x) given by Eq. 2.

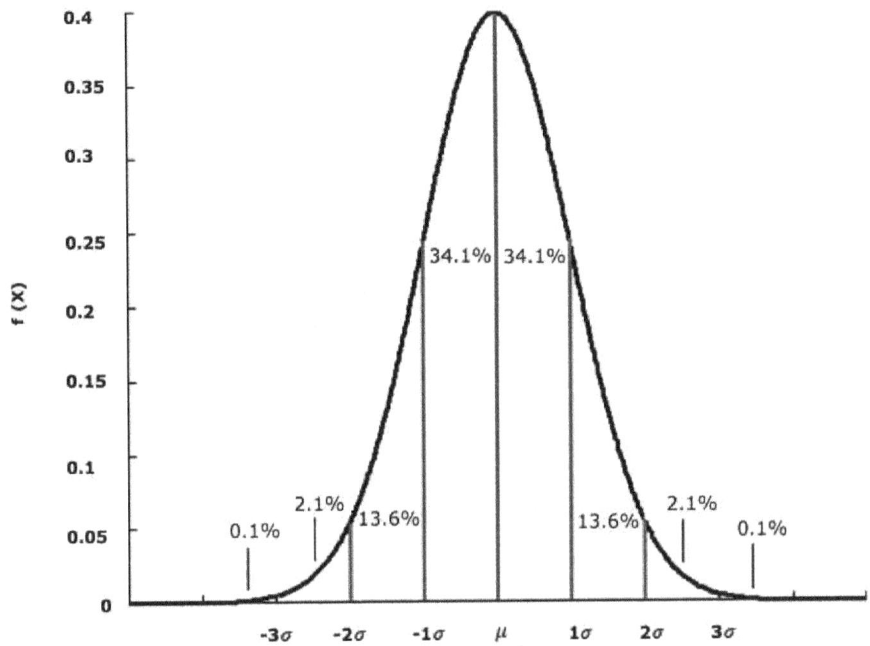

Fig. 2. The normal probability density function with standard deviations.

2.2 Accuracy, precision and errors

When doing measurements of some property of individuals, objects or samples the terms accuracy, precision and errors show up since they are intrinsic in doing any measure. Thus, the accuracy of a measurement or of an experiment is related to how closely the experimental results agree with a true or accepted value. Meanwhile precision is related to how reproducible the measurement or experiment is. To illustrate these two concepts, consider a set of data, the set of random variable $\{x_i\}$, which comes from the measurement of some property of an object. This set of data is distributed normally according to Eq. (2). The true or reference value might be on the left or right of the mean. Thus, the mean represents the peak of the distributed data and the standard deviation tells us how the data spreads around the mean. Meanwhile accuracy is the separation between the mean and the true value and, since each measurement might not agree well with each other, precision is expressed by quoting the standard deviation.

Systematic and random errors can easily be understood by considering two sets of data, related to two measurements, each defined by normal distribution. One set of data is reported with poor accuracy but very precise and the other with good accuracy but poor precision. For the first case, the difference between the mean and the true value is large;

meanwhile the bell curve of the distribution is very slender, see for example the case for $\mu=0$ and $\sigma^2=0.2$ in Fig. 1. That is, each measurement is very similar to each other but all measurements are not close to match the true value and all have a large error. This kind of error is the systematic error and it happens exactly in the same manner every time a new measurement is performed. For the second case, the peak of the bell curve, i.e. the mean, is very close to the true value but the shape of the bell curve is very broad, see for example the case for $\mu=0$ and $\sigma^2=4$ in Fig. 1. In other words, the measurements as a whole are correct but each measurement by itself is a poor measure of the true value. This is the case for random errors which change each time the measurement is repeated.

3. Methods based on chromatographic techniques

Chromatographic techniques have been widely used because they offer good information about sample composition. Their principal advantages are separation efficiency; identification of almost any type of molecule present in a food sample; and depending of which technique is employed, it is possible to obtain very low detection limits for a wide range of analytes. Liquid chromatography, in particular HPLC (*high performance liquid chromatography*), can detect compounds such as aldehydes, proteins, amino acids, phenolic compounds and carbohydrates (Ball 1990; De Zan et al., 2009; Francisco & Resurreccion 2009; Rubio Barroso et al., 2006; Schultheiss et al., 2000; Thoma et al., 2006). On the other hand, GC (*gas chromatography*) is more suited to the analysis of volatile or semi-volatile compounds; some substances must be extracted from the food sample, e.g., fatty acids from triglycerides; but others, such as alcohols, can be injected directly into the column (Petrovic et al., 2010; Wang et al., 2004). The most commonly detectors used for chromatographic techniques involve UV-Vis (*ultraviolet–visible*), fluorescence, electrochemical, MS (*mass spectroscopy*), FID (*flame ionization detector*), ECD (*electron capture detector*), electronic nose, etc. The methods developed through these techniques have established patterns of composition of several types of samples by monitoring the specific compounds. The principal disadvantage of chromatographic techniques is the complex operation which requires special training to ensure that the technique is performed correctly. False results are obtained when the laboratory equipment involved with the technique is not operated correctly. Besides, long analysis times are required.

3.1 Gas chromatography

Basically, chromatograph equipment consists of four systems: gas supply, the sampling, the column and the detector system. The gas supply system provides, depending on the kind of detector that is chosen, the necessary type of gas or gas mixture. The sampling system usually contains an automatic injector that is situated inside a thermostatically controlled enclosure and generally has its own oven, but sometimes shares the column oven for temperature control. The injector can have a complex transport system that can take samples, wash containers, prepare derivatives and, if necessary, carry out a very complex series of sample preparation procedures before injecting the sample onto the column. The column is the principal device that actually achieved the necessary separation, and has an oven to control the column temperature. Finally, for detection there is a wide range of detectors available each having unique operating parameters and its own performance characteristics. The best selection depends on the sample nature and this system also has its own oven (Holley et al., 1995). Table 1 shows an overview of GC detectors.

The analyzed substances through GC must be volatile and should be vaporized and moved through a long column by an inert carrier gas. The column is filled with a packing material covered with a not-volatile liquid. The molecules of each substance will be distributed into the gas and the liquid. The more volatile a substance is the longer it will be moving with the carrier gas, and the quicker it will emerge from the column (Otles et al., 2008). The sample pretreatment usually is complex and the compounds of importance, usually, must be extracted from the matrix but if they are not volatile then derivatization techniques must be used (Herraiz, 2000).

Detector	**Characteristics**	**Detection Limits**
Flame ionization detector (FID)	Non-selective	ng L^{-1}
Thermal conductivity detector (TCD)	Non-Selective	µg L^{-1} - ng L^{-1}
Electron capture detector (ECD)	Halogens	pg L^{-1}
Nitrogen–phosphorus detector (NPD)	Nitrogen and Phosphorous	ng L^{-1}
Photo-ionization detector (PID)	Aromatic compounds	ng L^{-1}
Flame photometric detector (FPD)	Sulfurous and phosphorous	ng L^{-1}
Pulsed flame photometric detector (PFPD)	Calibrating for several elements	ng L^{-1}
Atomic-emission detector (AED)	Calibrating for any element	ng L^{-1}
Electrolytic conductivity detector (ELCD)	Halogens, sulfurous, nitrogen,	ng L^{-1}
Mass spectrometric detector (MSD)	Selective	ng L^{-1} - pg L^{-1}

Table 1. GC detectors more common applicable for the determination of food components

The extraction of an analyte utilizes the partitioning of a material between two phases and it is based on solubility or insolubility in various solvents. Extraction is useful for sample preparation and purification, but is also often a first step in qualitative analysis. There are several kinds of extraction process such as liquid-solid, liquid-liquid, SPE (*solid phase extraction*) and SPME (*solid-phase microextraction*).

In liquid-solid extraction, a solvent (hydrophilic or hydrophobic, acidic, neutral or basic) is added to a solid. Insoluble material can be separated by gravity or vacuum filtration, and soluble material is extracted into the solvent. A sequence of solvents, by varying polarity or pH, can be used to separate complex mixtures into groups. Then, the filtered solution can be injected into the GC system. If the two phases are immiscible liquids the technique is called liquid-liquid extraction. Usually, one phase is aqueous (hydrophilic) and the other is a hydrophobic organic solvent. A sequence of extractions with more than one solvent can be used to separate, with considerable efficiency, relatively complex mixtures.

SPE uses the affinity of solutes dissolved or suspended in a liquid (known as the mobile phase) for a solid through which the sample is passed (known as the stationary phase) to separate a mixture into desired and undesired components. The result is that either the desired analytes of interest or undesired impurities in the sample are retained on the stationary phase. The portion that passes through the stationary phase is collected or discarded, depending on whether it contains the desired analytes or undesired impurities. If the retained portion on the stationary phase includes the desired analytes, they can then be removed from the stationary phase for collection in an additional step in which the stationary phase is rinsed with an appropriate eluent.

SPME involves the use of a fiber coated with an extracting phase, that can be a liquid (polymer) or a solid (sorbent), which extracts different kinds of analytes (including both volatile and non-volatile) from different kinds of media that can be in liquid or gas phase. The amount of extracted analyte by the fiber is proportional to its concentration in the sample as long as equilibrium is reached. Then the fiber is transferred to the injection port of the gas chromatograph where desorption and analysis of the analytes is carried out (Pawliszyn, 1997).

The most typical applications on GC for food analysis pertain to the quantitative and/or qualitative analysis of food composition, natural products, food additives, flavor and aroma components; a variety of transformation products, and contaminants, such as pesticides, fumigants, environmental pollutants, natural toxins, veterinary drugs, and packaging (Holley, 1995).

Among the natural products analyzed by GC one can highlight the analysis on olive oil samples. Recent studies are based on the determination of several kinds of analytes such as undesirable compounds, e.g. pesticides and herbicides (Dugo, 2005; Aramendia, 2007); monoaromatic volatile compounds (benzene, toluene and ethylbenzene) (Gilbert Lopez et al., 2010); beneficial health compounds such as phenolic compounds (Garcia Villalba et al., 2011); studies that involve the interpretation of the responsible compounds of oil aroma (Garcia Gonzalez & Aparicio, 2010) and so on. There are other works that analyze changes of patterns focused on comparison of their fatty acid composition through chemometric analysis (Lee et al., 1998). Chemometric analysis of the triacylglycerol and fatty acid composition is usually a media to determine their varietal and geographical authenticity (Luykx & van Ruth, 2008).

GC offers good information about distillated beverages composition and its utility has been proved on the analysis of spirit beverages like tequila, vodka, cognac, ron and brandy. Through a variety of detectors such as FID, MS, electronic nose, etc., coupled to GC equipment it has been possible to establish patterns of composition and concentration not only for white but for rested alcoholic beverages (aged in barrels) too. For these beverages aldehydes, phenols, terpenes, higher alcohols, volatile organic acids, esters, fatty acids, etc are monitored (Campo el at., 2007; Cardeal & Marriot, 2009; Peña Alvarez et al., 2006; Plutowska & Wardencki, 2008; Wang et al., 2004).

Other studies have been successfully applied to analyze and authenticate other food products. For example, coffee has been studied to detect dichloromethane, methylimidazole, adulterations of ground roasted coffee with roasted barley; other properties of coffee as fingerprint of coffee flavor and discrimination among several varieties has been done with the help of chemometric analysis (Casal et al., 2002; Hovell et al., 2010; Huang et al., 2007; Oliveira et al., 2009; Russo et al., 1989). Detection of pesticides, vitamins, sugars and organic acids on vegetables, fruits and fruit juices has been reported (Barden et al., 1997; Gonzalez et al., 2008; Pereira et al., 2006; Sanz & Martinez Castro, 2004; Wegener & Lopez Sanchez, 2010; Xiao et al., 2006; Yang et al., 2011). GC was used in conjunction with LDA (*linear discriminant analysis*) and PLS (*partial least squares*) to differentiate apple juices (Reid et al., 2004). The adulteration of strawberry puree with different levels of apple puree was detected using SPME-GC and PLS analysis at levels of 25% (Reid, O'Donnell, Downey, 2004). Sulfur compounds, fatty acids, flavor compounds and organochlorine components on milk (Luna & Juarez, 2005; Vazquez et al., 2005; Vazquez Landaverde et al., 2006; Vetter et al., 2000). Table 2 shows the typical conditions and applications when using GC for food analysis.

	Analytes	Sample pre-treatment and injection	Chromatographic conditions			
			Column Phase	Temperature Program	Flow/vol. (mLmin $^{-1}$/µL)	Detector
Contaminants	Pesticides	Splitless, PTV,	5% DPhe–95% DMPS	70 °C for 1 min, 10 °C min^{-1} ramp to	1,0 / 1,0	MS, ECD, NPD,
		DSI/DMI, SPME	50% DPhe–50% DMPS	130 °C. Then 6 °C min^{-1} to 230 °C, finally		FPD, PFPD, AED
			6% CyP-Phe–94% DMPS	by 8 °C min^{-1} to 250 °C and held for 13 min.		PID, ELCD
	Mycotoxins	Splitless, Drvt	5% DPhe–95% DMPS	120 °C for 2 min to 270 °C at 5°C min^{-1}. then to 290 °C at 10 °C min^{-1}	1,0 /2,0	MS, ECD
	Polychlorinated	Splitless, PTV	5% DPhe–95% DMPS	80 °c to 180 °C at 15 °C min^{-1}. then to 300 °C	1,0 / 2,0	ECD, MS
	Biphenyls		50% DPhe–50% DMPS	At 10 °C min^{-1} for 3 min		
	Polycyclic aromatic	Splitless, PTV	5% DPhe–95% DMPS	110 °C for 1 min to 240 °C at 20 °C min^{-1}.	1,0 / 1,0	MS, PID
	Hydrocarbons		50% DPhe–50% DMPS	Then 5 °C min^{-1} to 320 °C for 10 min		
	Veterinary drugs	Splitless, Drvt	100% DMPS	Depends of specific analyte	1,0 / 1,0	MS
			5% DPhe–95% DMPS			
	Chloropropanols	Splitless, PTV	5% DPhe–95% DMPS	50 °C for 1 min to 90 °C at 2 °C min^{-1}	1,0 / 10	MS
	Heterocyclic	Splitless, Drvt	5% DPhe–95% DMPS	70 °C for 1 min to 240 °C at 25 °C min^{-1} for	1,0 / 1,0	MS
	Amines		50% DPhe–50% DMPS	1 min. Then 10 °C min^{-1} to 300 °C		
	Epoxy-compounds	Splitless, Drvt	5% DPhe–95% DMPS	50°C for 5 min to 280°C at 4°Cmin^{-1} for 2min	1,0 / 1,0	MS
Natural components	Fatty acids	Split, Drvt	Polyethylene glycol	60 °C to 220 °C at 7 °C min^{-1}	1,0-1,5 / 1,0	FID, MS
			70% CyP-Phe–30% DMPS			
	Aroma	Split, splitless,	5% DPhe–95% DMPS	50 °C for 2 min. Then 5 °C min^{-1} to 210 °C	1,0 / 1,0	MS, FID
		SPME	Polyethylene glycol	for 40 min		
	Flavor	Split, splitless,	5% DPhe–95% DMPS	40 °C for 5 min. Then 3 °C min^{-1} to 230 °C	1,0 / 1,0	MS, FID
		SPME	Polyethylene glycol	for 15 min		

Abbreviations: SPME, solid-phase microextraction; FID, flame ionization detector; MS, mass spectroscopy; PTV, programmable temperature vaporization; DSI, direct sample introduction; DMI, difficult matrix introduction; ECD, electron capture detector; NPD, nitrogen-phosphorus detector; FPD, flame photometric detector; PFPD, pulsed flame photometric detector; AED, atomic-emission detector; PID, photo-ionization detector; ELCD, electrolytic conductivity detector; CyP-Phe, Cyanopropyl-phenyl; DMPS, dimethylpolysiloxane; DPhe, Diphenyl.

Table 2. Gas chromatographic conditions for most common compounds analyzed in food

3.2 HPLC

HPLC is a separation technique that involves the injection of a small volume of liquid sample into a tube packed with tiny particles (3 to 5 µm in diameter). Individual components of the sample are moved down the packed tube (column) with a liquid (mobile phase) forced through the column by high pressure delivered by a pump. For the case of LC (*liquid chromatography*) samples are transported along the column by a liquid moved by gravity.

In principle, LC and HPLC work in similar way but HPLC has some advantages over LC such as speed, efficiency, sensitivity and ease of operation, and they make it vastly superior to LC.

The compounds in a sample are separated one from the other by the column packing that involves various chemical and/or physical interactions among their molecules and the packing particles. These separated components are identified at the exit of the column by a flow-through device (detector) that measures them. The detector device can be based on several techniques such as a spectrophotometric, fluorescence or electrochemical detection. The output from the detector is called a chromatogram. The HPLC equipment is constituted by four principal components, i.e. the pump, the injector, the column and the detector systems.

Pump. The pump system forces a liquid (mobile phase) through the column at a specific flow rate and normal flow rates in HPLC are in the range of 1-to 2-mL/min. Typical pumps can reach pressures in the range of 6000-9000 psi (400-to 600-bar). During the chromatographic experiment a pump can deliver a constant mobile phase composition (isocratic) or an increasing mobile phase composition (gradient).

Injector. The injector serves to introduce the liquid sample into the flow stream of the mobile phase. Typical sample volumes are 5-to 20-microliters (µL) and the injector must also be able to withstand the high pressures of the liquid system. When the user has many samples to analyze or when manual injection is not practical then the use of an autosampler is recommended (this is an automatic version).

Column. The column system is considered the "heart of the chromatograph". The column's stationary phase separates the sample components of interest using various physical and chemical parameters. The pump must push hard to move the mobile phase through the column and this resistance causes a high pressure within the chromatograph. It is important to take into account that the correct selection of the column packing and the mobile phase are the most important factors in making the best performance with HPLC.

Detector. The detector can determine individual molecules that come out (elute) from the column. A detector serves to measure the amount of those molecules so that the chemist can quantitatively analyze the sample components. The detector provides an output to a recorder called chromatogram.

To separate most compounds there are four major separation modes, i.e. RPC (*Reversed-Phase Chromatography*), Normal Phase or Adsorption Chromatography, Ion Exchange Chromatography and SEC (*Size Exclusion Chromatography*).

For RPC the column packing is non-polar, e.g. C18, C8, C3, phenyl, etc. and the mobile phase is water (buffer) + water-miscible organic solvent, methanol and acetonitrile for example. RPC is by far the most popular mode (over 90%) and can be used for non-polar, polar, ionizable and ionic molecules. All this makes to RPC very versatile for samples containing a wide range of compounds; gradient elution is often used. One begins with a predominantly water-based mobile phase and then adds organic solvent as a function of time. The organic solvent increases the solvent strength and elutes compounds that are very strongly retained on the RPC packing.

The Normal Phase technique or Adsorption Chromatography is useful for water-sensitive compounds, geometric isomers, cis-trans isomers, class separations, and chiral compounds. The column packing is polar (e.g. silica gel, cyanopropyl-bonded, amino-bonded, etc.) and the mobile phase is non-polar (e.g. hexane, iso-octane, methylene chloride, ethyl acetate), normal phase separations are performed less than 10% of the time.

Ion Exchange Chromatography, in this mode the column packing contains ionic groups, e.g. sulfonic, tetraalkylammonium and the mobile phase is an aqueous buffer, for example phosphate or formate. Ion exchange is used for about 20% of the cases and it is well suited for the separation of inorganic and organic anions and cations in aqueous solution, Ionic dyes, amino acids, and proteins. In fact any salt compounds in brine water.

In Size Exclusion Chromatography there is no interaction between the sample compounds and the column packing material. Instead, molecules diffuse into pores within a porous medium and depending on their size (relative to the pore size) molecules can be separated. Thus, molecules larger than the pore opening do not diffuse while those smaller do and get separated. Large molecules elute first while smaller molecules elute later. The SEC technique is used by 10-15% of the cases, mainly for polymer characterization and for proteins.

Modern agriculture and food processing often involve the use of chemicals. Some of these chemicals and their functions are listed below:

- Fertilizers: increase production of agricultural plants
- Pesticides: protect crops against weeds and pests
- Antibiotics: prevent bacteria growth in animals during breeding
- Hormones: accelerate animal growth
- Colorants: increase acceptability and appeal of food
- Preservatives and antioxidants: extend product life
- Natural and artificial sweeteners and flavors: improve the taste of food
- Natural and synthetic vitamins: increase the nutritive value of food
- Carbohydrates: act as food binders

Such chemicals improve productivity and thus increase competitiveness and profit margins. However, if the amounts in the final product exceed certain limits some of these chemicals may prove harmful to humans. Therefore it is very important to have control of the right amounts of chemicals and on important technique is HPLC. The number of applications of this technique in food quality control is in continuous growth, and Table 3 shows some applications.

On the other hand, Fig. 3 shows the polarity and volatility characteristics of the most common compounds in food products. This figure gives a major idea about which technique is better between GC or HPLC for several kinds of compounds and which type of column or separation mode is the best choice according of the compound polarity.

It is possible to find several HPLC applications for many kinds of compounds in food products. For example the determination of vitamins B_6, K, B_2, D_3, and C in honey, animal products and in a wide range of fortified food products like fruit juices, in fruits directly and milk (Breithaupt, 2001; Ciulu et al., 2011; Fontannaz et al., 2006; Kall, 2003; Romeu Nadal et al., 2006; Salo et al., 2000). Analysis of the whey protein *b*-lactoglobulin has enabled detection of the adulteration of ovine and caprine cheese with bovine milk at levels as low as 2% v/v, and of caprine milk with bovine milk (Chen et al., 2004).

Several types of distilled beverages have been analyzed through HPLC such as tequila, rum, cognac, whisky and vodka for the determination of aldehydes (2-furaldehyde,

Sample type	Analytes	Sample pre-treatment	Chromatographic conditions				
			Column	Mobile phase	Gradient	Flow/vol. (mLmin $^{-1}$/µL)	Detector
Food aditives	Acidulants	SD, SPE, filtration	300 x 7,8 mm BioRad HPX 87-H, 9 µm	0,0035 M H2SO4	Non-gradient	0,6 / 10	UV-Vis
	antioxidants	LE-UB, SPE, LLE, SD	100 x 4 mm BDS, 3µm	A= Water + 0.2 mL H2SO4, pH=2,54; B=ACN	10-90% B	0,5 / 5	UV-DAD
	Preservatives	LE-UB, SPE, LLE, SD	125 x 4 mm Hypersil BDS, 5µm	A= Water + 0.2 mL H2SO4, pH=2,3; B=ACN	10-90% B 10% B	2,0 / 2,0	UV-DAD
	Artificial	LE low pH, UB, SPE	100 x 2,1 mm	A= 0,01 med mer sodium	5-95% B	0,35 / 1,0	UV-DAD;
	sweeteners	Drvt with OPA, MPA	Hypersil ODS, 5µm	acetate; B=methanol			Fluorescence
	colorants	Filtration, LSE	125 x 3 µm Hypersil BDS, 3mm	A = 0.01 M NaH2PO4+ 0.001 M TBADHP, pH=2 B = ACN	15-90% B 15% B	0,8 / 1,0	UV-DAD
	Flavors	filtration, LSE	100 x 4 mm Hypersil BDS, 3 µm	A=water+0.15ml H2SO4 conc pH = 2.3, B=ACN	10-90% B	0,8 /5	UV-DAD
contaminants	tetracyclines	TCD followed by	100 x 4 mm	A = water, pH = 2.1 with	15-60% B	0.5 / 5.0	UV-DAD
		LLE	Hypersil BDS, 3 µm	Sulfuric acid; B=ACN			
	Pesticides	LLE	100 x 3 mm Hypersil BDS, 3 µm	water/ACN (95:5)	10-100% ACN	0.5 / 5.0	UV-DAD
Natural components	Inorganic anions	Filtration	HP-IC	water/ACN (86:14) pH =8.6 by NaOH	Non-gradient	1.5 / 10	UV-VWD
	Lipids	LLE with THF	200 x 2.1 mm	A=water, B=ACN/methyl-	87-100% B	0.8 / 1.0	UV
			Hypersil MOS, 5 µm	terbutylether (9:1)			
	Fatty acids	Hyd by KOH followed by DVT	200 x 21 mm mos, 5 µm	A=water (70%) B=ACN + 1%THF (30%)	30-98% B	0.3 / 5.0	UV-DAD UV-VWD
	Carbo-hydrates	SDI	300 x 7.8 mm Bio-Rad HPXP, 9 µm	water	Non-gradient	0.7 / 5.0	Refractive index
	vitamins	LSE and Filtration	100 x 4 mm Hypersil BDS, 3 µm	A=water with pH=2.1 (H2SO4)=99%; B=ACN 1%	1-90% B	0.5 / 2.0	UV-DAD
	amino acids	Hyd by HCl	200 x 2.1 mm	A=0.03 M SA, pH=7.2 + 0.5%	0-100% B	0.6 / 1.0	UV-DAD
		Filtration	Hypersil ODS, 5 µm	THF; B=0.1 M SA/ACN (1:4)			Fluorescence

Abbreviations: SD, stem distillation; SPE, solid phase extraction; UV-Vis, ultraviolet-visible spectroscopy; LE-UB, Liquid Extraction with ultrasonic bath; LLE, liquid-liquid extraction; ACN, Acetonitrile; UV-DAD, ultraviolet-diode array detector; Drvt, derivatization; OPA, o-phthalaldehyde; MPA, mercapto-propionic acid; LSE, liquid-solid extraction; TDC, tetracycline dissociation; DVT online derivatization with bromophenacyl bromide; SDI, sample direct injection.

Table 3. HPLC conditions for most common compounds analyzed in food

5-hydroxymethyl-2-furaldehyde and furfural), amines, carbohydrates and toxic compounds like arsenic. However, there is poor information concerning methods for the identification of adulterate distilled beverages, see Sec. 4.3 below. Some authors have reported methods for determination of aging markers in tequila such as phenolic compounds (gallic acid, vanillin, syringaldehyde, sinapinaldehyde, so on) and through these compounds is possible to recognize adulterate tequilas (Alcazar et al., 2006; Coelho et al., 2005; Munoz Munoz et al., 2008; Soga, 2002; Vidal Carou et al., 2003).

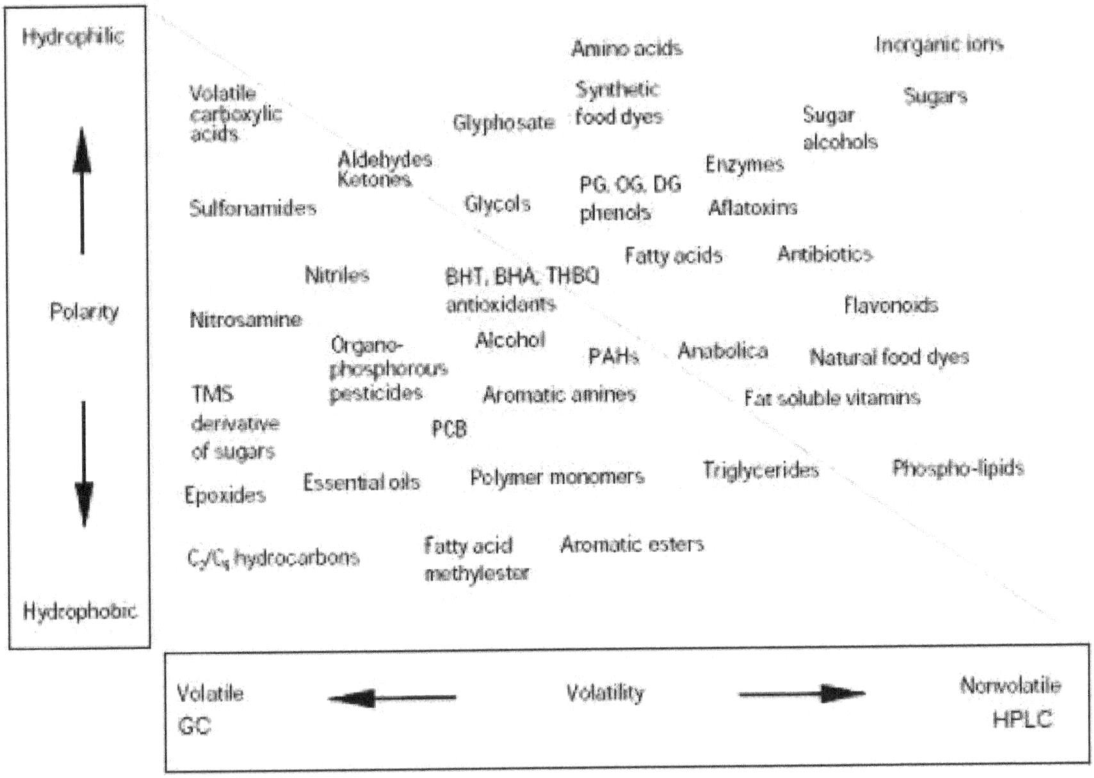

Fig. 3. Comparison of the physical and chemical properties of the main analytes of food products

Wines from different areas of origin in Canary Islands were correctly classified at levels as high as 100% using HPLC analysis. The study was on selected polyphenol compounds combined with PCA and LDA (Rodriguez Delgado et al., 2002). Spanish table wines were correctly differentiated at levels of 83–86% using PCA and LDA of the HPLC data obtained for selected biogenic amine compounds in the samples (Romero et al., 2002).

On the other hand, HPLC analysis of the triglyceride and tocopherol composition of coffee samples was combined with PCA and LDA to differentiate coffee samples on the basis of variety (Gonzalez et al., 2001). Another important food product that has been the subject of analysis by several techniques is the olive oil. The analysis of several phenolic acids is carried out by HPLC where the overlapped peaks are resolved by using chemometric tools such as MCR-ALS and PARAFAC2 (*parallel factor analysis*) (Marini et al., 2001). Other works are focused on the pre-treatment, Tasioula-Margari et. al. propose the simultaneous extraction and HPLC determination of phenols and tocopherols in virgin oil and an average recovery of 80% was achieved (Tasioula Margari & Okoger, 2001). Adulteration of olive oil with soybean oil can be detected by methods of triacylglycerol evaluation with HPLC-APCI-MS–MS (Fasciotti & Pereira Natto, 2010).

3.3 Electronic nose

Electronic nose technology is based on chemical gas-sensor array technology, i.e. the detection by an array of semi-selective gas sensors of the volatile compounds present in the headspace of a food sample. Some of the advantages of the electronic nose technology over other techniques are the high number of samples that can be analyzed in a short period of time, with good reproducibility and accuracy. However, this technique employs sensors that are not very selective for particular types of compounds, thus preventing any real identification or quantization of individual compounds present in a food sample.

Electronic nose technology in conjunction with chemometric analysis (PCA and ANN) has also been successfully applied to the analysis of changes of aroma, along days, released from a flavour encapsulated in a polysaccharide gel matrix, i.e. the time dependence of the aroma pattern emitted by an encapsulated essence (Rodriguez et al., 2010). Chemometric analysis is also applied to alcoholic beverages such as wine samples. Spanish white, red and rose wines were differentiated using a combination of electronic nose and principal components analysis (Guadarrama et al., 2001). On the other hand, authenticity studies have also been carried out for the differentiation of honey samples. Other applications include the determination of the geographical origins of food products and the differentiation of olive oils from adulterated samples with other kind of oils (Cerrato et al., 2002; Cosio et al., 2006).

Despite its drawbacks, electronic nose technology remains an area of research that holds much potential for future development in a higher number of applications related to food. Numerous electronic nose studies related to food already have been published. Many of them represent preliminary feasibility studies, but a limited number of them represent basic studies including long term validation of the technique on a specific application.

4. Spectroscopic techniques and chemometric tools

Spectroscopic techniques have the potential to simplify and reduce analytical times. This section reviews the use of some spectroscopic techniques which combined with chemometric assess food quality. Among the techniques that will be considered are Raman, NIR, MIR, NMR, UV-Vis and fluorescence.

Some of the main advantages of spectroscopic methods are simplicity, rapidity, and practically there is no use of sample pre-treatment. However, the capacity of simultaneous determination of several analytes in the same sample or the determination of a single analyte in complex matrices through direct spectroscopic measures diminishes because the spectral overlap. Chemometric tools such as the MVCM (*multivariate calibration models*) allow the spectral resolution and quantification in the presence of interferents. Further, the detection of discrepant samples of prediction is possible and recently, multiway chemometric techniques have been introduced for the analysis of complex samples (Bro, 2006; Culzoni et al., 2007; Ornelas, 2008; Rodriguez et al., 2008). The advantage of using data involving high-dimensional structured information is the higher stability towards interferents and matrix effects compared with first-order methodologies. There are several algorithms for analyzing second-order data, such as PARAFAC, BLLS (*bilinear least-squares*) and N-PLS (*multiway partial least-squares*) (Rodriguez et al., 2008).

PARAFAC is a decomposition method, which conceptually can be compared to bilinear PCA. The decomposition is made into triads or trilinear components, and each component consists of one score vector and two loading vectors. An advantage of PARAFAC is the uniqueness of the solution. This means that the true underlying spectra will be found if the right number of components is used and the signal-to-noise ratio is appropriate (Bro, 1997). The decomposition of EEMs (*excitation–emission matrices*) data into three-dimensional arrays, by PARAFAC, exploits the second-order advantage (Culzoni et al., 2006). This advantage allows direct extraction of the spectral profiles as well as the relative concentrations of individual sample components (Munoz de la Pena et al., 2006).
BLLS is a technique based on a direct least-squares procedure (Linder & Sundberg, 1998). It starts with a calibration step in which approximations to pure analyte matrices at unit concentration are found by direct least-squares. To estimate the pure analyte matrices, the calibration data matrices are first vectorised and grouped and, an analogous procedure to classical least-squares is then performed (Faber et al., 2002). Concentration estimation is usually carried out through the least-squares predictor (Linder & Sundberg, 1998).
A promising alternative is NPLS, which is a genuine multiway method. But these algorithms do not present the second-order advantage unless they are coupled with a procedure known as RBL (*residual bilinearisation*) (Cardeal & Marriott, 2009; Casal et al., 2002; Russo & Goretti, 1989). Recently, two reviews about the algorithms and applications of second- and third-order multivariate calibration have been published (Bro, 2006; Escandar et al., 2007).

4.1 The Raman, Mid-infrared (MIR 4000 to 400 cm^{-1}) and Near-infrared (NIR 14000-4000 cm^{-1}) spectroscopic techniques

The use of Raman, MIR and NIR spectroscopic techniques in chemical analysis has been broadened for the past two decades due to the advance of technological and scientific innovations. The involved instrumentation in these three techniques is easy to implement at any laboratory, for academic or industrial use, due to the increase of improved instruments in the market. Furthermore, for routine processes these techniques are very practical since special training is not required and the cost of the equipment would be much less than any of those use in chemical analysis. The main feature of these techniques when applied to any sample is that they are not destructive and the time to obtain results is short compared to wet analysis. Thus, if they are applied to food products for quality control the sample under study does not require any pre-treatment.
When Raman spectroscopy is compared against IR spectroscopy, it presents the advantage of low sensitivity to water; therefore lends itself for making measurements in liquid environments. On the other hand, it presents high sensitivity to C=C, C≡C and C≡N bonds and thus, the fatty acid composition in foods is easily determinate. Raman spectroscopy also gives high selectivity to inorganic compounds like salts.
The Raman spectroscopy has been employed for determination of food proteins. For this case Raman spectra of modified proteins trough analysis of a new C=O stretching vibrational band attributed to γ-carboxyl groups of aspartic and glutamic acids was used (Wong et al., 2004). For quantitative measurements of carotenoid, collagen and fat in fish muscle the Raman technique was also used (Marquard & Wold, 2004). In the case of edible oil analysis, the Raman technique allowed to investigate the chemical changes taking place during lipid oxidation in several edible oils through oxidative degradation of several vegetable oils by using heating at 160 °C (Muik et al., 2005).

Raman spectroscopy with chemometric analysis was successfully employed for determination of adulterants in honey. For this case honey is adulterated by using cheap invert sugars. Also, it was employed to successfully differentiate honeys of various botanical and geographical origins of the nectar which are related to the chemical composition of honey. Because of consumer preferences, prices of honeys from single plant species are much higher than those of common polyfloral honeys (Lema et al., 2010; Paradkar & Irudayaraj, 2002).

On the other hand, the analysis of food samples by using MIR or NIR gives information about molecular bonds and can therefore give details of the types of molecules present in food products. By using NIR spectroscopy one can easily quantify various properties of food such as online measurement of water, proteins, pigments and fat content. When these IR spectroscopic techniques are used jointly with multivariate analysis some results have been reported. For example, the quality control of potato chips was tested trough extraction of oil from potato chips with a carver press; the spectra were collected by using a temperature controlled ATR (*attenuated total reflection*) accessory (Shiroma & Rodriguez, 2009). These techniques were employed to differentiate between apple juice samples on the basis of apple variety; for this case chemometric procedures were applied to MIR and NIR data where PLS2 and LDA for varietal differentiation applied to PC (*principal component*) scores (Reid et al., 2005). For the detection of adulterate oil samples and classification of other vegetable oils according to their botanical origin the FTIR with chemometric analysis was used (Gurdeniz & Ozen, 2009; Wang & Li, 2011).

NIR and MIR have widely employed for meat quality control. Several works test the ability of both spectroscopic techniques to follow meat freshness decay in high-oxygen modified atmosphere packaged at different temperatures (Sinelli et al., 2010); determination of C22:5 and C22:6 for marine fatty acids analysis in pork adipose tissue (Flatten et al., 2005). FT-IR was exploited to measure biochemical changes within the fresh beef substrate, enhancing and accelerating the detection of microbial spoilage (Ellis et al., 2004). The potential of near infrared spectroscopy to predict texture and colour of dry-cured ham samples was investigated by analyzing of 117 boned and cross-sectioned dry-cured ham samples. The overall accuracy of the classification as a function of pastiness was 88.5%; meanwhile, according to colour was 79.7%. Partial least squares regression was used to formulate prediction equations for pastiness and color. The samples were classified into defective or no defective classes with a correct classification of 94.2% according to pasty texture evaluation and 75.7% as regard to colour evaluation (Garcia Rey et al., 2005).

4.2 NMR spectroscopy

NMR spectroscopy involves the analysis of the energy absorption by atomic nuclei with non-zero spins in the presence of a magnetic field. The energy absorptions of the atomic nuclei are affected by the nuclei of surrounding molecules, which cause small local modifications to the external magnetic field. NMR spectroscopy can therefore provide detailed information about the molecular structure of a food sample, given that the observed interactions of an individual atomic nucleus are dependent on the atoms surrounding it.

High-resolution NMR (HR-NMR; frequencies above 100 MHz) has been applied in many food products. NMR is conventionally used to obtain detailed chemical information on liquid-state systems. Recent advances in techniques and hardware now allow the routine acquisition of high-resolution ^{13}C NMR spectra from solid materials. Although ^{1}H is the most abundant NMR nucleus, there are technical difficulties in high-resolution solid-state ^{1}H NMR that make ^{13}C the nucleus of choice (Gidley, 1992).

The MNR studies are diverse such as the study of the acyl positional distribution on fish phospholipids in the carbonyl region. A selective enrichment of saturated and monounsaturated fatty acids in the *sn*-1 position, and a corresponding *sn*-2 location of polyunsaturated fatty acids (PUFA) was found (Medina & Sacchi, 1994). High resolution ^{1}H NMR has been applied to monitor the changes in the composition of natural mango juice subjected to spoilage and to microbial contamination with *Penicillium expansum;* this study was made through monitoring of typical fermentation products, organic acids, amino acids and less abundant components such as oligosaccharides and aromatic compounds (Duarte et al., 2006).

An important field for NMR analysis is to assess geographical origin of traditional food; diverse countries have adopted different denominations to label their typical food products in order to give them additional value (Consinni & Cagliani, 2010). The relative deuterium concentration and specific deuterium-site locations in a molecule can be determined using SNIFNMR (*Site-Specific Natural Isotope Fractionation-Nuclear Magnetic Resonance*). This can provide information about the chemical pathway of formation and, in some cases, information about the geographic origin of a sample can also be discerned (Cross et al., 1998). In this context, food products such as olive oil, dairy milk and cheese have been tested (Bescia et al., 2005; D'Imperio et al., 2007; Karoui & Baerdemaeker, 2007). The major disadvantage of HR-NMR is that it is one of the most expensive analytical techniques to employ.

4.3 Fluorescence and UV–Vis spectroscopy

Fluorescence spectroscopy has been used to assess different food proprieties by using different methods such as synchronous front-face fluorescence spectroscopy along chemometric methods. A review on this matter has been reported by Sadecka and Tothova, 2007. In particular some applications of such methods have been reported, for example for the determination of microbial load on chicken breast fillets stored aerobically (Shar et al., 2011). Studies of olive oil adulteration and classification of virgin olive oil from other types were also made (Guimet et al., 2004; Guimet et al., 2005). Similar to other spectroscopic techniques, fluorescence spectroscopy has a large potential for being used in food research and this potential has been increasing during last years. Fluorescence spectroscopy can determinate some properties of food products without sample preparation since it is a non-destructive technique; there is no use of chemicals; food can be solid or liquid and the time of performance to obtain results can be very short when compared against those wet techniques; it can be used to analyze compounds at concentration as low as parts per billion, and among anything many food products contain intrinsic compounds that emit light when excited with the proper light-wavelength.

Other food products that have been studied under different techniques are alcoholic beverages, e.g. beers, table wines and spirits. Some works have shown the effectiveness of applying chemometric methods to different spectroscopic techniques. For example, NIR spectra to estimate the ripeness of wine grapes (Herrera et al., 2003), and to FT-IR and UV spectra for the characterization and classification of wine (Guillén et al., 2005). The alcohol content in beverages has also been done through spectroscopic techniques (Barboza & Poppi, 2003). Differentiation between brandies and wine distillates has been achieved and reported through luminescence (Tothova et al., 2009). Thus, it can be claimed that multivariate data analysis has played a good rule jointly with chromatographic and spectroscopic methods when applied to food products, in particular, for alcoholic beverages (Barbosa Garcia et al., 2007; Edelmann et al., 2001; Mattarucci et al., 2010; Navas & Jimenez 1999; Savchuk et al., 2001).

On the other hand, with UV-Vis spectroscopy table wines have also been classified and differentiated (Urbano et al., 2006) and the authentication of whiskeys through absorption spectroscopy has been reported (MacKenzie & Aylott, 2004). The UV–Vis spectroscopy with chemometric analysis is a simple way to distinguish the types of the popular spirit made from the juice of the agave plant, i.e. tequila (Barbosa Garcia et al, 2007). Two kinds of tequilas are produced, the 100% blue agave and the mixed which is only 51% of blue agave. Mezcal is another spirit made from different type of agave and also could be distinguished from tequila with similar methodology. The quality control of these spirits, along the process of production, could be possible *in situ*. Another result from these studies is the differentiation among different brands of tequila and all these results can be extended to other spirits. Therefore, adulteration and authentication of tequilas is possible to be recognized though a simple method. These results were made through the UV-Vis absorption spectroscopy and validate through HPLC (Contreras et al., 2010; Munoz Munoz et al., 2010).

5. Conclusions

In addition to sensory parameters such as aroma, colour or taste, the quality of food all over the world is based on measurable factors such as chemical and nutritional composition (percentage of sugar, fatty acids, antioxidants, protein, fibre etc.), as well as microbiological control. In this chapter, an overview of some of the most used methodologies for quality control of food products has been shown. It is clear that chemical analysis plays an important role in this matter and the choice of appropriate analytical method should be treated as an essential aspect. This is so since the chosen method for analysis should be adequate to the purpose for which results are required, e.g., determination of forbidden and permitted substances (application of food laws and official regulations) or monitoring of key compounds that enhance the food value. Besides the suitable method of analysis, it was pointed out in this chapter that sampling and pre-treatment of food products play an important rule in the quality control process for food products. A short review of sampling procedures was given and the pre-treatment on food was pointed out along the presented analytical method.

New trends on the quality control processes are clearly seen nowadays. Industry needs to reduce costs and time during the test of food products. Besides high levels of specificity and accuracy, analysis along the line of production is needed. Pre-treatment of samples should be minimized to reduce costs and times for testing food products. Thus, in this chapter it was shown that there are a great variety of analytical methods for food quality control. However those based on chromatography are the best bet since new methodologies with chemometric analysis are rising up. The main developments in chromatographic methods are focused on the reductions of analysis times. Nowadays there are chromatographic runs lasting only a few minutes. These improvements increase the industrial potential of chromatography, although the use of MS detection would vastly increase the cost. The electronic nose technology has the advantage of being relatively cheap, quick and easy to operate. On the other hand, spectroscopic methodologies are the newest that are becoming stronger in the field. They have some interesting features not seen in other analytical methods, e.g. no-pretreatment of samples, the cost of laboratory equipment for routine analysis is low, can be fast compared to other methods, can be performed *in situ* along the line of production and so on. Moreover, some other techniques as NMR spectroscopy, despite its high level of specificity and accuracy in food characterization, have disadvantages in cost terms for online applications like chromatographic techniques.

6. Acknowledgment

Authors thank Dr. Meneses Nava for some technical support and to the Group of Optical Properties of Matter at Centro de Investigaciones en Optica for their comments and suggestions.

7. References

Alcázar, A., Jurado, J.M., Pablos, F., González, A.G., Martín, M.J. (2006). HPLC determination of 2-furaldehyde and 5-hydroxymethyl-2-furaldehyde in alcoholic beverages. *Microchemical Journal*, Volume 82, Issue 1, January 2006, pp. 22-28.

Aramendía, M.A., Borau, V., Lafont, F., Marinas, A., Marinas, J.M., Moreno, J.M., Urbano, F.J., (2007). Determination of herbicide residues in olive oil by gas chromatography–tandem mass spectrometry. *Food Chemistry*, Volume 105, Issue 2, 2007, pp. 855-861.

Ball, G.F.M. (1990). The application of HPLC to the determination of low molecular weight sugars and polyhydric alcohols in foods: A review. Food *Chemistry*, Volume 35, Issue 2, 1990, pp. 117-152.

Barbosa-Garcia, O., Ramos-Ortiz, G., Maldonado, J.L., Pichardo-Molina, J., Meneses-Nava, M.A., Landgrave, J., Cervantes-Martinez., J. (2007). UV–vis absorption spectroscopy and multivariate analysis as a method to discriminate tequila. *Spectrochimica Acta Part A* 66 (2007) 129–134.

Barboza, F.D., Poppi R.J., (2003). Determination of alcohol content in beverages using short-wave nearinfrared spectroscopy and temperature correction by transfer calibration procedures. *Analytical and Bioanalytical Chemistry*, 377, pp. 695–701.

Barden, T.J., Croft, M.Y., Murby, E.J., Wells, R.J., (1997). Gas chromatographic determination of organic acids from fruit juices by combined resin mediated methylation and extraction in supercritical carbon dioxide. *Journal of Chromatography A*, Volume 785, Issues 1-2, 17 October 1997, pp. 251-261.

Breithaupt, D.E., (2001). Determination of folic acid by ion-pair RP-HPLC in vitamin-fortified fruit juices after solid-phase extraction. *Food Chemistry*, Volume 74, Issue 4, September 2001, pp. 521-525.

Brescia, M.A., Monfreda, M., Buccolieri, A., Carrino, C., (2005). Characterisation of the geographical origin of buffalo milk and mozzarella cheese by means of analytical and spectroscopic determinations Original. *Food Chemistry*, Volume 89, Issue 1, January 2005, pp. 139-147.

Bro R., (2006). Review on Multiway Análisis in Chemistry -2000-2005. *Crit. Rev. Anal. Chem.* 36 (2006) pp. 279 293.

Bro, R., (1997). PARAFAC: Tutorial & applications. *Chemom Intell Lab Syst*, 1997, 38, pp. 149-171.

Campo, E., Cacho, J., Ferreira, V. (2007). Solid phase extraction, multidimensional gas chromatography mass spectrometry determination of four novel aroma powerful ethyl esters: Assessment of their occurrence and importance in wine and other alcoholic beverages. *Journal of Chromatography A*, Volume 1140, Issues 1-2, 26 January 2007, pp. 180-188.

Cardeal, Z.L., Marriott, P.J. (2009). Comprehensive two-dimensional gas chromatography-mass spectrometry analysis and comparison of volatile organic compounds in Brazilian *cachaça* and selected spirits. *Food Chemistry*, Volume 112, Issue 3, 1 February 2009, pp. 747-755.

Casal, S., Fernandes, J.O.,Oliveira, M.B.P.P., Ferreira, M.A., (2002). Gas chromatographic-mass spectrometric quantification of 4-(5-)methylimidazole in roasted coffee after ion-pair extraction. *Journal of Chromatography A*, Volume 976, Issues 1-2, 8 November 2002, pp. 285-291

Cerrato Oliveros, M.C., Pérez Pavón, J.L., García Pinto, C., Fernández Laespada, M.E., Moreno Cordero, B., Forina M., (2002). Electronic nose based on metal oxide semiconductor sensors as a fast alternative for the detection of adulteration of virgin olive oils. *Analytica Chimica Acta*, Volume 459, Issue 2, 22 May 2002, pp. 219-228.

Chen, R. K., Chang, L.W., Chung, Y. Y., Lee, M. H., & Ling, Y. C., (2004). Quantification of cow milk adulteration in goat milk using high-performance liquid chromatography with electrospray ionization mass spectrometry. *Rapid Communications in Mass Spectrometry*, 18, pp. 1167–1171.

Ciulu, M., Solinas, S., Floris, I., Panzanelli, A., Pilo, M.I., Piu, P.C., Spano, N., Sanna, G., (2011). RP-HPLC determination of water-soluble vitamins in honey. *Talanta*, Volume 83, Issue 3, 15 January 2011, pp. 924-929.

Cochran, W.G., 1997. *Sampling Techniques*. Third edition, John Wiley & Sons, ISBN 0-471-16240-X, U.S.A.

Coelho, N.M.M., Coelho, L.M., de Lima, E.S., Pastor, A., de la Guardiã, M., (2005). Determination of arsenic compounds in beverages by high-performance liquid chromatography-inductively coupled plasma mass spectrometry. *Talanta*, Volume 66, Issue 4, 15 May 2005, Pages 818-822.

Consonni, R., Cagliani, L.R., (2010). Nuclear Magnetic Resonance and Chemometrics to Assess Geographical Origin and Quality of Traditional Food Products. *Advances in Food and Nutrition Research*, Volume 59, 2010, Chapter 4, pp. 87-165.

Contreras, U., Barbosa Garcia, O., Pichardo Molina, J.L., Ramos Ortiz, G., Maldonado Rivera, J.L., Meneses Nava, M.A., Ornelas Soto, N.E., López-de-Alba, P.L. (2010). Screening method for identification of adulterate and fake tequilas by using UV-VIS spectroscopy and chemometrics. *Food Research International*, Volume 43, Issue 10, December 2010, pp. 2356-2362.

Cosio, M.S., Ballabio, D., Benedetti, S., Gigliotti, C., (2006). Geographical origin and authentication of extra virgin olive oils by an electronic nose in combination with artificial neural networks. *Analytica Chimica Acta*, Volume 567, Issue 2, 17 May 2006, pp. 202-210.

Cross, J.L., Gallaher, T., Leary, J., and Schreiner, S., (1998). The application of site-specific natural isotope fractionation-nuclear magnetic resonance (snif-nmr) to the analysis of alcoholic beverages. *The C h e m i c a l Educator.* 1 / vol. 3, n o . 5, i s sn 1 4 3 0 - 4 1 7 1. 1998.

Culzoni, M.J., Damiani, P.C., García-Reiriz, A., Goicoechea, H.C. and Olivieri, A.C., (2007). Experimental study of non-linear second-order analytical data with focus on the second-order advantage. *Analyst*, 2007, 132, pp. 654-663.

Culzoni, M.J., Goicoechea, H.C., Pagani, A.P., Cabezon, M.A., Olivieri, A.C., (2006). Evaluation of partial least-squares with second-order advantage for the multi-way spectroscopic analysis of complex biological samples in the presence of analyte-background interactions. *Analyst* 131, 2006, pp. 718–732.

D'Imperio, M., Mannina, L., Capitani, D., Bidet, O., Rossi, E., Bucarelli, F.M., Quaglia, G.B., Segre, A., (2007). NMR and statistical study of olive oils from Lazio: A geographical, ecological and agronomic characterization. *Food Chemistry,* Volume 105, Issue 3, 2007, pp. 1256-1267.

De Zan, M.M., Cámara, M.S., Robles, J.C., Kergaravat, SV., Goicoechea, H.C., (2009). Development and validation of a simple stability-indicating high performance liquid chromatographic method for the determination of miconazole nitrate in bulk and cream formulation. *Talanta,* 79, 2009, pp. 762-767.

Duarte, I.F., Delgadillo, I., Gil., A.M., (2006). Study of natural mango juice spoilage and microbial contamination with penicillium expansum by high resolution ^{1}H NMR spectroscopy. *Food Chemistry*, Volume 96, Issue 2, May 2006, pp. 313-324.

Dugo G., Di Bella, G., La Torre, L., Saitta, M. (2005). Rapid GC-FPD determination of organophosphorus pesticide residues in Sicilian and Apulian olive oil. *Food Control,* Volume 16, Issue 5, June 2005, pp. 435-438.

Edelmann, A., Diewok, J., Schuster,K., and Lend, B., (2001). Rapid Method for the Discrimination of Red Wine Cultivars Based on Mid-Infrared Spectroscopy of Phenolic Wine Extracts. *J. Agric. Food Chem.* 49, 2001, pp. 1139-1145.

Ellis, D.I., Broadhurst, D., Goodacre, R., (2004). Rapid and quantitative detection of the microbial spoilage of beef by Fourier transform infrared spectroscopy and machine learning. *Analytica Chimica Acta,* Volume 514, Issue 2, 1 July 2004, 193-201.

Escandar, G.M., Faber N.M., Goicoechea H.C., Muñoz de la Peña A., Olivieri A.C., Poppi, R.J. (2007). Second and third-order multivariate calibration: data, algoritms and applications. *TrAC Trends Anal. Chem.* 26 (2007) pp. 752-765.

Faber N.M., Ferré J., Boqué R., Salivas J.H., (2002). *Chemom Intell Lab Syst* 63, 2002, pp. 107–116.

Fasciotti, M., Pereira Netto, A.D. (2010). Optimization and application of methods of triacylglycerol evaluation for characterization of olive oil adulteration by soybean oil with HPLC–APCI-MS–MS. *Talanta,* Volume 81, Issue 3, 15 May 2010, pp. 1116-1125.

Flåtten, A., Bryhni, E.A., Kohler, A., Egelandsdal, B., Isaksson, T., (2005). Determination of C22:5 and C22:6 marine fatty acids in pork fat with Fourier transform mid-infrared spectroscopy. *Meat Science,* Volume 69, Issue 3, March 2005, pp. 433-440.

Fontannaz, P., Kilinç T., Heudi, O., (2006). HPLC-UV determination of total vitamin C in a wide range of fortified food products. *Food Chemistry*, Volume 94, Issue 4, March 2006, pp. 626-631.

Francisco, M.L., Resurreccion, A.V.A., (2009). Development of a reversed-phase high performance liquid chromatography (RP-HPLC) procedure for the simultaneous determination of phenolic compounds in peanut skin extracts. Food *Chemistry*, Volume 117, Issue 2, 15 November 2009, Pages 356-363.

Gallardo Velazquez, T., Osorio Revilla, G., Zuñiga de Loa, M., Rivera Espinoza, Y. (2009). Application of FTIR-HATR spectroscopy and multivariate analysis to the quantification of adulterants in Mexican honeys. *Food Research International*, Volume 42, Issue 3, April 2009, pp. 313-318.

García Gonzalez, D.L., Aparicio, R. (2010). Coupling MOS sensors and gas chromatography to interpret the sensor responses to complex food aroma: Application to virgin olive oil. *Food Chemistry*, Volume 120, Issue 2, 15 May 2010, pp. 572-579.

García Villalba, R., Pacchiarotta, T., Carrasco Pancorbo, A., Segura Carretero, A., Fernández Gutierrz, A., Deelder, A.M., Mayboroda, O.A. (2011). Gas chromatography–atmospheric pressure chemical ionization-time of flight mass spectrometry for profiling of phenolic compounds in extra virgin olive oil. *Journal of Chromatography A*, Volume 1218, Issue 7, 18 February 2011, pp. 959-971.

García-Rey, R.M., García-Olmo, J., De Pedro, E., Quiles-Zafra, R., Luque de Castro, M.D., (2005). Prediction of texture and colour of dry-cured ham by visible and near infrared spectroscopy using a fiber optic probe. *Meat Science*, Volume 70, Issue 2, June 2005, pp. 357-363.

Gidley, M.J., (1992). High-resolution solid state NRM of food materials. Review Article. *Trends in Food Science & Technology*, Volume 3, 1992, Pages 231-236.

Gilbert Lopez, B., Robles Molina, J., García Reyes, J., Molina Diaz, A. (2010). Rapid determination of BTEXS in olives and olive oil by headspace-gas chromatography/mass spectrometry (HS-GC-MS). *Talanta*, Volume 83, Issue 2, 15 December 2010, pp. 391-399.

González Rodriguez, R.M., Rial Otero, R., Cancho Grande, B., Simal Gandara, J. (2008). Determination of 23 pesticide residues in leafy vegetables using gas chromatography–ion trap mass spectrometry and analyte protectants. *Journal of Chromatography A*, Volumes 1196-1197, 4 July 2008, pp. 100-109.

Gonzalez, A. G., Pablos, F., Martin, M. J., Leon-Camacho, M., & Valdenebro, M. S., (2001). HPLC analysis of tocopherols and triglycerides in coffee and their use as authentication parameters. *Food Chemistry*, 73, pp. 93–101.

Guadarrama, A., Rodriguez-Mendez, M. L., Sanz, C., Rios, J. L., & de Saja, J. A. (2001). Electronic nose based on conducting polymers for the quality control of the olive oil aroma – Discrimination of quality, variety of olive and geographic origin. *Analytica Chimica Acta*, 432, pp. 283–292.

Guillén, D. A., Palma, M., Natera, R., Romero, R., Barroso, C. G., (2005). Determination of the Age of Sherry Wines by Regression Techniques Using Routine Parameters and Phenolic and Volatile Compounds. *J. Agric. Food Chem.*. 53, 2005, pp. 2412-2417.

Guimet, F., Ferre, J., Boque, R., & Rius, F. X. (2004). Application of unfold principal component analysis and parallel factor analysis to the exploratory analysis of olive oils by means of excitation-emission matrix. *Analytica Chimica Acta*, 515 (1), 2004, pp. 75–85.

Guimet, F., Ferré, J., Boqué, R., (2005). Rapid detection of olive-pomace oil adulteration in extra virgin olive oils from the protected denomination of origin "Siurana" using excitation–emission fluorescence spectroscopy and three-way methods of analysis . *Analytica Chimica Acta*, Volume 544, Issues 1-2, 15 July 2005, pp. 143-152.

Gurdeniz, G., Ozen, B., (2009). Detection of adulteration of extra-virgin olive oil by chemometric analysis of mid-infrared spectral data. *Food Chemistry*, Volume 116, Issue 2, 15 September 2009, pp. 519-525.

Herrera, J., Guesalaga, A., Agosin, E., (2003). Shortwave–near infrared spectroscopy for non-destructive determination of maturity of wine grapes. *Meas. Sci. Technol.* 14, 2003, pp. 689–697.

Herraiz, T. (2000). Analysis of the bioactive alkaloids tetrahydro-β-carboline and β-carboline in food. *Journal of Chromatography A*, Volume 881, Issues 1-2, 9 June 2000, pp. 483-499.

Hinkelmann, K., & Kempthorne, O., (1994). *Design and analysis of experiments: an introduction to experimental design*. Wiley interscience. ISBN-10: 0471551783. U.S.A.

Holley, K., Pennington, M., Phillips, P., (1995). Gas chromatography in food analysis: an introduction, *Nutrition & Food Science*, Vol. 95 Iss: 5.

Hovell, A.M.C., Pereira, E.J., Arruda, N.P., Rezende, C.M., (2010). Evaluation of alignment methods and data pretreatments on the determination of the most important peaks for the discrimination of coffee varieties Arabica and Robusta using gas chromatography–mass spectroscopy. *Analytica Chimica Acta*, Volume 678, Issue 2, 30 September 2010, pp. 160-168.

Huang, L.F., Wu, M.J., Zhong, K.J., Sun, X.J., Liang, Y.Z., Dai, Y.H., Huang, K.L., Guo, F.Q., (2007). Fingerprint developing of coffee flavor by gas chromatography–mass spectrometry and combined chemometrics methods. *Analytica Chimica Acta*, Volume 588, Issue 2, 11 April 2007, pp. 216-223.

Kall, M. A., (2003). Determination of total vitamin B_6 in foods by isocratic HPLC: a comparison with microbiological analysis. *Food Chemistry*, Volume 82, Issue 2, August 2003, pp. 315-327.

Karoui, R., and Baerdemaeker, J., (2007). A review of the analytical methods coupled with chemometric tools for the determination of the quality and identity of dairy products. Review Article.

Food Chemistry, Volume 102, Issue 3, 2007, pp. 621-640.

Lee, D.S., Noh, B.S., Bae, S.Y., Kim, K. (1998). Characterization of fatty acids composition in vegetable oils by gas chromatography and chemometrics. *Analytica Chimica Acta*, Volume 358, Issue 2, 20 January 1998, pp. 163-175.

Lerma-García, M.J., Ramis-Ramos, G., Herrero-Martínez, J.M., Simó-Alfonso, E.F., (2010). Authentication of extra virgin olive oils by Fourier-transform infrared spectroscopy. *Food Chemistry*, Volume 118, Issue 1, 1 January 2010, pp. 78-83.

Linder M., Sundberg R. (1998). *Chemom Intell Lab Syst* 42, 1998, pp. 159–178.

Luna P., Juárez, M. de la Fuente, M., (2005). Validation of a Rapid Milk Fat Separation Method to etermine the Fatty Acid Profile by Gas Chromatography. *Journal of Dairy Science*, Volume 88, Issue 10, October 2005, pp. 3377-3381.

Luykx, D., van Ruth, S. (2008). An overview of analytical methods for determining the geographical origin of food products. *Food Chemistry*, Volume 107, Issue 2, 15 March 2008, pp. 897-911.

MacKenzie, W.M., Aylott, R.I., (2004). Analytical Strategies to confirm Scotch Whisky Authenticity, Part II: Mobile brand authentication. *Analyst* 129, 2004, pp. 607-6012.

Marcos, I.M., Pérez Pavon, J.L., Fernández Laespada, M.E., García Pinto, C., Moreno Cordero, B. (2002). Detection of adulterants in olive oil by headspace-mass spectrometry. *Journal of Chromatography A*, Volume 945, Issues 1-2, 1 February 2002, Pages 221-230.

Marini, F., D'Aloise, A., Bucci, R., Buiarelli, F., Magrì, A.L., Magrì, A.D., (2011). *Chemometrics and Intelligent Laboratory Systems*, Volume 106, Issue 1, 15 March 2011, pp. 142-149.

Marquardt, B.J., Wold, J.P., (2004). Raman analysis of fish: a potential method for rapid quality screening. *Lebensmittel-Wissenschaft und-Technologie*, Volume 37, Issue 1, February 2004, pp. 1-8.

Mattarucchi, E., Stocchero, M., Moreno-Rojas, J., Giordano, G., Reniero, F., and Guillou, C., (2010). Authentication of Trappist Beers by LC-MS Fingerprints and Multivariate Data Analysis. *J. Agric. Food Chem.*, 58 (23), 2010, pp. 12089–12095.

Medina, I., Sacchi, R., (1994). Acyl stereospecific analysis of tuna phospholipids via high resolution^{13}C-NMR spectroscopy. *Chemistry and Physics of Lipids*, Volume 70, Issue 1, 31 March 1994, pp. 53-61.

Muik, B., Lendl, B., Molina-Díaz, A., Ayora-Cañada, M.J., (2005). Direct monitoring of lipid oxidation in edibl e oils by Fourier transform Raman spectroscopy. *Chemistry and Physics of Lipids*, Volume 134, Issue 2, April 2005, pp. 173-182.

Muñoz de la Peña A., Espinosa Mansilla A., Mora Díez N., Bohoyo, G.D., Olivieri A.C., Escándar G.M., (2006). Second-order calibration of excitation-emission matrix fluorescence spectra for the determination of N-phenylanthranilic acid derivatives. *Appl Spectrosc* 60, 2006, pp. 330–338.

Muñoz-Muñoz, A., Pichardo-Molina, J., Gabriel Ramos-Ortíz, G., Barbosa-García, O., Maldonado, J., Meneses-Nava, M., Ornelas-Soto, N., Escobedo, A., and López-de-Alba, P. (2010). Identification and Quantification of Furanic Compounds in Tequila and Mezcal using Spectroscopy and Chemometric Methods. *J. Braz. Chem. Soc.*, Vol. 21, No. 6, 2010, pp. 1077-1087.

Muñoz-Muñoz, A.C., Charles Grenier, A., Gutiérrez-Pulido, H., Cervantes-Martínez, J., (2008). Development and validation of a High Performance Liquid Chromatography-Diode Array Detection method for the determination of aging markers in tequila. *Journal of Chromatography A*, Volume 1213, Issue 2, 12 December 2008, pp. 218-223.

Navas, M. and Jimenez, A., (1999). Chemiluminescent Methods in Alcoholic Beverage Analysis. *J. Agric. Food Chem.* 47, 1999, pp. 183-189.

Oliveira, R., Oliveira, L., Franca, A., Augusti, R. (2009). Evaluation of the potential of SPME-GC-MS and chemometrics to detect adulteration of ground roasted coffee with roasted barley. *Journal of Food Composition and Analysis*, Volume 22, Issue 3, May 2009, pp. 257-261.

Ornelas N., (2008). Desarrollo de nuevas metodologías analíticas para la determinación de compuestos de interés médico y medioambiental. Ph. D. Thesis. Universidad de Guanajuato, Gto., Mexico, 2008.

Otles, S.; Hajslova, J. and Cajka T., (2008). Handbook of Food Analysis Instruments. 2008 Taylor & Francis Group, LLC. ISBN-10: 1420045660.

Paradkar, M.M., Irudayaraj, J., (2002). Discrimination and classification of beet and cane inverts in honey by FT-Raman spectroscopy. *Food Chemistry*, Volume 76, Issue 2, February 2002, pp. 231-239.

Pawliszyn, J. (1997). Solid Phase Microextraction: Theory and Practice, Wiley-VCH, 1997. ISBN-10: 0471190349

Peña Alvarez, A., Capella, S., Juárez, R., Labastida, C. (2006). Determination of terpenes in tequila by solid phase microextraction-gas chromatography–mass spectrometry. *Journal of Chromatography A*, Volume 1134, Issues 1-2, 17 November 2006, pp. 291-297.

Pereira C.C., Ribeiro, C.P., Nobrera, R., Borges, C.P., (2006). Pervaporative recovery of volatile aroma compounds from fruit juices Review Article. *Journal of Membrane Science*, Volume 274, Issues 1-2, 5 April 2006, pp. 1-23.

Petrović, M., Kezić, N., Bolanča, V. (2010). Optimization of the GC method for routine analysis of the fatty acid profile in several food samples. Food *Chemistry*, Volume 122, Issue 1, 1 September 2010, pp. 285-291.

Plutowska, B., Wardencki, W. (2008). Application of gas chromatography–olfactometry (GC–O) in analysis and quality assessment of alcoholic beverages- A review. *Food Chemistry*, Volume 107, Issue 1, 1 March 2008, pp. 449-463.

Reid, L. M., O'Donnell, C. P., & Downey, G. (2004). Potential of SPME-GC and chemometrics to detect adulteration of soft fruit purees. *Journal of Agricultural and Food Chemistry*, 52, pp. 421- 427.

Reid, L. M., O'Donnell, C. P., Kelly, J., Daniel, J., & Downey, G. (2004). Preliminary studies for the differentiation of apple juice samples on the basis of heat-treatment using chemometric analysis of chromatographic data. *Journal of Agricultural and Food Chemistry*, 52, pp. 6891–6896.

Reid, L.M., Woodcock, T., O'Donnell, C.P., Kelly, J.D., Downey, G. (2005). Differentiation of apple juice samples on the basis of heat treatment and variety using chemometric analysis of MIR and NIR data. *Food Research International*, Volume 38, Issue 10, December 2005, pp. 1109-1115.

Rodríguez, M., Durán, I., Ornelas, N., López de Alba, P.L., López L., (2008). Determination of anticarcinogenic and rescue therapy drugs in urine by photoinduced spectrofluorimetry using multivariate calibration: comparison of several second-order methods. *Anal. Bioanal. Chem.*, 391 (2008) pp. 1119-1127.

Rodriguez, S.D., Monge, M.E., Olivieri, A.C., Negri, R.M., Bernik, D.L., (2010). Time dependence of the aroma pattern emitted by an encapsulated essence studied by means of electronic noses and Chemometric analysis. *Food Research International*, Volume 43, Issue 3, April 2010, pp. 797-804.

Rodriguez-Delgado, M. A., Gonzalez-Hernandez, G., Conde-Gonzalez, J. E., & Perez-Trujillo, J. P., (2002). Principal component analysis of the polyphenol content in young red wines. *Food Chemistry*, 78, pp. 523–532.

Romero, R., Sanchez-Vinas, M., Gazquez, D., & Bagur, M. G., (2002). Characterization of selected Spanish table wine samples according to their biogenic amine content from liquid chromatographic determination. *Journal of Agricultural and Food Chemistry*, 50, pp. 4713–4717.

Romeu-Nadal, M., Morera-Pons S., Castellote, A., López-Sabater, M.C., (2006). Rapid high-performance liquid chromatographic method fo vitamin C determination in human milk versus an enzymatic method. *Journal of Chromatography B*, Volume 830, Issue 1, 2 January 2006, pp. 41-46.

Rubio Barroso, S., Santos Delgado, M.J., Martín Olivar, C., Pólo Diez, L.M., (2006). Indirect Chiral HPLC determination and Fluorimetric Detection of D-Amino acids in Milk and Oyster Samples. *Journal of Dairy Science*, Volume 89, Issue 1, January 2006, pp. 82-89.

Russo, M.V., Goretti,G., Libert, A., (1989). Direct headspace gas chromatographic determination of dicholoromethane in decaffeinated green and roasted coffee. *Journal of Chromatography A*, Volume 465, Issue 3, 1989, pp. 429-433.

Sadecka J., Tothova J., (2007): Fluorescence spectroscopy and chemometrics in the food classification-a review. *Czech Journal of Food Sciences*, 25, 1989, pp. 159-173.

Sahar, A., Boubellouta, T., Dufour, E., (2011). Synchronous front-face fluorescence spectroscopy as a promising tool for the rapid determination of spoilage bacteria on chicken breast fillet. *Food Research International*, Volume 44, Issue 1, January 2011, pp. 471-480.

Salo Väänänen, P., Ollilainen, V., Mattila, P., Lehikoinen, K., Salmela Molsa, E., Piironen, V. (2000). Simultaneous HPLC analysis of fat-soluble vitamins in selected animal products after small-scale extraction. *Food Chemistry*, Volume 71, Issue 4, December 2000, pp. 535-543.

Sanz, M.L.,Villamiel, M., Martínez Castro, I. (2004). Inositols and carbohydrates in different fresh fruit juices. *Food Chemistry*, Volume 87, Issue 3, September 2004, pp. 325-328.

Savchuk, S., Vlasov, V., Appolonova, S., Arbuzov, V., Vedenin, A., Mezinov, A., and Grigor'yan, B., (2001). Application of Chromatography and Spectrometry to the Authentication of Alcoholic Beverages. *Journal of Analytical Chemistry*, Vol. 56, No. 3, 2001, pp. 214–231.

Schultheiss, J., Jensen, D., Galensa, R. (2000). Determiantion of aldehydes in food by high-performance liquid chromatography with biosensor coupling and micromembrane suppressors. *Journal of Chromatography A*, Volume 880, Issues 1-2, 2 June 2000, pp. 233-242.

Shiroma, C., Rodriguez-Saona, L., (2009). Application of NIR and MIR spectroscopy in quality control of potato chips. *Journal of Food Composition and Analysis*, Volume 22, Issue 6, September 2009, pp. 596-605.

Sinelli, N., Limbo, S., Torri, L., Di Egidio, V., Casiraghi, E., (2010). Evaluation of freshness decay of minced beef stored in high-oxygen modified atmosphere packaged at different temperatures using NIR and MIR spectroscopy. *Meat Science*, Volume 86, Issue 3, November 2010, pp. 748-752.

Soga, T., (2002). Chapter 14. Analysis of carbohydrates in food and beverages by HPLC and CE. *Journal of Chromatography Library*, Volume 66, 2002, Pages 483-502.

Tasioula-Margari, M., Okoger, O., (2001). Simultaneous determination of phenolic compounds and tocopherols in virgin olive oil using HPLC and UV detection. *Food Chemistry, Volume 74, Issue 3, August 2001, pp. 377-383.*

Thomä, C., Krause, I., Kulozik, U. (2006). Precipitation behaviour of caseinomacropeptides and their simultaneous determination with whey proteins by RP-HPLC. *International Dairy Journal*, Volume 16, Issue 4, April 2006, pp. 285-293.

Tothova, J., Sádecká, J. and Májek, P., 2009. Total Luminescence Spectroscopy for Differentiating Between Brandies and Wine Distillates. *Czech J. Food Sci.*, Vol. 27, 6, 2009, pp. 425–432.

Urbano, M., Luque de Castro, M. D., Perez, P. M., Garcia-Olmo, J., Gomez-Nieto, M. A., (2006). Ultraviolet-visible spectroscopy and pattern recognition methods for differentiation and classification of wines. *Food Chemistry* 97, (1), 2006, pp. 166-175.

Vazquez Landaverde, P.A., Torres, J.A., Qian, M.C., (2006). Quantification of Trace Volatile Sulfur Compounds in Milk by Solid-Phase Microextraction and Gas Chromatography–Pulsed Flame Photometric Detection. *Journal of Dairy Science,* Volume 89, Issue 8, August 2006, pp. 2919-2927.

Vazquez, P.A, Velazquez, G., Torres, J.A, Qian, M.C., (2005). Quantitative Determination of Thermally Derived Off-Flavor Compounds in Milk Using Solid-Phase Microextraction and Gag Chromatography. *Journal of Dairy Science,* Volume 88, Issue 11, November 2005, Pages 3764-3772.

Vetter W., Alder, L., Kallenborn, R., Schlabach, M. (2000). Determination of Q1, an unknown organochlorine contaminant, in human milk, Antarctic air, and further environmental samples. *Environmental Pollution,* Volume 110, Issue 3, December 2000, pp. 401-409.

Vidal-Carou, M.C., Lahoz-Portolés, F., Bover-Cid, S., Mariné-Font, A., (2003). Ion-pair high-performance liquid chromatographic determination of biogenetic amines and polyamines in wine and other alcoholic beverages. *Journal of Chromatography A,* Volume 998, Issues 1-2, 23 May 2003, pp. 235-241.

Wang, J., Li, Q.X., (2011). Chemical Composition, Characterization, and Differentiation of Honey Botanical and Geographical Origins. *Advances in Food and Nutrition Research,* Volume 62, 2011, Chapter Chapter 3, pp. 89-137.

Wang, M.L., Wang, J.T., Choong Y.M., (2004). A rapid and accurate method for determination of methanol in alcoholic beverage by direct injection capillary gas chromatography. *Journal of Food Composition and Analysis,* Volume 17, Issue 2, April 2004, pp. 187-196.

Wang, M.L., Wang, J.T., Choong, Y.M., (2004). Simultaneous quantification of methanol and ethanol in alcoholic beverages using a rapid gas chromatographic method coupling with dual internal standards. *Food Chemistry,* Volume 86, Issue 4, August 2004, pp. 609-615.

Wegener, J.W., López Sanchez, P. (2010). Furan levels in fruit and vegetables juices, nutrition drinks and bakery products. *Analytica Chimica Acta,* Volume 672, Issues 1-2, 5 July 2010, pp. 55-60.

Wong, H.W., Choi, S.M., Lee Phillips D., Ma, C.Y., (2004). Raman spectroscopic study of deamidated food proteins Original Research Article. Food *Chemistry,* Volume 113, Issue 2, 15 March 2009, pp. 363-370.

Xiao, Q., Hu, B., Yu, C., Xia, L., Jiang, Z. (2006). Optimization of a single-drop microextraction procedure for the determination of organophosphorus pesticides in water and fruit juice with gas chromatography-flame photometric detection Original Research Article *Talanta*, Volume 69, Issue 4, 15 June 2006, pp. 848-855.

Yang, X., Zhang, H., Liu, Y., Wang, J., Zhang, Y.C., Dong, A.D., Zhao, H.T., Sun, C.H., Cui, J., (2011). Multiresidue method for determination of 88 pesticides in berry fruits using solid-phase extraction and gas chromatography–mass spectrometry: Determination of 88 pesticides in berries using SPE and GC-MS. *Food Chemistry*, Volume 127, Issue 2, 15 July 2011, pp. 855-865.

Zhang, J., Zhang, X., Dediu, L., Victor, C. (2011). Review of the current application of fingerprinting allowing detection of food adulteration and fraud in China. *Food Control*. Vol. 22, Issue 8, August 2011, pp. 1126-1135.

Zhu, X., Li, S., Shan, Y., Zhang, Z., Li, G., Su, D., Liu, F. (2010). Detection of adulterants such as sweeteners materials in honey using near-infrared spectroscopy and chemometrics. *Journal of Food Engineering*, Volume 101, Issue 1, November 2010, pp. 92-97.

3

Quality Control of *Panax* Species by Monoclonal Antibody and DNA Analysis

Hiroyuki Tanaka
Faculty of Pharmaceutical Sciences, Kyushu University Japan

1. Introduction

Almost all *Panax* spp. (family Araliaceae) have been used in folk medicine. The most famous variety is *P. ginseng*, which was recorded in Chinese Materia Medica 2000 years ago. It is used to enhance stamina and capacity to cope with fatigue and physical stress, and in tonics against cancers, disturbances of the central nervous system (memory, learning, and behavior), hypothermia, carbohydrate and lipid metabolism, immune function, the cardiovascular system and radioprotection. Meanwhile, *P. notoginseng*, cultivated extensively in Kumming province in China, is also an important crude drug used as an astringent and tonic. *P. japonicus* grows mainly in Japan and China and is used as a stomachic and a hair-growth tonic in Japan. In ginseng markets worldwide, *P. quinquefolius* usually commands a much higher price than *P. ginseng*. Since the roots of these ginseng products are similar in appearance and many commercial ginseng products are in the form of a powder or shredded slices, identification of the origins of ginseng products is not an easy task. Authentication of the sources of ginseng and ginseng products based on scientifically profiling has aroused much interest.

Ginsenosides (ginseng saponins) are known to be bioactive components of ginseng. According to the difference in aglycon in these saponins, ginsenosides are classified into three types: the 20(*S*)-protopanaxadiol type [e.g., ginsenosides Rb1 (G-Rb1), -Rc (G-Rc), -Rb2 (G-Rb2), -Rd (G-Rd); malonylginsenosides Rb1 (MG-Rb1), -Rb2 (MG-Rb2) and -Rc (MG-Rc)], the 20(*S*)-protopanaxatriol type [e.g., ginsenosides Rg1 (G-Rg1), -Rf (G-Rf), and -Re (G-Re)], and the oleanolic acid type [e.g., ginsenoside Ro (G-Ro)] (see Figure 1). Ginsenosides have been shown to affect various biological processes: e.g., tumor metastasis and anti-diabetes effects (Wu *et al.*, 1992; Newman *et al.*, 1992), the central nervous system (Kim *et al.*, 1990; Kim *et al.*,1996; Tokuyama *et al.*, 1996;), and retardation of the aging process (Metori *et al.*, 1997). It is well known that the content of ginsenosides varies in ginseng root or root extract depends on the method of extraction, subsequent treatment, or even the season of collection (Kim *et al.*, 1981); therefore, standardization of quality is essential.

Many analytical approaches have been used to identify ginsenosides in ginseng extract (Sticher and Soldati, 1979; Soldati and Sticher, 1980; Tani *et al.*, 1981; Kitagawa *et al.*, 1987; Yamaguchi *et al.*, 1988; Samukawa *et al.*, 1995; Wang *et al.*, 1999; Chan *et al.*, 2000; Li *et al.*, 2000). We have prepared monoclonal antibodies (MAbs) against major active compounds of *P. ginseng*, G-Rb1 (Tanaka *et al.*, 1999) and G-Rg1 (Fukuda *et al.*, 2000a), and established an

ELISA and an immunoaffinity concentration for ginsenosides (Fukuda *et al.*, 1999; Fukuda *et al.*, 2000b; Fukuda *et al.*, 2001); however, no formation of MAb against the crude drug of *P. ginseng* has been reported, although immunological approaches for analyses of *P. ginseng* using a polyclonal antibody against *P. ginseng* have been investigated (Kitagawa *et al.*, 1996). The present study describes the establishment of two MAbs against *P. ginseng* protein component, and the application of an ELISA for the qualitative analysis and classification of *Panax* spp. using the anti-*P. ginseng* MAbs.
Previously, we used RAPD analysis for the homogeneity of regenerated *Panax* plants in vitro (Shoyama *et al.*, 1995); however, we have not yet succeeded in distinguishing individual *Panax* spp. using their crude drugs. Therefore, we planned to perform a combination of RAPD and new double staining for ginsenosides by Eastern blotting using anti-G-Rb1, -Rg1 MAbs and to standardize the quality of ginseng.

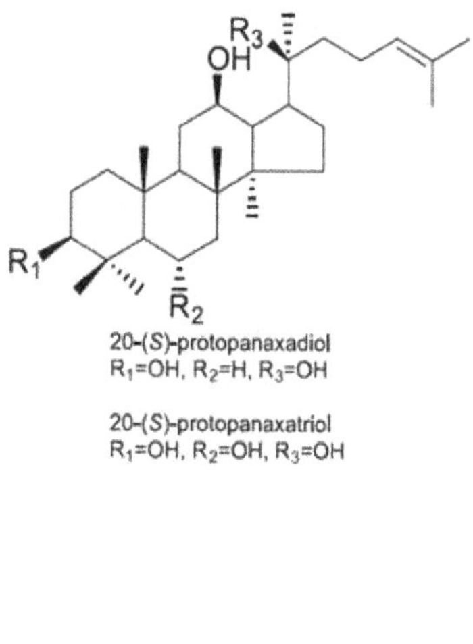

20-(*S*)-protopanaxadiol
R_1=OH, R_2=H, R_3=OH

20-(*S*)-protopanaxatriol
R_1=OH, R_2=OH, R_3=OH

Aglycone	Ginsenoside	R1	R2	R3
Protopanaxadiol	G-Rb1	-O-Glc[2->1]Glc	H	-O-Glc[6->1]Glc
	G-Rb2	-O-Glc[2->1]Glc	H	-O-Glc[6->1]Ara(p)
	G-Rc	-O-Glc[2->1]Glc	H	-O-Glc[6->1]Ara(f)
	G-Rd	-O-Glc[2->1]Glc	H	-O-Glc
	MG-Rb1	-O-Glc[2->1]Glc[6]->Ma	H	-O-Glc[6->1]Glc
	MG-Rb2	-O-Glc[2->1]Glc[6]->Ma	H	-O-Glc[6->1]Ara(p)
	MG-Rc	-O-Glc[2->1]Glc[6]->Ma	H	-O-Glc[6->1]Ara(f)
Protopanaxatriol	G-Rg1	OH	-O-Glc	-O-Glc
	G-Rh1	OH	-O-Glc	OH
	G-Re	OH	-O-Glc[2->1]Rha	-O-Glc
	G-Rf	OH	-O-Glc[2->1]Glc	OH
	20-Gluco-G-Rf	OH	-O-Glc[2->1]Glc	-O-Glc

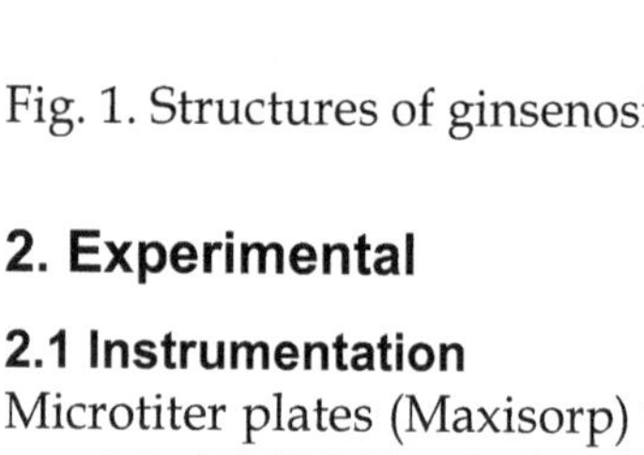

Aglycone	Ginsenoside	R1	R2
Oleanolic acid	G-Ro	-O-GlcA[2->1]Glc	-O-Glc

Glc, glucose; Ma, malonyl; Ara (p), arabinose in pyranose form; Ara (f), arabinose in furanose form; Rha, rhamnose.

Fig. 1. Structures of ginsenosides

2. Experimental

2.1 Instrumentation

Microtiter plates (Maxisorp) were purchased from Nalge Nunc (NY). The microplate reader was Model 450 (Bio-Rad Laboratories, CA). The PCR thermal cycler was a 1605 Air Thermo-Cycler (Idaho Technology, UT).

2.2 Chemicals and immunochemicals

Five kinds of commercial ginseng roots and other crude drugs were obtained from Nakai Koshindo (Kobe, Japan). Standards of ginsenosides were purchased from Wako Pure Chemical Ind., Ltd. (Osaka, Japan). Bovine serum albumin (BSA) and human serum albumin (HSA) were provided by Pierce (Rockford, IL). Polyvinylidene difluoride (PVDF) membranes were purchased from Millipore Corporation (Bedford, MA). A glass microfiber filter sheet (GF/A) was purchased from Whatman International Ltd. (Maidstone, UK). Peroxidase (POD)-labeled goat IgG fraction to mouse IgG was provided by ICN Pharmaceuticals Inc. (Aurora, OH). All other chemicals were standard commercial products of analytical grade.

2.3 Immunization and hybridization

Powdered white ginseng (*P. ginseng*) was suspended in phosphate-buffered saline (PBS), and extracted under sonication for 2 min. The white ginseng water-soluble fraction (WSF) obtained was immediately used as the immunogen. Mice were immunized by a protocol modified from Kitagawa (Kitagawa *et al.*, 1996). First, BALB/c male mice were injected intraperitoneally with an initial injection of 500 µg WSF in PBS emulsified with an equal volume of Freund's complete adjuvant (Difco Laboratories, MI). Two boosts of 500 µg WSF in Freund's incomplete adjuvant (Difco Laboratories, MI) were performed intraperitoneally at intervals of 2 weeks. The final immunization (1 mg) was injected as a PBS solution. On the third day after the final immunization, splenocytes were isolated and fused with a hypoxanthine-thymidine-aminopterin (HAT)-sensitive mouse myeloma cell line, P3-X63-Ag8-U1, by the polyethylene glycol (PEG) method (Galfre and Milstein, 1981). Hybridoma-producing MAb reactive to *P. ginseng* WSF were selected in enriched RPMI 1640-Dulbecco's-Ham's F12 (eRDF; Kyokuto Pharmaceutical Industrial Co., Ltd., Tokyo, Japan) medium containing HAT, and cloned twice by the limited dilution method (Goding, 1980).
Another hybridoma-producing MAb reactive to *P. ginseng* was prepared using red ginseng (*P. ginseng*) WSF as an immunogen by the above procedure.

2.4 ELISA using MAbs against ginseng

Dried samples (2.0 mg) of various ginseng and other crude drugs were powdered, suspended in 50 mM carbonate buffer at pH 9.6 (1.0 ml) under sonication for 10 min. The suspensions of ginseng WSF were diluted with 50 mM carbonate buffer at pH 9.6 and then assayed using ELISA.
Reactivities of MAbs to various kinds of ginseng WSFs were determined by ELISA. The wells of a 96 well-immunoplate were coated with a suspension of 100 µl/well of various concentrations of ginseng WSF for 1 hr. The plate was washed three times with PBS containing 0.05% Tween 20 (TPBS), and then treated with 300 µl PBS containing 5% skim milk (SPBS) for 1 hr to reduce non-specific adsorption. The plate was again washed three times with TPBS and reacted with 100 µl test MAb for 1 hr. Again, the plate was washed three times with TPBS, and then incubated with 100 µl of 1,000 times dilution of POD-labeled goat IgG fraction to mouse IgG for l hr. After washing a further three times with TPBS, 100 µl substrate solution [0.1 M citrate buffer (pH 4) containing 0.003% H_2O_2 and 0.3 mg/ml of 2,2'-azino-bis(3-ethylbenzothiazoline-6-sulfonic acid) diammonium salt (ABTS)] was added to each well and incubated for 20 min. Absorbance was measured by a microplate reader at 405 nm. All reactions were carried out at 37 °C.
The cross-reactivities (CR %) of various ginseng and other crude drugs were determined as follows:

$$CR\% = \frac{A - A_o}{A_{PG} - A_o} \times 100$$

where A is the absorbance of the test crude drug, A_{PG} is the absorbance of white ginseng, and Ao is the absorbance of the blank.

2.5 Western blot analyses of *P. ginseng* WSFs

Western blot analysis was carried out according to a reported method (essentially the method of Towbin) (Towbin *et al.*, 1979). Reduced protein WSFs contained in suspensions of various ginseng (20 μg) in electrophoresis sample buffer were separated by SDS-polyacrylamide electrophoresis (SDS-PAGE) (Laemmli, 1970) on 10% polyacrylamide gel, and electroblotted onto a PVDF membrane (Immobilon-P), which was then incubated with MAb to *P. ginseng* for 3 hr. The membrane was then incubated with 1,000 times dilution of POD-labeled goat IgG fraction to mouse IgG in PBS containing 0.2% gelatin (GPBS) for 1 hr. The POD-labeled secondary antibody bound to the membrane was then developed to blue bands with a substrate solution (4-chloro-1-naphthol soln.).

2.6 Competitive ELISA using anti-G-Rb1, -Rg1 MAbs

Dried samples (50 mg) of various ginseng were powdered and extracted with MeOH (5.0 ml) under sonication five times. The combined extract was filtered and then evaporated to dryness. To eliminate the malonyl group from malonylated ginsenosides, the extracts were treated with 0.1% KOH in MeOH at room temperature for 1 hr. The combined extracts were diluted with 20% methanol suitable for competitive ELISA.

G-Rb1-HSA (100 μl, 1 μg/ ml) dissolved in 50 mM carbonate buffer (pH 9.6) was adsorbed to the wells of a 96 well-immunoplate, and then treated with 300 μl SPBS for 1 hr to reduce non-specific adsorption. Fifty microliters of various concentrations of G-Rb1 or samples dissolved with 20% methanol were incubated with 50 μl MAb solution (83 μg/ml) for 1 hr. The plate was washed three times with PBS containing TPBS, and then incubated with 100 μl of 1,000 times dilution of POD-labeled goat IgG fraction to mouse IgG for 1 hr. After washing the plate three times with TPBS, 100 μl substrate solution (ABTS soln.) was added to each well and incubated for 15 min. The absorbance was measured by a microplate reader at 405 nm. Quantitative analysis of G-Rg1 was performed by a similar competitive ELISA procedure as above.

2.7 Double-stained Eastern blotting

Ginsenosides and the extract of various ginseng were applied to TLC plates and developed with *n*-BuOH-EtOAc-H_2O (15:1:4). One developed TLC plate was dried and sprayed with H_2SO_4. Another TLC plate was dried and then sprayed with blotting solution mixture of isopropanol-methanol-H_2O (1:4:16, by volume). It was placed on a stainless steel plate and then covered with a PVDF membrane sheet. After covering with a glass microfiber filter sheet, it was pressed evenly for 50 s with a 120°C hot plate as previously described with modification (Fukuda *et al.*, 2000b). The PVDF membrane was separated from the plate and dried. The blotted PVDF membrane was dipped in water containing $NaIO_4$ (10 mg/ml) under stirring at room temperature for 1 hr. After washing with water, 50 mM carbonate buffer solution containing BSA was added and stirred for 3 hr. The PVDF membrane was washed with TPBS for 5 min twice and then washed with water. The PVDF membrane was immersed in anti-G-Rb1 MAb and stirred at room temperature for 1 hr. After washing the

PVDF membrane twice with TPBS and water, 1,000 times dilution of POD-labeled goat IgG fraction to mouse IgG in GPBS was added and stirred at room temperature for 1 hr. The POD-labeled secondary antibody bound to the membrane was then developed to blue bands with a substrate solution (4-chloro-1-naphthol soln.).

In the experiment of the immunocytolocalization of G-Rb1, a sliced fresh *P. ginseng* root was placed on the PVDF membrane and they were pressed together evenly for 6 hr. The blotted PVDF membrane was stained using the same procedure as described for the Eastern blotting method.

For staining with anti-G-Rg1 MAb, the blotted PVDF membrane was treated in the same way as anti-G-Rb1 MAb except that it was exposed to 2 mg of 3-amino-9-ethylcarbazole in 10 ml of 50 mM acetate buffer (pH 5.0) containing 0.03% H_2O_2 and 5% *N,N*-dimethylformamide.

2.8 RAPD analysis

DNA for RAPD analysis was extracted from the crude drug powder (100 mg) by the method of Murray and Thompson (1980) with some modification (Nakai *et al.*, 1996). The obtained crude DNA was further purified by the Geneclean II kit (Bio 101, Illkirch, France) as follows: to the DNA solution, 6 M NaI at three times the volume of the DNA solution, plus Glass milk (5 μl) were added and mixed using a vortex mixer. The mixture was incubated at 0 °C for 10 min, with mixing every 1 min. After 10 min incubation, the mixture was centrifuged at 6,000 rpm at 2 °C for 30 s. The supernatant was removed and then washed with New Wash 3 times. Finally, the DNA fraction was centrifuged at 14,000 rpm at 2 °C for 30 s. The supernatant was removed. After the addition of sterile pure water (50 μl), the DNA solution was incubated at 55 °C for 5 min. The mixture was again centrifuged at 15,000 rpm at room temperature for 20 min. A 45 μl supernatant sample was recovered and the DNA concentration was determined using a U-3210 Spectrophotometer (Hitachi, Tokyo, Japan). Amplifications were carried out in 10 μl reaction volumes composed of 1.5 ng/μl plant DNA, 50 mM Tris/HCl (pH 8.5), 5 mM $MgCl_2$, 500 μg/ml BSA, 2.0 % Ficol, 4 mM tartrazine, 10 μM EDTA, and 0.04 units/μl *Tth* DNA polymerase (Toyobo, Osaka, Japan) (Nei and Li, 1979).

The Air Thermo-Cycler was programmed for 60 s at 94 °C, followed by 60 cycles of 10 s at 94 °C, 30 s at 36 °C, and 60 s at 72 °C, followed by 120 s at 72 °C for amplification. Amplification products were separated in 1% agarose gels in 0.5 Tris/borate/EDTA (TBE) buffer. Gels containing ethidium bromide (5 μl/100 ml) were developed at 120 V for 3 hr. Gels were detected and photographed by a DNA transilluminator Model NTM-20 (UVP Inc., Upland, CA) at 302 nm. The sizes of the amplification products were estimated using a 100 bp (100 bp-2.0 kb) ladder (Amersham Pharmacia Biotech, Buckinghamshire, UK). The random primers consisted of ten base sequences from a kit purchased from QIAGEN Operon Technologies Inc. (Chatsworth, CA). The OPB and OPO series, having ten base sequences that had been synthesized previously (Nakai *et al.*, 1996), were as follows:

OPB-01 (5′-GTTTCGCTCC-3′), OPB-02 (5′-TGATCCCTGG-3′),
OPB-03 (5′-CATCCCCCTG-3′), OPB-04 (5′-GGACTGGAGT-3′),
OPB-05 (5′-TGCGCCCTTC-3′), OPB-06 (5′-TGCTCTGCCC-3′),
OPB-07 (5′-GGTGACGCAG-3′), OPB-08 (5′-GTCCACACGG-3′),
OPB-09 (5′-TGGGGGACTC-3′), OPB-12 (5′-CCTTGACGCA-3′),
OPB-13 (5′-TTCCCCCGCT-3′), OPB-14 (5′-TCCGCTCTGG-3′),
OPB-18 (5′-CCACAGCAGT-3′), OPB-19 (5′-ACCCCCGAAG-3′),

OPO-03 (5′-CTGTTGCTAC-3′), OPO-04 (5′-AAGTCCGCTC-3′),
OPO-08 (5′-CCTCCAGTGT-3′), OPO-09 (5′-TCCCACGCAA-3′),
OPO-10 (5′-TCAGAGCGCC-3′), OPO-12 (5′-CAGTGCTGTG-3′),
OPC-18 (5′-CTCGCTATCC-3′)
Genetically similar (*F*) values were determined by Nei and Li's method (1979).

3. Results and discussion

3.1 ELISA using MAbs against ginseng

This paper demonstrated ELISA for *Panax* spp. using two kinds of MAbs against *P. ginseng* protein components. Hyperimmunized BALB/c mice with ginseng WSF yielded splenocytes which were fused with P3-X63-Ag8-U1 myeloma cells by a routine procedure established in our laboratory (Sakata *et al.*, 1994). After additional testing with ELISA employing various ginseng, two hybridoma-producing MAbs were cloned and expanded. MAb 3H4 was produced from white ginseng WSF as an immunogen, whereas MAb 5H8 was produced from red ginseng WSF as an immunogen. Two MAbs reactive to *P. ginseng* were classified into IgG1 with *k* light chains.
MAbs that bound to the ginseng protein components on the surface of the wells were then reacted with POD-labeled goat anti-mouse IgG as the secondary antibody in ELISA using MAbs 3H4 and 5H8. First, the reactivity of IgG-type MAbs 3H4 and 5H8 to various concentrations of *P. ginseng* protein components was tested by varying antibody concentrations and by performing a dilution curve. In general, the color development intensity was regulated at around 1 for a highly reliable ELISA result. Optical antibody concentrations (MAb 3H4; 0.01 μg/ml, MAb 5H8; 5 μg/ml) of absorbance of approximately 1 were selected for the determination of cross-reactivities against crude drugs by ELISA.

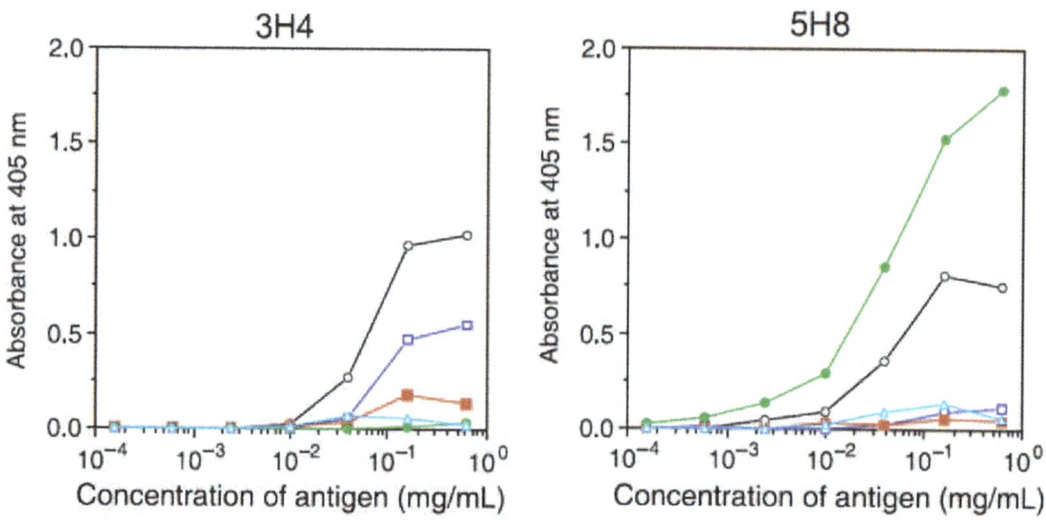

Fig. 2. Typical dose-response curves for five types of ginsengs measured by ELISA using MAbs 3H4 and 5H8. In order to examine the specificity of the ELISA, MAbs reactive to *P. ginseng* (MAb 3H4, 0.01 μg/mL; MAb 5H8, 5 μg/mL) were added to each well of a 96-well immunoplate coated with various concentrations of powdered drug material from white ginseng (○), red ginseng (●), *Panax notoginseng* (□), *P. quinquefolius* (■) and *P. japonicus* (Δ). Values plotted are means ($n = 3$)

3.2 Cross-reactivity of MAbs 3H4 and 5H8 against various crude drugs

Figure 2 shows typical dose response curves of five kinds of ginseng measured by ELISA using MAbs 3H4 and 5H8. ELISA using MAb 3H4 was not specific to *P. ginseng* and showed cross-reactivity with *P. notoginseng* and *P. quinquefolius*, but did not react with other crude drugs. This wide cross-reactivity is the major advantage of the antibody reagent used in this ELISA. Although both MAbs 3H4 and 5H8 cross-reacted with the *P. ginseng* protein components, the cross-reactivity against other *Panax* spp. varied, as shown in Table 1. The most important property of this MAb 3H4 is its ability to distinguish ginseng produced from *P. ginseng* by processing, since 3H4 did not react with red ginseng. MAb 5H8 has weak cross-reactivity with *P. notoginseng*, *P. quinquefolius* and *P. japonicas*; however, since MAb 5H8 cross-reacted with Scopoliae rhizoma, other assay methods such as our ELISA using anti-G-Rb1 and -Rg1 MAbs might be needed.

Crude drug	Cross-reactivity (%)[a]	
	3H4	5H8
White ginseng (*Panax ginseng*)	100	100
Red ginseng (*P. ginseng*)	<1	204
San-chi ginseng (*P. notoginseng*)	53.4	4.4
American ginseng (*P. quinquefolius*)	43.1	2.4
Japanese ginseng (*P. japonicus*)	1.4	3.2
Scopoliae Rhizoma	<1	20.2
Gardeniae Fructus	<1	4.5
Glycyrrhizae Radix	<1	3.0
Uvae Ursi Folium	<1	2.7
Phellodendri Cortex	<1	2.7
Sennae Folium	<1	2.1
Paeoniae Radix	<1	1.5
Bupleuri Radix	<1	1.3
Senegae Radix	<1	1.3
Rhei Rhizoma	<1	1.2
Aurantii Pericarpium	<1	<1
Coptidis Rhizoma	<1	<1
Cinnamomi Cortex	<1	<1
Scutellariae Radix	<1	<1

[a]Values are means ± standard deviation ($n = 3$).

Table 1. Cross-reactivity (CR%) of MAbs against various ginseng and other crude drugs assayed using the ELISA method

3.3 Detection of protein specific to MAbs against ginseng

Blot analysis demonstrated that MAb 3H4 reacted with two major bands, M_r 24 kDa and 29 kDa, contained in 3 kinds of ginseng, as indicated in Figure 3. This observation suggests that the epitope is common to the two proteins. Judging from these results, MAb 3H4 might recognize common ginseng protein components contained in all *Panax* spp. On the other hand, MAb 5H8 selectively reacted with a broad band which roughly corresponds with bands at approximately M_r 24-29 kDa in *P. ginseng*, shown in Figure 3. This does not correspond to the result of the ELISA where MAb 5H8 reacted with *P. ginseng* and red ginseng, suggesting that the immunogenic proteins were probably denatured during the manufacturing process and might not have been separated by SDS-PAGE.

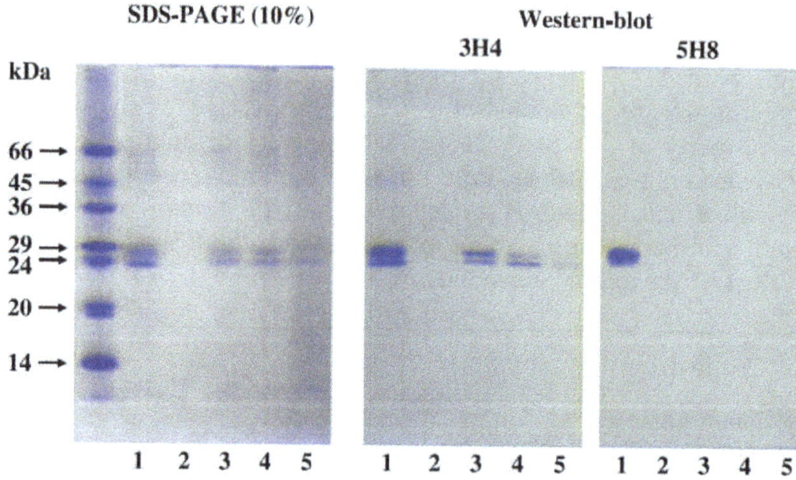

Fig. 3. SDS-PAGE and western blotting analyses of various ginsengs using MAbs 3H4 and 5H8. Samples were resolved by electrophoresis on a 10% acrylamide gel. Proteins were stained with Coomassie Brilliant Blue. Proteins separated by SDS-PAGE were transferred onto the PVDF membranes and incubated with MAbs 3H4 and 5H8. The bound MAb was reacted with PODlabelled secondary antibody, followed by reaction with substrate in order to develop blue protein bands. Lane 1, white ginseng (*Panax ginseng*; lane 2, red ginseng (*P. ginseng*), lane 3, sanchi-ginseng (*P. notoginseng*); lane 4, American ginseng (*P. quinquefolius*); lane 5, Japanese ginseng (*P. japonicus*). Molecular weights are as indicated by arrows

We established two MAbs that reacted predominantly with *P. ginseng* protein components to develop new immunological methods for analysis of *Panax* spp., resulting in two ELISAs using two MAbs. MAb 3H4, showing specific reactivity against ginseng, is predicted to be a probe for immunochemical discrimination between *Panax* spp. and other crude drugs. In addition, ELISA using MAb 5H8 can distinguish *P. ginseng* and red ginseng from other *Panax* spp. It became evident that the discrimination between white ginseng and red ginseng was could be performed by Western blotting. This assay is also technically easy to perform and allows small amounts of sample to be analyzed, as demonstrated by this study. The ELISA developed in this paper can be utilized for a homogeneity assay of *Panax* spp., therefore making it possible to study in the phytochemical field.

3.4 G-Rb1 and -Rg1 concentrations in *Panax* spp. measured by ELISA

G-Rb1 and -Rg1 were quantitatively determined by the competitive ELISA that we developed previously (Tanaka *et al.*, 1999; Fukuda *et al.*, 2000a). Kitagawa et al. isolated malonyl ginsenosides from white ginseng, finding that non-processed ginseng contents are higher than in processed ginseng (Kitagawa *et al.*, 1983). It is thought that MG-Rb1 influences ELISA since it is suggested that MG-Rb1 has similar cross-reactivity with G-Rb1. Therefore, G-Rb1 concentrations in various *Panax* spp. were measured after MG-Rb1 had been converted into G-Rb1 by mild alkaline conditions. The concentrations of G-Rb1 and -Rg1 are shown in Table 2 and vary according to species. Fibrous ginseng, which is made from the actively growing part of *P. ginseng*, showed the highest G-Rb1 concentration, 64.4 ±

3.6 mg/g dry wt. *P. notoginseng* and *P. quinquefolius* also showed high concentrations, 47.1 ± 3.3 and 48.5 ± 1.8 mg/g dry wt., respectively; however, the G-Rb1 concentration in *P. japonicus* analyzed by ELISA must be inaccurate since a very high S.D. of the G-Rb1 concentration in *P. japonicus* is shown in Table 2. In the present study, *P. notoginseng* showed the highest G-Rg1 concentration, 22.9 ± 3.2 mg/g dry wt. Also fibrous ginseng showed a high concentration, 4.98 ± 0.04 mg/g dry wt. The concentrations determined by ELISA agreed well with those determined by HPLC (Kitagawa *et al.*, 1987). ELISA was more sensitive than TLC (Tani *et al.*, 1981) or HPLC (Sticher and Sticher, 1979; Soldati and Sticher, 1980). Moreover, Yamaguchi et al. (1988) and Samukawa et al. (1995) reported the comparative concentrations of ginsenosides in various commercial ginseng radices analyzed by HPLC. The results obtained in this investigation indicate that the determination of ginsenoside concentrations could be carried out semi-quantitatively by ELISA, which might become a promising tool for the standardization of ginseng samples.

Sample	G-Rb1 content (mg/g dry weight) [a]	G-Rg1 content (mg/g dry weight) [a]
Ginseng (*Panax ginseng*)	5.49 ± 0.75	2.28 ± 0.02
Red Ginseng (*P. ginseng*)	3.57 ± 0.62	1.34 ± 0.08
Fibrous Ginseng (*P. ginseng*)	64.4 ± 3.6	4.98 ± 0.04
San-chi Ginseng (*P. notoginseng*)	47.1 ± 3.3	22.9 ± 3.2
American Ginseng (*P. quinquefolius*)	48.5 ± 1.8	3.15 ± 0.23
Janpanese Ginseng (*P. japonicus*)	1.37 ± 0.34	0.12 ± 0.01

[a] Values are means ± standard deviation (n = 3).

Table 2. Quantitative determination of ginsenosides Rb1 and Rg1 in various ginsengs using the ELISA method

3.5 Double-stained Eastern blotting of ginsenosides using anti-G-Rb1 and anti-G-Rg1 MAbs

Direct detection of small molecular compounds on a TLC plate by immunostaining is impossible because they are easily washed out by buffer solution without fixing. We therefore designed a system in which ginsenosides were blotted onto a PVDF membrane from the developed TLC plate for immunostaining. After ginsenosides had been transferred to the PVDF membrane, it was treated with $NaIO_4$ solution, followed by the addition of BSA. This reaction enhanced the fixation of ginsenosides via ginsenoside-BSA conjugate on the PVDF membrane. Figure 4-B indicates the Eastern blotting patterns of ginsenosides using anti-G-Rb1 MAb in three kinds of *Panax* spp., *P. ginseng, P. notoginseng* and *P. quinquefolius.*

Figure 4-C shows the Eastern blotting of double staining using anti-G-Rb1 and -Rg1 MAbs for ginsenoside standards. When the mixture of anti-G-Rg1 and -Rb1 MAbs and the pair of substrates were tested for staining of ginsenosides, all ginsenosides, G-Rg1, -Re, -Rd, -Rc and -Rb1, stained blue (data not shown), although purple staining for G-Rg1 was expected because 3-amino-9-ethylcarbazole was used as the substrate. It can therefore be suggested that the sensitivities of the substrate between 3-amino-9-ethylcarbazole and 4-chloro-1-naphtol might be different, so we performed successive staining of the PVDF membrane using anti-G-Rg1 and then anti-G-Rb1. Finally, we succeeded in the double staining of ginsenosides, indicating that G-Rg1 and -Re were stained purple and the other blue, separately, as indicated in Fig. 4-C. From these results, both antibodies could distinguish individual aglycons, 20(*S*)-protopanaxatriol and 20(*S*)-protopanaxadiol. For this application, crude extracts of three *Panax* spp. were analyzed by the newly developed double-staining system. Major ginsenosides could be determined clearly by this double-staining method. G-Rb1, -Rc and -Rd possessing 20(*S*)-protopanaxadiol as an aglycon stained as blue bands, and G-Re and -Rg1 as purple, depending on the substrate (4-chloro-1-naphtol). Figure 4-D shows the double staining of Eastern blotting for three *Panax* spp. When compared to the single staining of Eastern blotting by anti-G-Rb1 MAb (Fig. 4-B), it became evident that the quality of *Panax* spp. regarding ginsenosides varied. *P. notoginseng* contained a higher amount of G-Rg1, but G-Rc disappeared (Fig. 4-D, lane 4). A higher amount of G-Re and trace amounts of G-Rd and -Rg1 were observed in *P. quinquefolius*, as indicated in Fig. 4-D, lane 5. Three bands stained red by anti-G-Rg1 MAb were found, as indicated by arrows, although they could not be detected by staining with anti-G-Rb1 MAb. It is suggested that these bands might be related to G-Rg1 and G-Re having 20(*S*)-protopanaxatriol as an aglycon in the molecule. A survey of previous papers (Shoji, 1990) suggested that the three unknown bands could be determined as G-Rh1, G-Rf and 20-gluco G-Rf, which are mono-, di- and triglycosides of 20(*S*)-protopanaxatriol, respectively, depending upon individual Rf values. This finding suggests that the structures of aglycon can be recognized from the band color, and the Rf value is reflected by the sugar number. Using this result, we determined two bands under G-Rb1 as MG-Rb1 (Kitagawa *et al.*, 1983) and 20-*O*-gentiobiosyl-chikusetsusaponin III (Shoji, 1990), which has five sugars in a molecule of *P. ginseng*, in good agreement with the Rf value previously reported (Kitagawa *et al.*, 1983; Shoji, 1990). Finally, these two compounds were identified by comparing with authentic samples (data not shown).

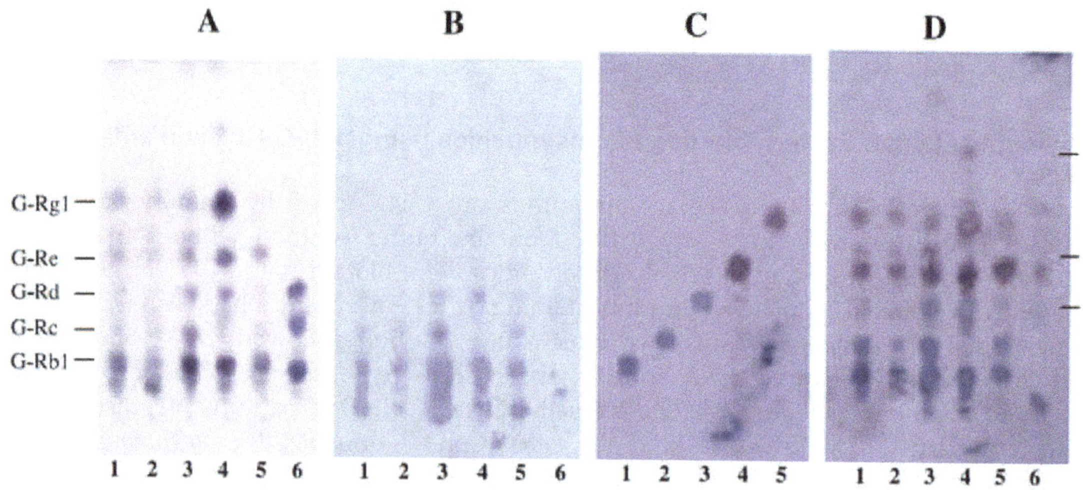

Fig. 4. Staining of various *Panax* samples. (A) Sulphuric acid staining; (B) eastern blotting using anti-G-Rb1 MAb; and (D) double-stain eastern blotting using anti-G-Rb1 and –Rg1 MAbs. Lanes 1–6 show white ginseng, red ginseng, fibrous ginseng, *P. notoginseng*, *P. quinquefolius* and *P. japonicus* (60 μg), respectively. (C) Double-stain eastern blotting of ginsenoside standards using anti-G-Rb1 and -G-Rg1 MAbs. Lanes 1–5 show G-Rb1, -Rc, -Rd, -Re and –Rg1 (3 μg), respectively

Figure 5 illustrates the immunocytolocalization of G-Rb1 in fresh *P. ginseng* roots. The phloem contained a higher concentration of G-Rb1 than the xylem. We conducted a controlled study with a slice of fresh *Glycyrrhiza* root using the same procedure to evaluate the specific detection of ginsenosides in the *P. ginseng* root with this system. In consequence, the *Glycyrrhiza* root, although it contained saponins structurally related to G-Rb1, was not immunostained by the Eastern blotting method using anti-G-Rb1 MAb 9G7, indicating the high specificity for *Panax* spp. of this method (data not shown).

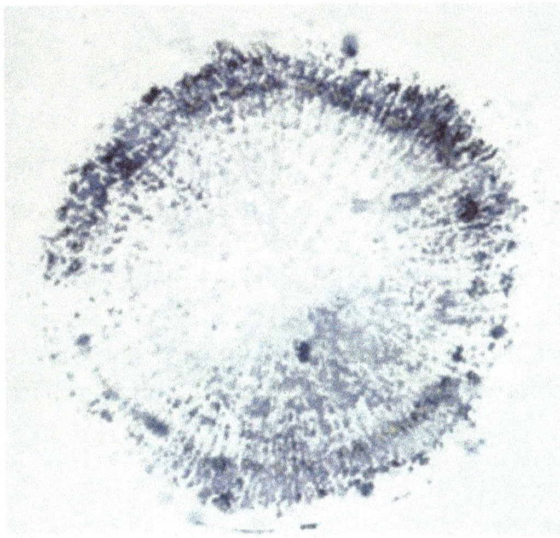

Fig. 5. Immunocytolocalisation of G-Rb1 in *Panax ginseng* root using anti-G-Rb1 MAb

3.6 RAPD analysis

The total DNA extracted from the crude drugs of *Panax* spp. was analyzed by RAPD using 21 random primers, resulting in 113 total bands. Figure 6 shows a representative amplified band pattern identified by primers.

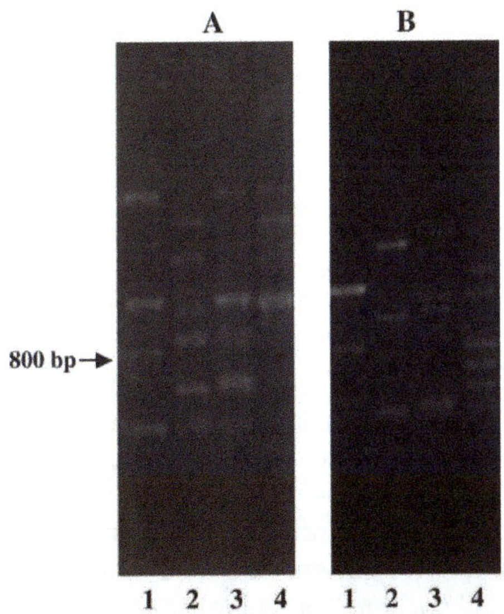

Fig. 6. Detection of polymorphic bands among *Panax* species using primer (A) OPO-08 (5'-CCTCCAGTGT-3') and (B) OPB-05 (5'-TGCGCCCTTC-3'). Lanes 1–4 show *P. notoginseng*, *P. japonicus*, *P. ginseng* and *P. quinquefolius*, respectively

The genetic distance matrix between individual species was calculated according to Nei and Li's method (1979). The degree of similarity among their fingerprints confirmed that *P. ginseng* is more closely related to *P. quinquefolius* than to *P. japonicus*. This result corresponds to the conclusions based on morphological taxonomic studies (Hara, 1970). It is suggested that RAPD analysis may be a useful method for determining the quality and homogeneity of *Panax* spp. as previously reported for regenerated plants of *Panax* spp. in vitro (Shoyama *et al.*, 1988).

4. Conclusion

The combination of RAPD and the developed double-stained Eastern blotting method can authenticate *P. notoginseng* and *P. japonicus*. Double-stained Eastern blotting indicated that *P. notoginseng* roots did not contain G-Rc, although the TLC profile was unclear. These results therefore suggest that a combination system of ELISA using MAbs, double-stained Eastern blotting and RAPD could identify four *Panax* spp. Moreover, a newly established immunocytolocalization method clearly shows not only the distribution of ginsenosides in ginseng roots, but also differentiates ginseng from other crude drugs.

5. Acknowledgment

This research was supported by a Grant-in-Aid for Scientific Research from the Ministry of Education, Culture, Sports, Science and Technology of Japan, the Uehara Memorial Foundation, a Sasakawa Scientific Research Grant from the Japan Science Society, the research fund from Kyushu University Foundation, and the research fund from Japan Kampo Medicine Manufacturers.

6. References

Chan, T.W.D. et al. (March 2000). Differentiation and Authentication of *Panax ginseng, Panax quinquefolius,* and Ginseng Products by Using HPLC/MS. *Analytical Chemistry,* Vol.72, No.6, pp. 1281-1287, ISSN 0003-2700

Fukuda, N. et al. (July 1999). Western Blotting for Ginseng Saponins, Ginsenosides Using Anti-ginsenoside Rb1 Monoclonal Antibody. *Biological & Pharmaceutical Bulletin,* Vol.22, No.2, pp. 219-220, ISSN 0918-6158

Fukuda, N.; Tanaka, H. & Shoyama, Y. (November 2000a). Formation of Monoclonal Antibody against a Major Ginseng Component, Ginsenoside Rg1 and its Characterization. Monoclonal antibody for a Ginseng Saponin. *Cytotechnology,* Vol.34, No.3, pp. 197-204, ISSN 0920-9069

Fukuda, N.; Tanaka, H. & Shoyama, Y. (July 2000b). Applications of ELISA, Western blotting and Immunoaffinity Concentration for Survey of Ginsenosides in Crude Drugs of *Panax* Species and Traditional Chinese Herbal Medicines. *Analyst,* Vol.125, No.8, pp. 1425-1429, ISSN 0003-2654

Fukuda, N.; Tanaka, H., Shoyama, Y. (October 2001). Double Staining of Ginsenosides by Western Blotting Using Anti-ginsenoside Rb1 and Rg1 Monoclonal Antibodies. *Biological & Pharmaceutical Bulletin,* Vol. 24,No.10, (2001), pp. 1157-1160, ISSN 0918-6158

Galfre, G. & Milstein, C. (1981). Preparation of Monoclonal Antibodies: Strategies and Procedures. *Methods in Enzymology,* Academic Press Inc., Vol.73, pp. 3-46, ISBN 0-12-181973-6, London, UK.

Goding, J.W. (August 1980). Antibody Production by Hybridomas. *Journal of Immunological Methods, Vol.*39, No.4, Sp. Iss. Si, pp. 285-308. ISSN 0022-1759

Hara, H. (1970). On the Asiatic Species of the Genus *Panax*. *The Journal of Japanese Botany*, Vol.45, pp. 197-212, ISSN 00222062

Kim, S.K. et al. (January 1981). Seasonal-Variation of Saponin, Sucrose and Monosaccharides in Cultivated Ginseng Roots. *Planta Medica,* Vo. 42, No.2, pp. 181-186, ISSN 0032-0943

Kim, H.S.; Jang, C.G. & Lee, M.K. (April 1990). Antinarcotic Effects of the Standardized Ginseng Extract G115 on Morphine. *Planta Medica,* Vol.56, No.2, pp. 158-163, ISSN 0032-0943

Kim, H.S. et al. (January 1996). Effects of Ginseng Total Saponin on Cocaine-induced Hyperactivity and Conditioned Place Preference in Mice. *Pharmacology Biochemistry Behavior,* Vol. 53, No.1, pp. 185-190, ISSN 0091-3057

Kitagawa, I. et al. (September 1983). Malonyl-ginsenoside-Rb1, Malonyl-ginsenoside Rb2, Malonyl-insenoside Rc, and Malonyl-ginsenoside Rd, 4 New Malonylated Dammarane-type Triterpene Oligoglycosides from Ginseng Radix. *Chemical & Pharmaceutical Bull*etin, Vol. 31, No.9, pp. 3353-3356. ISSN 00092363

Kitagawa, I. et al. (July 1987). Chemical Studies on Crude Drug Processing 5, On the Constituents of Ginseng Radix Rubra-(2) Comparison of the Constituents of White Ginseng and Red Ginseng Prepared from the Same Panax-ginseng Root. *Yakugaku Zasshi* Vol.107, No.7, pp. 495-505, ISSN 0031-6903

Kitagawa, T.; Bai, G. & Fujiwara, K. (March 1996). Specificities of Five Kinds of Antisera Produced against Crude Drugs, Pinellia Tuber, Hoelen, Glycyrrhizae Radix, Trichosanthes Root and Panax Ginseng. *Biological & Pharmaceutical Bulletin,* Vol.19, No.3, pp. 335-340, ISSN 0918-6158

Laemmli, U.K. (August 1970). Cleavage of Structural Proteins during Assembly of Head of Bacteriophage-T4. *Nature* Vol.227, pp. 680-685, ISSN 0028-0836

Li, W. et al. (November 2000). Use of High-Performance Liquid Chromatography-Tandem Mass Spectrometry To Distinguish *Panax ginseng* C. A. Meyer (Asian Ginseng) and Panax quinquefolius L. (North American Ginseng). *Analytical Chem*istry, Vol. 72, No.21, pp. 5417-5422, ISSN 0003-2700

Metori, K.; Furutsu, M. & Takahashi, S. (March 1997). The Preventive Effect of Ginseng with Du-Zhong Leaf on Protein Metabolism in Aging. *Biological & Pharmaceutical Bulletin,* Vol. 20, No. 3, pp. 237-242, ISSN 0918-6158

Murray, M.G. & Thompson, W.F. (August 1980). Rapid Isolation of High Molecular-weight Plant DNA. *Nucleic Acids Res Vol.* 8, No. 19, pp. 4321-4325, ISSN 0305-1048

Nakai, R.; Shoyama, Y. & Shiraishi, S. (January 1996). Genetic Characterization of *Epimedium* Species Using Random Amplified Polymorphic DNA (RAPD) and PCR-restriction fragment length polymorphism (RFLP) diagnosis. *Biological & Pharmaceutical Bulletin*, Vol, 19, No. 1, pp. 67-70, ISSN 0918-6158

Nei, M. & Li, W.H. (October 1979). Mathematical-model for Studying Genetic-variation in Terms of Restriction Endonucleases. *Proceedings of the Natural Academy of Sciences of the United States of America,* Vol. 76, No. 10, pp. 5269-5273, ISSN 0027-8424

Newman, M.J. et al. (April 1992). Saponin Adjuvant Induction of Ovalbumin-specific CD8+ Cytotoxic Lymphocyte-T Responses. *Journal of Immunology,* Vol. 148, No. pp. 2357-2362, ISSN 0022-1767

Sakata, R.; Shoyama, Y. & Murakami H. (July 1994). Production of Monoclonal Antibodies and Enzyme Immunoassay for Typical Adenylate Cyclase Activator. *Cytotechnology*, Vol. 16, No.2, pp. 101-108, ISSN 0920-9069

Samukawa, K. et al. (March 1995). Simultaneous Analysis of Ginsenosides of Various Ginseng Radixes by HPLC. *Yakugaku Zasshi*, Vol. 115, No.3 pp. 241-249, ISSN 0031-6903

Shoji, J. (1990). In: *Recent Advances in Ginseng Studies*, S. Shibata, Y. Ohtsuka, H. Saito, (Ed), Hirokawa Publications, 11-13, ISBN 4-567-42200-7 Tokyo, Japan

Shoyama, Y.; Kamura, K. & Nishioka, I. (April 1988). Somatic Embryogenesis and Clonal Multiplication of *Panax ginseng*. *Planta Medica, Vol.* 16, No. 2, pp. 155-156, ISSN 0032-0943

Sticher, O. & Soldati, F. (June 1979). HPLC Separation and Quantitative-Determination of Ginsenosides from *Panax ginseng, Panax quinquefolium* and from Ginseng Drug Preparations. *Planta Medica* Vol.36, No. 1, pp. 30-42, ISSN 0032-0943

Soldati, F. & Sticher, O. (August 1980). HPLC Separation and Quantitative-Determination of Ginsenosides from *Panax ginseng, Panax quinquefolium* and from Ginseng Drug Preparations 2. *Planta Med* Vol. 39, No. 8, pp. 348-357, ISSN 0032-0943

Tanaka, H.; Fukuda, N. & Shoyama, Y. (February 1999). Formation of Monoclonal Antibody against a Major Ginseng Component, Ginsenoside Rb1 and its Characterization. *Cytotechnology*, Vol.29, No. 2, pp. 115-120, ISSN 0920-9069

Tani, T. et al. (April 1981). Histochemistry 2, Ginsenosides in Ginseng (*Panax ginseng*, root). *Journal of Natural Producgts*, Vol. 44, No. 4, pp. 401-407, ISSN 0163-3864

Tokuyama, S.; Takahashi, M. & Kaneto, H. (August 1996). The Effect of Ginseng Extract on Locomotor Sensitization and Conditioned Place Preference Induced by Methamphetamine and Cocaine in Mice. *Pharmacology Biochemistry and Behavior* Vol. 54, No. 4, pp. 671-676, ISSN 0091-3057

Towbin, H.; Staehelin, T. & Gordon, J. (September 1979). Electrophoretic Transfer of Proteins from Polyacrylamide Gels to Nitrocellulose Sheets-Procedure and Some Applications. *Proceedings of the Natural Academy of Sciences of the United States of America*, Vol. 76, No. 9, pp. 4350-4354, ISSN 0027-8424

Wang, X. et al. (April 1999). Determination of Ginsenosides in Plant Extracts from *Panax ginseng and Panax quinquefolius* L. by LC/MS/MS. *Analytical Chemistry*, Vol. 71, No. 8, pp. 1579-1584, ISSN 0003-2700

Wu, J.Y. et al. (March 1992). Saponin Adjuvant Enhancement of Antigen-specific Immune-Responses to an Experimental HIV-1Vaccine. *Journal of Immunology*, Vol. 148, No. pp. 1519-1525, ISSN 0022-1767

Yamaguchi, H. et al. (September 1988). High-performance Liquid-chromatographic Analysis of Acidic Saponins of Ginseng and Related Plants. *Chemical & Pharmaceutical Bulletin*, Vol. 36, No. 9, pp. 3468-3473. ISSN 0009-2363

4

Quantitative Determination of Drugs in Dosage Forms as a Tool of Quality Control Studies

Sigrid Mennickent, Marta de Diego,
Mario Vega and Carmen Gloria Godoy
Faculty of Pharmacy,
University of Concepción, Concepción
Chile

1. Introduction

Pharmaceutical stability may be defined as the capability of a particular formulation, in a specific container/closure system, to remain within its physical, chemical, microbiological, therapeutic, and toxicological specifications, during transport, storage and use. Chemical degradation may results in a loss of potency or an increase in drugs toxicity, so that clinical use of a medicine must be unacceptable if the degradation is relatively great. When a drug dosage form is altered (by dissolution, pulverization, or addition to other materials) or the environment of the drug is modified by changes in storage conditions, the stability of a drug may be affected [1-5]. Although there are exceptions, 90% of labeled potency generally is recognized as the minimum acceptable potency level (Gennaro, 2000).

Stability testing forms an important part of the process of drug development; it provides evidence on how the quality of drug substance or drug product varies with time under the influence of a variety of environmental factors, such as humidity, temperature, and light. The stability studies of drugs can be performed at the original product ("real-time" tests or long-term tests at specific temperatures and relative humidity representing storage conditions experienced in the distribution chain of the climatic zone(s) of the country or region of the world concerned; accelerated stability tests; pharmacies storage tests) or at remainder doses of these products. The chemical stability is evaluated by testing quantity of drug at different time during the storage (Lund, 1994; USP, 2007).

The aim of the stability studies is to determine the shelf life of the product and its optimum storage conditions (Connors et al., 1986; Lund, 1994; The Sixth ICH International Conference on Armonization of Technical Requirements for Registration of Pharmaceuticals for Human Use [ICH], 2003; The United States Pharmacopeia [USP], 2007; Watson, 2005; Yoshioka, 2000).

Therefore, the authors have been developing and validating HPTLC methods with the aim of quantification of drugs in dosage forms, suitable for stability and quality control studies, as at original products as at its remainder doses.

2. Drugs

Some drugs analyzed by HPTLC developed methods had been Fluphenazine, Haloperidol and L-DOPA.

2.1 Fluphenazine

Fluphenazine is a phenotiazine antipsychotic agent. The drug is a propylpiperazine derivative of phenotiazine (Delgado et al., 1998; Hardman & Limbird, 2006; Mc Evoy, 2006; Sweetman, 2003).

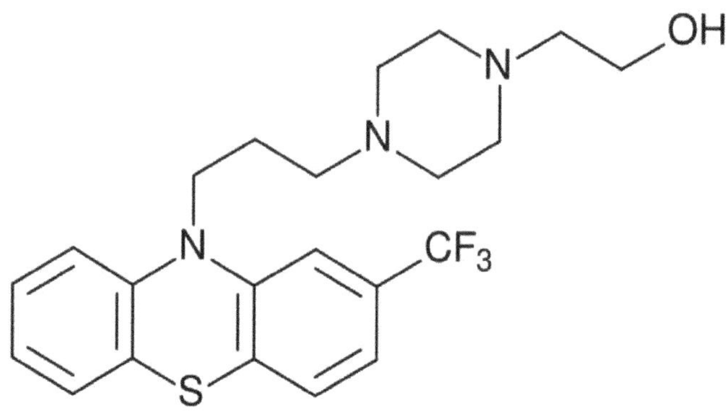

Fig. 1. Chemical structure of Fluphenazine

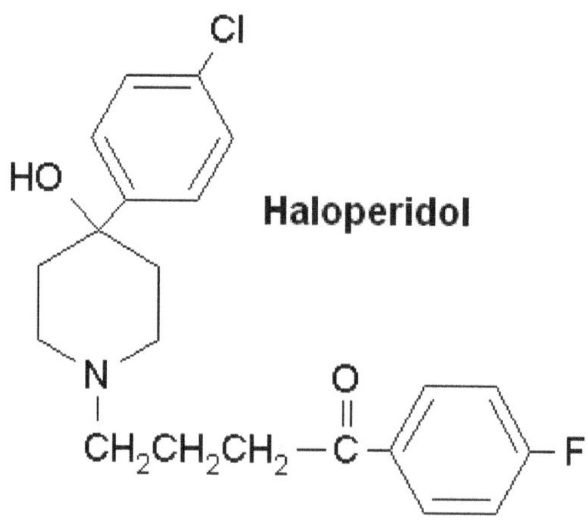

Fig. 2. Chemical structure of Haloperidol

Drug therapy with fluphenazine is integral for the management of acute psychotic episodes with violent behavior in patients with schizophrenia and generally is required for long-term stabilization to improve symptoms between episodes and to minimize the risk of recurrent acute episodes (Hardman & Limbird, 2006; Mc Evoy, 2006; Sweetman, 2003).

Fluphenazine hydrochloride, decanoate, and enantate are all sensitive to light. Therefore, it is very important to determine the quantity of fluphenazine in its dosage forms because in the presence of light, photolysis occur rapidly, resulting in drug loss and potency reduction (Delgado et al., 1998; Hardman & Limbird, 2006; Mc Evoy, 2006; Moffat el al, 2004; Sweetman, 2003).

2.2 Haloperidol

Haloperidol, a butyrophenone derivative, is used for the symptomatic management of psychotic disorders, in the same way that fluphenazine (Delgado et al., 1998; Hardman & Limbird, 2006; Mc Evoy, 2006; Sweetman, 2003).

When haloperidol injection is used, dose is depending on the severity of the illness, the age of the patient and on their response to the pharmacotherapy. Therefore, sometimes the dose corresponed only to a portion of the injection. The portion which is not used is stored for the next administration or is discarded (Delgado et al., 1998; Hardman & Limbird, 2006; Mc Evoy, 2006). The stability of this portion is unknown.

2.3 L-DOPA

L-DOPA, the levorotatory isomer of dihydroxyphenylalanine, a natural amino acid, is the precursor of the neurotransmitter dopamine.

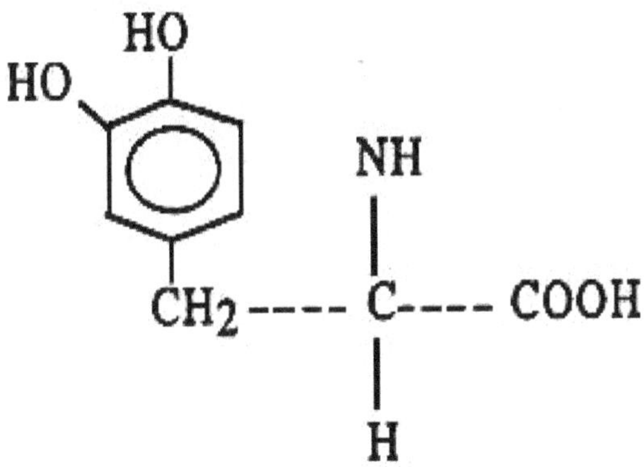

Fig. 3. Chemical structure of L-DOPA

The actions of L-DOPA are mainly those of dopamine. Unlike dopamine, L-DOPA can readily enter the Central Nervous System and is used in the treatment of conditions, such as Parkinson´s disease, which are associated with depletion of dopamine in the brain (Delgado et al., 1998; Hardman & Limbird, 2006; Mc Evoy, 2006, Sweetman, 2003). L-DOPA is considered by many clinicians the drug of choice in the management of idiopathic parkinsonian syndrome (Mc Evoy, 2006).

It is very important to determine the quantity of L-DOPA in its dosage forms, because, in the presence of moisture or atmospheric oxygen, it is rapidly oxidized resulting in drug loss and potency reduction (Carstensen, 1990; Mc Evoy, 2006; USP, 2007; Sweetman, 2003).

3. Methods

Some methods have been reported for the analysis of fluphenazine, haloperidol and L-DOPA in pharmaceutical preparations or in biological fluids. These methods include: spectrophotometry (Blanco et al., 2000; Damiani et al., 2005; Karpinska et al., 2005; Madrakian et al., 2004; Madrakian et al., 2006; Marcolino-Junior et al., 2001; Nagaraja et al., 2001; Nagaralli et al., 2002; Nour El-Dien et al., 2005; Pistonesi et al., 2004; Talebpour et al., 2005), gas chromatography (Jemal et al., 2005), liquid chromatography (Ali & Aboul-Enein, 2005; Chaná et al., 2004; Crevoisier et al., 2003; Fernández et al., 2001; Karimi et al., 2006; Kircherr & Kühn-Velten, 2006; Lea et al., 1982; Nyholm et al., 2002; Sagar & Smyth, 2000;

Saxer et al., 2004; Trabelsi et al., 2002; Wang & Fang, 2006), electrophoresis (Zhang et al., 2001) and voltammetry (Maia et al., 2005). Nevertheless, these methods have often suffered from diverse disadvantages with regard to cost or selectivity, with complex sample preparation procedures, and long analysis time.

Also, one method by TLC was found for determination of fluphenazine hydrochloride in coated tablets, but not in ampoules (Maslanka & Krzek, 2005). Only one paper of stability of haloperidol in injections is discussed in literature, but this paper deals whit the stability of haloperidol in 5% dextrose injection (Das Gupta & Stewart, 1982).

3.1 High performance thin layer chromatography (HPTLC)

High performance of HPTLC is due to it fastness, solvent economy and high throughput of samples. Chromatography of samples simultaneously with standards it is another advantage, allowing to run up to 60 spots simultaneously (27 samples plus standards by each side of the plate). Sensitivity of HPTLC is normally in the range of nanograms in absorbance and picograms in fluorescence mode.

The authors have performed some works using HPTLC for quantitative determination of drugs in biological fluids (Mennickent et al., 2003,2007a, 2007b, 2009, 2010a, 2010b) and in dosage forms (de Diego et al., 2007a, 2007b, 2010a, 2010b; Mennickent et al., 2007a, 2007b, 2007c, 2010), with exact and reliable results.

The HPTLC methods developed are simples, rapids, with low LOD and LOQ values, with very good accuracy and precision, with robustness, and economical.

3.1.1 Method for fluphenazine injections

For the quantification of fluphenazine in injections, the method was linear in the range of 100 ng/band to 500 ng/band (r=0.998).The limit of detection (LOD) and limit of quantification (LOQ) were 1.45 ng/band and 4.40 ng/band, respectively. The intra-assay and inter-assay precision, expressed as the relative standard deviation (RSD),

were in the range of 0.73%-1.77% (n=3) and 1.18%-1.86% (n=9), respectively. The recovery of fluphenazine hydrochloride was in the range 98.29% and 101.53%, with a RSD not higher than 1.87%. The method was selective for fluphenazine hydrochloride from the preservatives of the injections (Rf for fluphenazine hydrochloride was 0.33, whereas parabens run to the solvent front) (Fig. 4 and Fig. 5).

Stability-indicating capability of the HPTLC assay was studied by forced decomposition of 5 mL of a solution of fluphenazine 1 mg/mL, with 10 mL of 0.1 N hydrochloric acid, 10 mL of 0.1 N sodium hydroxide and 10 mL of 3% H_2O_2. The mixtures with NaOH and with HCl were heated on hot plates at 60°C for 60 minutes. The mixture with H_2O_2 was storage at room temperature (25°C) for 60 minutes. Then, each mixture was diluted to 100 ng/uL with ethanol and analyzed.

Also, stability-indicating capability of the assay was proved by conducting forced degradation conditions of UV and VIS radiation on fluphenazine standard, as solution of 100ng/uL.

One degradation product was found after treatment of fluphenazine with HCl, and two degradation products were found after treatment with NaOH. Rf for fluphenazine was 0.30, whereas Rf for degradation product with HCl was 0.01, and Rf for degradation products with NaOH were 0.03 and 0.23 respectively. None degradation product was found with H_2O_2 (Fig.6).

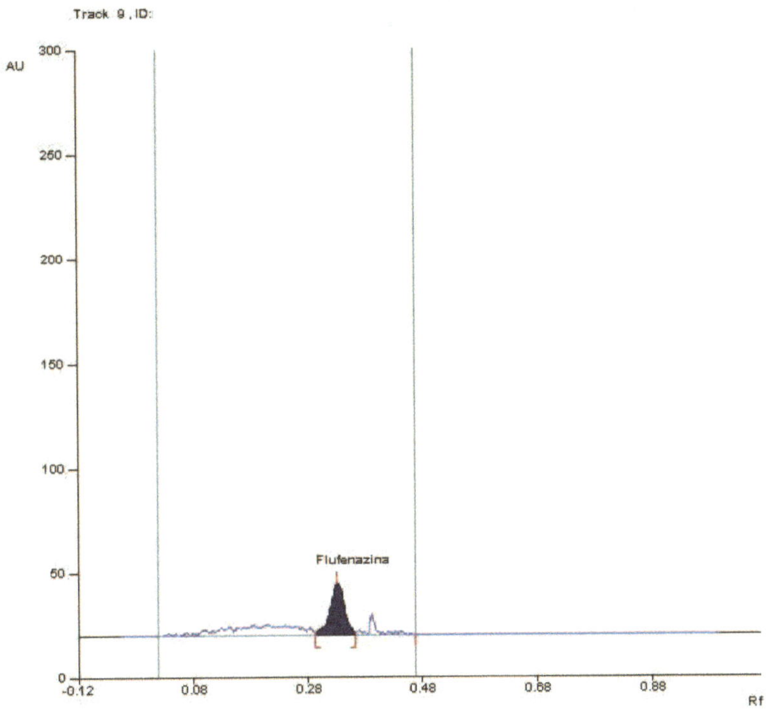

Fig. 4. Selectivity of the method. Study with parabens. Peak observed: fluphenazine. Rf: retarding factor. AU: absorbance unit

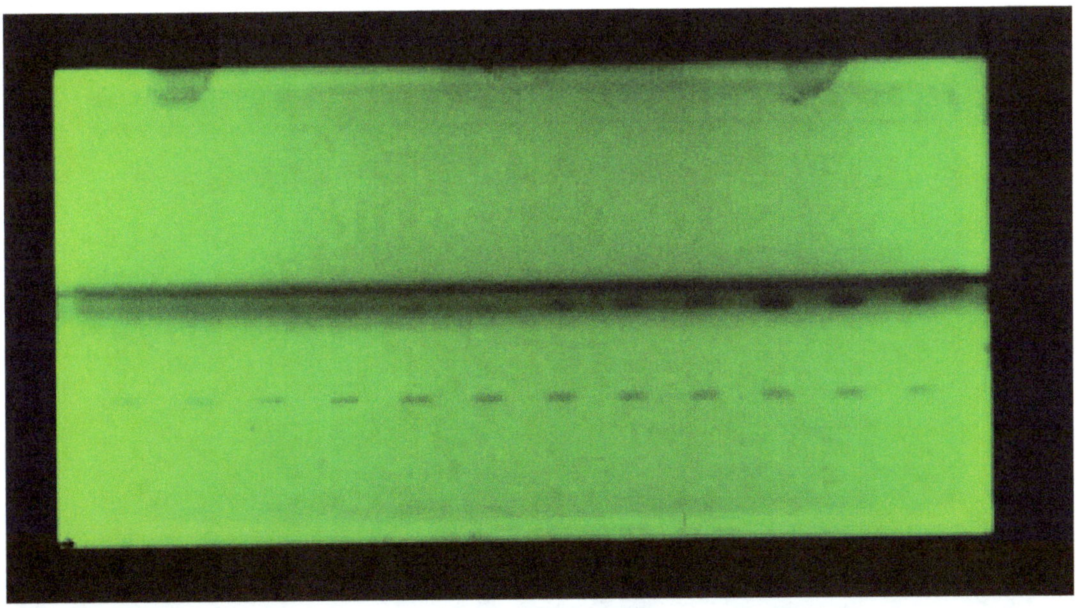

Fig. 5. Picture (video store, CAMAG) of plate at selectivity with parabens. Tracks 1-3 (from left to right of the plate) : fluphenazine hydrochloride; tracks 4-6: fluphenazine hydrochloride + methylparaben; tracks 7-9: fluphenazine hydrochloride + propylparaben; tracks 10-12: fluphenazine hydrochloride + methylparaben + propylparaben. Bands of parabens can be observed at the solvent front

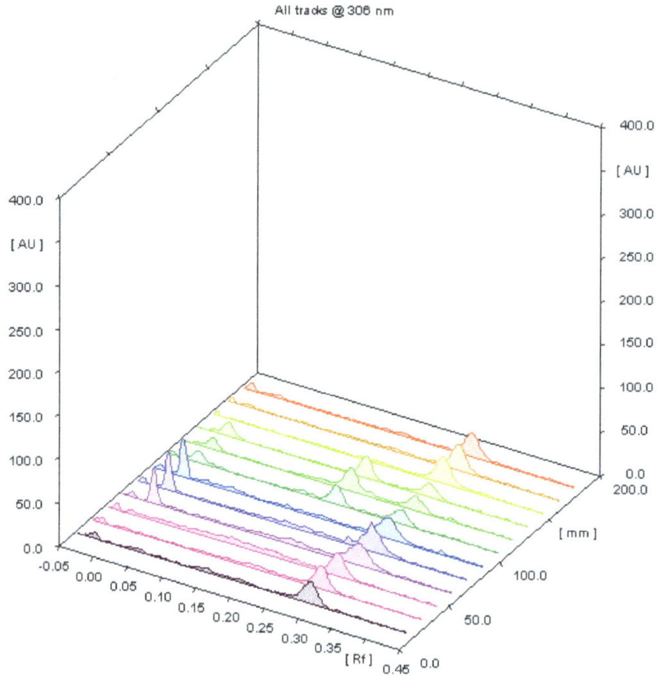

Fig. 6. Degradation study of fluphenazine with HCl, with NaOH and with H_2O_2. Tracks 1-3 (from bottom side to the upper side): fluphenzine; tracks 4-6: fluphenazine + HCl; tracks 7-9: fluphenazine + NaOH; track 10-12: fluphenazine + H_2O_2. Rf peak pluphenazine = 0.30. Other peaks at tracks 4-9: degradation products. Rf: retarding factor. AU: absorbance unit

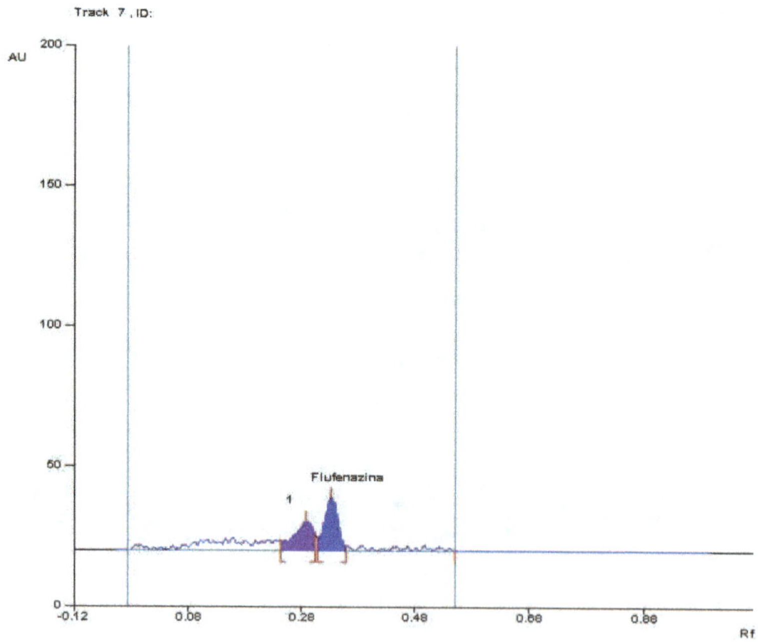

Fig. 7. Degradation study of fluphenazine with VIS radiation. Peak 1 (from left to right): fluphenazine; peak 2: degradation product. Rf: retarding factor: AU: absorbance unit

When the drug was exposed to forced degradation with VIS radiation, another peak different to the peak of fluphenazine was found, therefore it could be a degradation product. Rf for fluphenazine = 0.30 and Rf for degradation product = 0.56 (Fig. 7). One of the products of photolysis mentioned in literature is a sulphoxide (Lund, 1994).
Values for precision study of the method can be observed at the Table 1.

	Relative standard deviation (RSD), %	
Concentration (ng/uL)	Intraassay precision[a]	Intermediate precision[b]
100	1.77	1.86
300	1.64	1.47
500	0.73	1.18

[a] n= 3; analyzed on the same day (for each concentration)
[b] n= 9; analyzed on three different days (for each concentration)

Table 1. Precision of the HPTLC method for fluphenazine injections

Values founded for the accuracy of the method are presented at the Table 2.

Added concentration (ng/uL)	Found concentration (ng/uL) [a]	Accuracy, % [b]	RSD, % [c]
	Intraassay (n=9)		
80	79.90 ± 1.31	99.87	1.64
100	100.45 ± 1.10	100.45	1.10
120	121.84 ± 2.28	101.53	1.87
	Interassay (n=27)		
80	78.63 ± 1.34	98.29	1.71
100	99.74 ± 1.65	99.74	1.65
120	120.90 ± 1.83	100.75	1.52

[a] Each value is the mean ± standard deviation.
[b] (Founded concentration/ added concentration) x 100.
[c] Relative standard deviation (coefficient of variation).

Table 2. Method accuracy

3.1.2 Method for haloperidol injections

For the quantification of haloperidol in injections, the method was linear between 10ng/band to 100 ng/band (r = 0.999), the method was selective between haloperidol and the parabens, the preservatives in haloperidol lactate injection (Rf for haloperidol was 0.70, whereas parabens run to the solvent front) (Fig. 8-10). RSD for precision was ≤ 1.92%, and accuracy was from 98.59% to 101.90% of recovery. LOD was 0.89 ng/band and LOQ was 2.71 ng/band.
Stability-indicating capability of the HPTLC assay was established by forced decomposition of 5 mL of a solution of haloperidol lactate 1 mg/mL, with 10 mL of 0.1 N hydrochloric acid and 10 mL of 0.1 N sodium hydroxide. The mixture was heated on a hot plate at 60°C for 60 minutes, cooled to room temperature, diluted to 100 ng/uL with methanol and analyzed.
Also, stability-indicating capability of the assay was proved by conducting forced degradation conditions of VIS radiation on haloperidol standard.

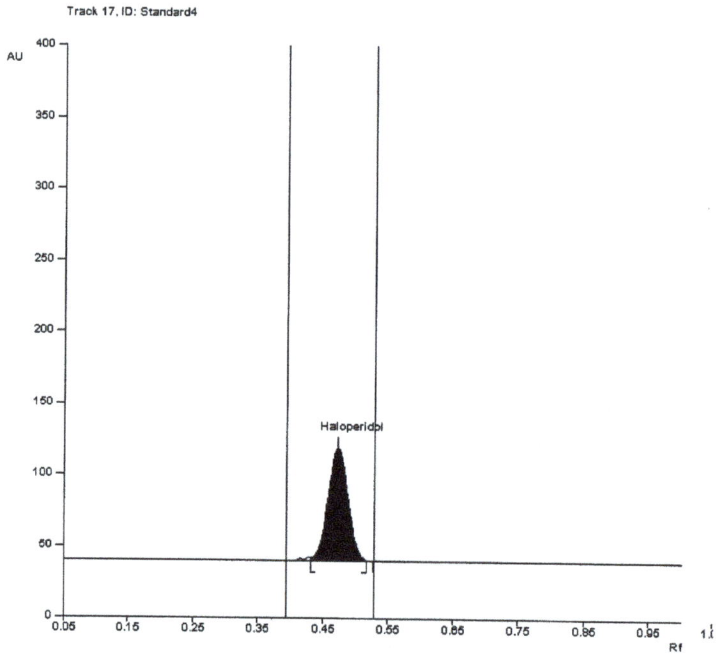

Fig. 8. Peak of haloperidol. Rf: retarding factor: AU: absorbance unit. Solution concentration: 80 ng/uL

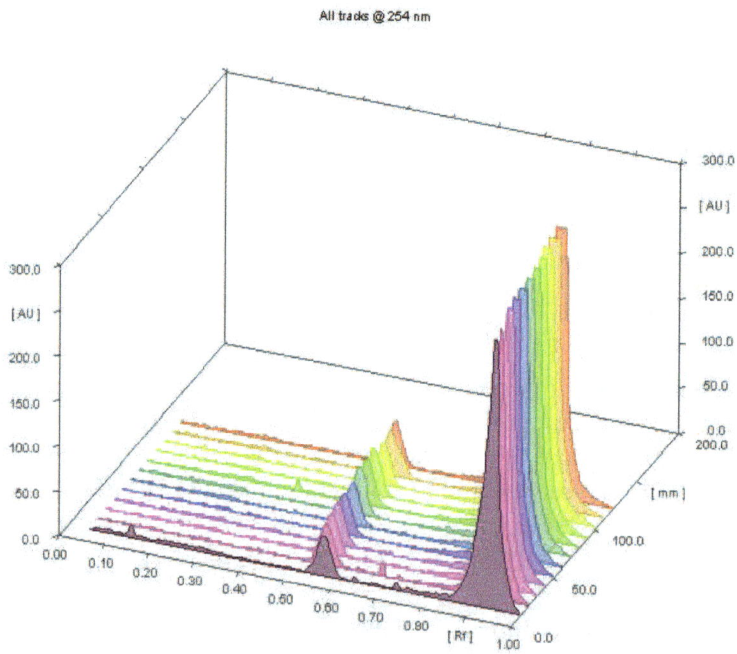

Fig. 9. Selectivity of the method. Study with parabens. Tracks 1-3 (from the bottom side to the upper side): haloperidol; tracks 4-6: haloperidol + methylparaben; tracks 7-9: haloperidol + propylparaben; tracks 10-12: haloperidol + methylparaben + propylparaben. Peak 1(from left to right): haloperidol; peak 2: solvent front. Rf: retarding factor. AU: absorbance unit

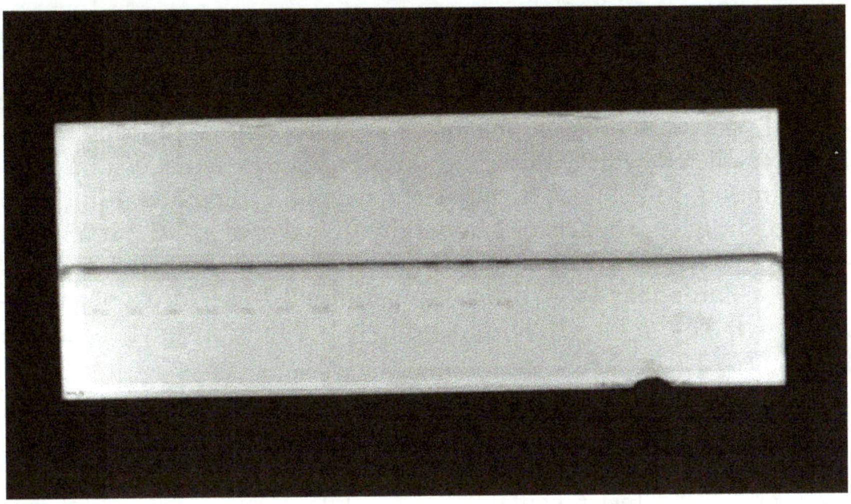

Fig. 10. Picture (video store, CAMAG) of plate at selectivity between haloperidol and parabens. Tracks 1-3: haloperidol; tracks 4-6: haloperidol + methylparaben; tracks 7-9: haloperidol + propylparaben; tracks 10-12: haloperidol + methylparaben + propylparaben. Bands of parabens can be observed at the solvent front

After treatment of haloperidol lactate with acid none degradation product was found. However, after treatment with basic, one minor peak was found, which probably correspond to a degradation product, with a resolution of 2.4 between haloperidol and another peak (Fig. 11)

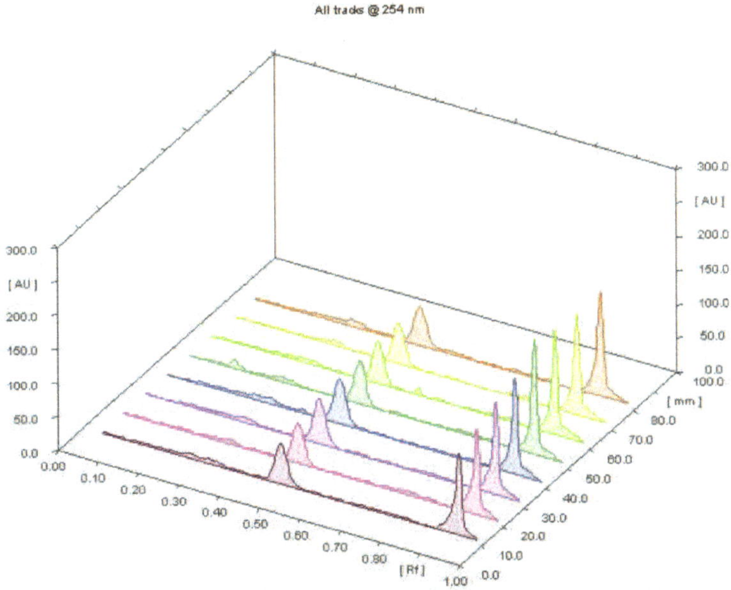

Fig. 11. Selectivity of the method. Study at forced degradation of haloperidol with 0.1 N HCl and 0.1 N NaOH. Tracks 1,2,7,8 (from the bottom side to the upper side): haloperidol; tracks: 3-4: haloperidol + HCl; tracks 5-6: haloperidol + NaOH. Peak 1 (from left to right): haloperidol; peak 2: solvent front. Minor peak at tracks 5-6: degradation products. Rf: retarding factor: AU: absorbance unit

When the drug was exposed to forced degradation with VIS radiation, no degradation product was found.

The degradation products for haloperidol mentioned in literature are acrolein, chlorobenzene, p-fluorobenzaldehyde, p-fluoroacetophenone, p-fluorophenyl propenyl ketone, when haloperidol was irradiated with a sterilising dose of gamma radiation (Lund et al., 1994). Another studies found 4-(4-chlorophenyl)-4-hidroxypiperydine and 4-fluorobenzoic acid, presumed to be hydrolytic products of haloperidol (Jemal et al., 2005; Karipnska et al., 2005) and 4-[4-(4-chlorophenyl)-4-hydroxy-1-piperidinyl]-1-(4-fluorophenyl)-1-butanone N-oxide; and 4-[4-(4-chlorophenyl)-4-hydroxy-1-piperidinyl]-1-(4-hydroxyphenyl)-1-butanone; 4-[4-(4-chlorophenyl)-3,6-dihydro-1(2H)-piperidinyl]-1-(4-fluorophenyl)-1-butanone (Lund et al., 1994).

Values for the precision study are shown at the Table 3.

	Relative standard deviation (RSD), %		
Concentration (ng/uL)	Instrumental precision[a]	Intraassay precision[b]	Intermediate precision[c]
10	0.81	1.31	1.92
50	0.37	1.74	1.53
100	0.51	0.38	1.11

[a] n= 10; analyzed on the same day

[b] n= 5; analyzed on the same day (for each concentration)

[c] n= 9; analyzed on three different days (for each concentration)

Table 3. Precision of the method

Values for the accuracy of the method can be observed at the Table 4.

Added concentration (ng/uL)	Found concentration (ng/uL) [a]	Accuracy, % [b]	
	Intraassay (n=9)		
80	78.87 ± 2.98	98.59	3.78
100	101.21 ± 3.78	101.21	3.74
120	119.05 ± 1.75	99.21	1.47
	Interassay (n=27)		
80	81.52 ± 3.59	101.90	4.40
100	99.74 ± 4.41	99.74	4.42
120	119.35 ± 5.37	99.46	4.50

[a] Each value is the mean ± standard deviation.;

[b] (Founded concentration/ added concentration) x 100;

[c] Relative standard deviation (coefficient of variation).

Table 4. Method accuracy

Stability study of haloperidol lactate injection 5mg /mL was realized at the following conditions: 25 ± 2 °C, because it is the more common temperature founded at hospitals in Chile and is the temperature mentioned by ICH guidelines for stability studies at dosage forms; and refrigeration temperature (8 ± 1 °C) in its original glass ampoules after it was opened, removed a portion of drug, and sealed with Teflon. The samples at room temperature were stored under light exposure and light protection. The study was performed over 15 days.

Samples were taken at appropriate time intervals (0, 3, 5, 7, 10 and 15 days), and analyzed in duplicate by HPTLC to determine haloperidol concentration. For stability study, 100 uL of the haloperidol lactate injection 5 mg/mL was transferred to a 10 mL volumetric flask and diluted with methanol to volume (final concentration of 50 ng/uL).
The percentage of haloperidol remaining after each interval was determined by comparing the concentration at that time with the initial haloperidol concentration, measured before storage (t = 0) at the different conditions. Haloperidol lactate injections, when stored at 25 ± 2 °C under light exposure and light protection, and when stored at refrigeration temperature (8 ± 1 °C) in original glass ampoules opened and after closed with Teflon retained at least 90% of the initial concentration over 15 days (Table 5).

Storage time (days)	**Initial concentration remaining** (%) (Mean ± SD)		
	23 ± 2 °C		**8 ± 1 °C**
	Exposed to light		**Protected from light**
0	100 .00	100.00	100.00
3	94.77 ± 0.6	96.20 ± 2.1	98.99 ± 0.3
5	93.64 ± 1.4	94.79 ± 0.8	98.75 ± 1.2
7	93.26 ± 2.1	93.20 ± 1.8	96.99 ± 1.4
10	91.87 ± 0.3	92.88 ± 2.0	94.75 ± 2.1
15	90.69 ± 1.7	91.71 ± 0.5	92.53 ± 0.8

Table 5. Stability of injectable haloperidol

3.1.3 Method for L-DOPA tablets

For the quantification of L-DOPA in tablets, the method was linear between 100 ng/band to 500 ng/ band (r = 0.999). The intra-assay variation was between 0.26% and 0.65% and the inter-assay was between 0.52% and 2.04%. LOD was 1.12 ng, and LOQ was 3.29 ng. The accuracy ranged from 100.40 % to101.09%, with a coefficient of variation not higher than 1.40%. The method was selective for L-DOPA (Rf = 0.37) and carbidope (Rf = 0.79) (Fig. 12).
Table 6 shown the values for the precision study of the method.
The values found for the accuracy of the method can be observed at Table 7.
At Table 8 can be observed the values found for the determination of L-DOPA in tablets by the proposed HPTLC method and by the USP HPLC method.
Accelerated stability study was performed on commercial tablets of L-DOPA. The temperature used was 40±2°C and the relative humidity was 75±5 (Zone II, OMS). The study was carried out by three months, taking samples to t=0 and one time each month.

	Relative standard deviation (RSD), %		
Concentration (ng/µL)	Instrumental precision[a]	Intraassay precision[b]	Intermediate precision[c]
100	0.45	0.48	2.04
300	0.68	0.65	0.77
500	0.23	0.26	0.52

[a] n= 10; analyzed on the same day; [b] n= 5; analyzed on the same day (for each concentration) [c] n= 9; analyzed on three different days (for each concentration)

Table 6. Precision of the method

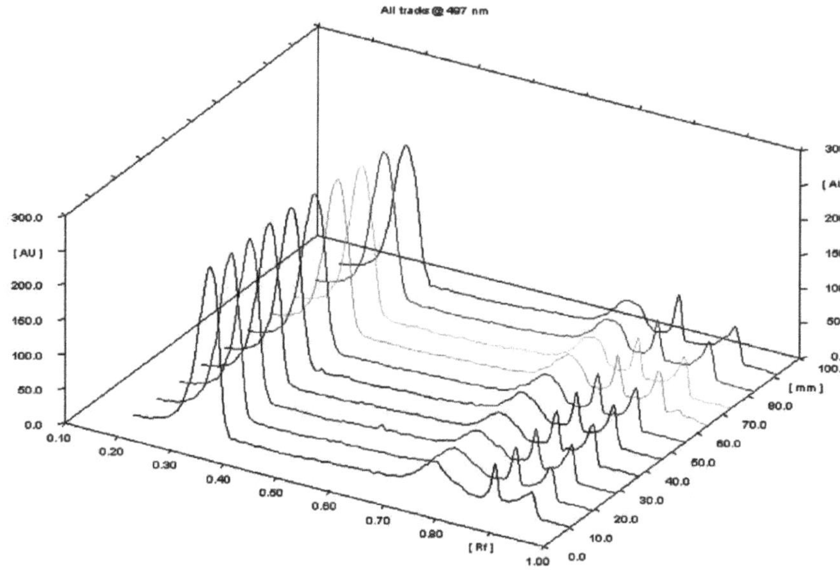

Fig. 12. Selectivity of the method. Peak 1 (from left to right): L-DOPA; peak 2: Carbidope (dopa-decarboxilase inhibitor)

Added concentration (ng/µL)	Found concentration (ng/µL) [a]	Accuracy, % [b]	RSD, %
	Intraassay (n=9)		
320	322.10 ± 4.20	100.66	1.30
400	404.22 ± 3.70	101.06	0.92
480	485.25 ± 1.20	101.09	0.25
	Interassay (n=27)		
320	321.27 ± 4.50	100.40	1.40
400	402.30 ± 3.80	100.58	0.94
480	482.83 ± 2.35	100.60	0.49

[a] Each value is the mean ± standard deviation; [b] (Found concentration/ added concentration) x 100.

Table 7. Method accuracy

Parameter	HPTLC	HPLC
Labelled claim (mg per tablet)	100.00	100.00
Amount found[a] (mg per tablet)	90.99	90.00
RSD (%)	2.40	1.53
F calc.: 11.86; *F* theoretical[b]: 13.61		

[a] Each result is the mean of nine experiments (three solutions, three determinations of each of them).
[b] $\alpha = 0.05$

Table 8. Comparison for determination of L-DOPA in tablets by the proposed method and by HPLC

Tablets were processed as follow (USP, 2007): 20 tablets were weighed and ground into fine powder and an accurately weighed portion equivalent to 30 mg of L-DOPA was diluted to 100 mL with water: methanol (7:3, v/v) . The solution was centrifuged and then, 1 mL of the supernatant was diluted to a 10 mL with the mixture solvent.

Results of the accelerated stability study can be observed at Table 9.

t(months)	Percentage L-DOPA per tablet	Quantity L-DOPA per tablet (mg)
0	100.00	90.99
1	96.65	87.94
2	87.21	79.35
3	85.60	77.89

Table 9. Results for the accelerated stability study of L-DOPA tablets

Therefore, at the second month of accelerated stability study, L-DOPA tablets don't have a change significant at the percentage of active principle per tablet, but at the third month of the study, the change at the percentage is more than a 5% (ICH, 2003).

4. Conclusion

The proposed HPTLC methods are a new analytical alternative for quantification of the mentioned drugs in these dosage forms. None HPTLC method for quantitative analysis of fluphenazine hydrochloride in injections, haloperidol in injections and L-DOPA in tablets were found in literature before our methods.

These methods are simple, fast, precise, sensitive (low LOD and LOQ values), accurate and specifics for the quantification of these drugs in the dosage forms studied. Moreover, HPTLC allows for a large number of samples to be measured simultaneously, very important, especially in quality control.

The procedure works without separation steps, only centrifugation, because the excipients are not dissolved by the working solvents.

Therefore, the proposed HPTLC methods are very good methods for quantitative analysis of fluphenazine hydrochloride in injection, haloperidol lactate in injections, and L-DOPA in tablets, being appropriates to stability studies.

By the other side, the results indicate that haloperidol lactate injection (glass ampoules) could be stored for at least 15 days and use when needed, reducing wastage and unnecessary expenses. This could result in substantial money savings for some institutions.

5. Acknowledgment

The authors would like to thank the Research Council at the University of Concepción (Project DIUC 201.074.034-1.0 and Project DIUC 204.074.034-1.0), and to Pharmacists Miss Loreto Pino, Mr. Mario Nail, Mr. Jonathan Contreras and Mr. Cristobal Reyes.

6. References

Ali, I., & Aboul-Enein, H. (2005). Fast determination of haloperidol in pharmaceutical preparations using HPLC in monolithic silica column. *J.Liq. Chromatogr. Relat. Tecnol.*, 28, 3169-3179.

Blanco, M; Coello, M., Iturriaga, H., Maspoch, S., & Villegas, N. (2000) Simultaneous spectrophotometric determination of levodopa and benserazide in a pharmaceutical. *Anal. Lett.* , 33 (13), 2701-2718.

Carstensen, J. (1990). *Drug Stability. Principles and Practices,* Marcel Dekker, Inc., New York, USA.

Chaná, P., Kunstmann, C., Reyes-Parada, M., & Sáez-Briones, P.(2004). Delayed early morning turn „ON" in response to a single dose of levodopa in advanced Parkinson´s disease: pharmacokinetics should be considered. *J. Neurol. Neurosurg. Psychiatrie*, 75, 1782-1783

Connors, K; Amidon, G., & Stella, V.(1986). *Chemical Stability of Pharmaceuticals*, John Wiley & Sons, New York, USA.

Crevoisier, C., Monreal, A., Metzger, B., & Nilsen, T.(2003). Comparative single- and multiple-dose pharmacokinetics of levodopa and 3-O-methyldopa following a new dual-release and a conventional slow-release formulation of levodopa and benserazide in healthy volunteers. *Eur.Neurol.*, 49, 39-44.

Damiani, P., Moschetti, A., Rovetto, A., Benavente, F., & Olivieri, A.(2005). Design and optimization of a chemometrics-assisted spectrophotometric method for the simultaneous determination of levodopa and carbidopa in pharmaceutical products. *Anal. Chim. Acta*, 543 (1-2), 192-198.

Das Gupta, V., & Stewart, K.R. (1982). Stability of haloperidol in 5% dextrose injection. *Am.J.Hosp.Pharm.*, 1982, 39(2), 292-294.

de Diego, M..,Godoy, C.G., & Mennickent, S.(2007). Chemical stability of midazolam injection for high performance liquid chromatography. *J.Sep.Sci.*, 30 (12), 1833-1838.

de Diego, M., Avello, M., Mennickent, S., Fernández, M., & Fernández., P. (2007). Validated liquid chromatographic method for the quantification of allicin in garlic powder and tablets.. *J.Sep.Sci.*, 30(16),2703-2707.

de Diego, M.,Godoy, C.G., & Mennickent, S.(2010). Chemical stability of ceftriazone by a validated stability-indicating liquid chromatographic method. *J.Chil.Chem.Soc.*, 55 (3): 335-337.

de Diego, M., Godoy, R., Godoy, C.G., & Mennickent, S. (2010). "Chemical stability of enalapril maleate drug substance and tablets by a stability-indicating liquid chromatographic method".*Quimica Nova*. In press, 2010.

Delgado, J., & Remers, W. (1998). *Wilson and Gisvolds. Textbook of Organic Medicinal and Pharmaceutical Chemistry*, Lippincott-Raven, Philadelphia, USA.

Fernández, M., Fernández, T., García, B., Gutiérrez, J., & Iraizoz, A. (2001). Accelerated stability of levodopa-carbidopa tablets. *Rev. Cubana Farm.*, 35 (2),1-5.

Gennaro, A. (2000). *Remington: the Science and Practice of Pharmacy*, Lippincott Williams /Wilkins, Philadelphia, USA.

Hardman, J., & Limbird, L. (2006).*Las Bases Farmacológicas de la Terapéutica*, Mc Graw-Hill, Mexico, Mexico.

Jemal, M., Ivanshiv, E., Both, D., Koski, R., & Cohen, A. (2005). Picogram level determination of fluphenazine in human plasma by automated gas chromatography/mass selective detection. *Biomed. Environ. Mass Spectrom.*, 14, 699-704.

Karimi, M., Carl, J.L., Loftin, S., & Perlmutter, J.S. (2006). Modified high-performance liquid chromatography with electrochemical detection method for plasma measurement of levodopa, 3-0 methyldopa, dopamine, carbidope and 3,4-dihydroxyphenyl acetic acid. *J.Chromatogr. B.*, 19 (1-2), 120-123.

Karpinska, J., Smyk, J., & Wolyniec, E. (2005). A spectroscopic study on applicability on spectral analysis for simultaneous quantificatin of l-dopa, benserazide and ascorbic acid in batch and flow systems. *Spectrochim. Acta A Mol Biomol. Spectrosc.*, 62 (1-3), 213-220.

Kircherr, H., & Kühn-Velten, W. (2006). Quantitative determination of forthy-eight antidepressants and antipsychotics in human serum by HPLC tandem mass spectrometry: a multi level, single sampling approach. *J.Chromatogr.B*, 843,100-113.

Lea, A.R., Haley, D.M., & Daguid, P.R. (1982). Analysis of haloperidol tablets by high-performance liquid chromatography –an inter-laboratory study. *J.Chromatogr.*, 250, 35-42.

Lund, W. (1994) *The Pharmaceutical Codex*, The Pharmaceutical Press, London, UK.

Maia, M.S., Yamashita, M., & Angnes, L. (2005). Voltammetric studies and determination of levodopa and carbidopa in pharmaceutical products. *Electroanalysis*, 18 (7), 656-661.

Madrakian, T., Afkhami, M., Borazjani, M., & Bahram, M. (2004). Simultaneous derivative spectrophotometric determination of levodopa and carbidopa in pharmaceutical preparations. *Bull. Korean Chem. Soc.*,25 (12), 1764-1767.

Madrakian, T., Afkhami, A., Khalafi, L., & Mohammadnejad, M.(2006). Spectrophotometric determination of cathecolamines based on their oxidation reaction followed by coupling with 4 -aminobenzoic acid. *J.Braz. Chem. Soc.*, 17 (7), 1-20.

Marcolino-Junior, L.H., Teixeira, M.F., Pereira, A.V., & Fatibello-Filho (2001). Flow injection determination of levodopa in tablets using a solid-phase reactor containing lead (IV) dioxide immobilized. *J.Pharm.Biomed.Anal.*, 25 (3-4), 393-398.

Maslanka, A., & Krzek, J. (2005). Densitometric high performance thin-layer chromatography identification and quantitative analysis of psychotropic drugs. *JAOAC Inter.*, 88, 70-79.

Mc Evoy, G. (2006). *AHFS Drug Information*, American Society of Health- System Pharmacists, Bethesda, USA.

Moffat, A., Osselton, M.D., & Widdop, B. (2004).*Clarke´s Analysis of Drugs and Poisons*, Pharmaceutical Press, London, UK.

Mennickent, S., Vega, M., & Godoy, C.G. (2003). Development and validation of a method using instrumental planar chromatography for quantitative analysis of carbamazepine in saliva. *J.Chil.Chem.Soc.*, 48, (3), 71-73.

Mennickent, S., Sobarzo, A., Vega, M., Godoy, C.G., & de Diego, M. (2007). Quantitative determination of clozapine in serum by instrumental planar chromatography. *J.Sep.Sci.*, 30, 2167 -2172.

Mennickent, S.,Vega, M.,Godoy, C.G., & León, M.D. (2007). Relación entre niveles de carbamazepina en saliva y plasma: un estudio piloto. *Rev.Méd.Chile*, 135: 335-340.

Mennickent, S., Pino, L., Vega, M., Godoy, C.G., & de Diego, M. (2007). Quantitative determination of haloperidol in tablets by high performance thin-layer chromatography. *J. Sep. Sci.*, 30, 772-777.

Mennickent, S., Pino, L., Vega, M., & de Diego, M. (2007). Chemical stability of haloperidol injection by high performance thin - layer chromatography. *J.Sep.Sci.*, 31, 201-206.

Mennickent, S., Nail, M., Vega, M., & de Diego, M. (2007). Quantitative determination of L-DOPA in tablets by high performance thin-layer chromatography. *J.Sep.Sci.*, 30, 1893-1898.

Mennickent, S., Fierro, R.,Vega, M.. ,de Diego, M., & Godoy, C.G. (2009) Instrumental planar chromatographic method for determination of carbamazepine in human serum.*J.Sep.Sci.*,32, 1454 -1458.

Mennickent, S., Sobarzo, A., Vega, M., de Diego, M., Godoy, C.G., Rioseco, P., & Saavedra, L.(2010). Determination of clozapine in serum of patients with schizophrenia as a measurement of medication compliance. *International Journal of Psychiatry in Clinical Practice*, 14, 41-46.

Mennickent, S., Fierro, R., Vega, M., .de Diego, M., & Godoy, C.G. (2010). Quantitative determination of fluoxetine in human serum by high performance thin layer chromatography. *J.Sep.Sci.*, 33, 2206 -2210.

Mennickent;, S.,Contreras, J., Reyes, C.,Vega, M., & de Diego, M. (2010). Validated instrumental planar chromatographic method for quantification of fluphenazine hydrochoride in injections. *J.Planar Chromatogr.*, 23, 1-13.

Nagaraja, P., Vasantha, R.A., & Sunitha, K.R. (2001). A new sensitive and selective spectrophotometric method for determination of cathecol derivatives and its pharmaceutical preparations. *J.Pharm.Biomed.Anal.*, 25 (3-4), 417-424.

Nagaralli, B.S., Seetharamappa, J., Melwanki, M.B., Ramesh, K.C., & Keshavayya, J. (2002). Spectrophotometric investigations of the assay physiologically active cathecolamines in pharmaceutical formulations. *J.AOAC Inter.*, 85 (6), 1288-1292.

Nour El-Dien, F.A., Zayed, M.A., Mohamed, G., & El-Nahas, R. (2005). Two spectrophotometric assays for dopamine derivatives in pharmaceutical products and in biological samples of schizophrenic patients using copper tetramine complex and tri-iodide reagent. *J.Biomed. Biotecnol.*, 205 (1), 9.

Nyholm, D., Lennernans, H., Gomes-Trolin, C., & Aquilonious, S-M. (2002). Levodopa pharmacokinetics and motor performance during activies of daily living in patients with Parkinson´s disease on individual drug combinations. *Clin.Neuropharmacol.* ,25 (2), 89-96.

Pistonesi, M., Centurión, M.E., Fernández, B., Damiani, P., & Olivieri, A. (2004). Simultaneous determination of levodopa and benserazide by stopped-flow injecrion analisys and three-way multivariate calibration of kinetic-spectrophotometric data. *J. Pharm. Biomed.Anal.*, 36, 541-547.

Sagar, K.A., & Smyth, M.R. (2000). Bioavailability studies of oral dosage forms containing levodopa and carbidopa using column-switching chromatography followed by electrochemical detection. *Analyst*, 125, 439-445.

Saxer, C., Nilna, M., Nakashima, A., Nagae, Y., & Masude, N.(2004). Simultaneous determination of levodopa and 3-O-methyldopa in human plasma by liquid chromatography with electrochemical detection. *J.Chromatogr. B.*, 802 (2), 299-305.

Sweetman, S. (2003). Martindale. *Guía Completa de Consulta Farmacoterapéutica*, Pharma Editores S.L, Barcelona, Spain.

Talebpour, Z., Haghgoo, S., & Shamsipur, M. (2005). HNMR spectroscopy analysis for simultaneous determination of levodopa, carbidopa and methyldopa in human serum and pharmaceutical formulations. *Anal. Chim. Acta*, 506 (1), 97-104.

The Sixth ICH International Conference on Armonization of Technical Requirements for Registration of Pharmaceuticals for Human Use (2003). Osaka, Japan.

The United States Pharmacopeia (USP 30) (2007). United States Pharmacopeial Convection, Inc., Rockville, USA.

Trabelsi, H., Bouzouita,K., & Safta, F.(2002). Determination and degradation study of haloperidol by high performance liquid chromatography. *J.Pharm.Biomed.Anal.*, 29 (4), 649-657.

Wang, J., & Fang, Y (2006). Determination, purity assessment and chiral separation of levodopa methyl ester in bulk and formulation pharmaceuticals. *Biomed. Chromatogr.*, 20 (9), 904-910.

Watson, D. (2005).*Pharmaceutical Analysis*, Elsevier, Edinburgh, UK.

Yoshioka, S., & Stella, V. (2000). *Stability of Drugs and Dosage Forms*, Kluwer Academic Plenum Publishers, New York, USA.

Zhang, L., Chen, G., Hu, Q., & Fang, Y. (2001). Separation and determination of levodopa and carbidopa in composite tablets by capillary zone electrophoresis with amperometric detection. *Anal. Chim. Acta*, 43(2), 287-292.

5

Manufacture, Structure Confirmation and Quality Control of the Chiral Drugs

Zhang Zhen[1,2] and Bi Kaishun[2]
[1]*Center for Drug Evaluation, State Food and Drug Administration, Beijing*
[2]*Shenyang Pharmaceutical University, Shenyang, Liaoning,*
China

1. Introduction

The general thinking of quality control of the chiral drugs is that we need to conduct the research following the characteristic of the chiral drug besides principles already existing[1]. During the research, according to the way by which the chiral center being introduced, we should adopt the effective measurement to control the optical purity of chiral material and each step resultant; choose the appropriate way (direct or indirect) to prove the absolute configuration according to compound's unique feature as well as research foundation already existing such as its preparation craft, the comparison of structure confirmation, the literature data and so on.

2. Synthesizing technology for chiral drugs

Chiral drug is a kind of special chemical drug. Its particularity must be considered in the research except the guideline for chemical drug[2]. We need to pay more attention to the change of chiral center and the optical purity in the process momentarily.
During the research, both the optical purity of the starting material and the control of the process are important, which may have effect to the final product. So the internal control standard should be established especially the control of the optical purity. According to the way by which the chiral center being introduced, we should adopt different method to control the optical purity of each intermediate material. Moreover, we should monitor the change of the configuration in the reaction by establishing the appropriate process control target.

2.1 Route analysis for synthesizing technology of chiral drug

As it was said in the guideline[3], both asymmetrical synthesis and the resolution have superiority to obtain chiral drug - although the selectivity is better and the optical purity of final product is higher, asymmetrical synthesis has more steps; on the contrary, the route of resolution method is shorter, but the chiral purity is not meet the requirement sometimes, especially when there are more than one chiral center exist in the drug. We can choose the rational method according to the feature in the actual application.
For the process of asymmetric synthesis, we consult the relevant literature as much as possible before establishing the process, and adequately understand the mechanism, reaction conditions and stereoselectivity about the different reactions, then find out the corresponding

reaction. Because the steric hindrance of materials, some reactions have larger stereoselectivity, and the needed configuration may be the one that is obtained from the reaction. If the needed is not the predominance configuration or that is not ideal proportion, some measurement should be adopted to improve the reaction selectivity, introducing a large group into the starting material such as salt or ester, then improve greatly the stereoselectivity. For example, some chiral drug evaluating needs to form two chiral carbons, the researchers induce a tert-butyl group to the starting material, after forming the chiral center, the inducing group is eliminated, the result confirm the inducing group that will improve the stereoselectivity from 60% to 98%, then get high yield, and the sequent purification process had been simplified synchronously. The strategy to the synthesis such as figure 1.

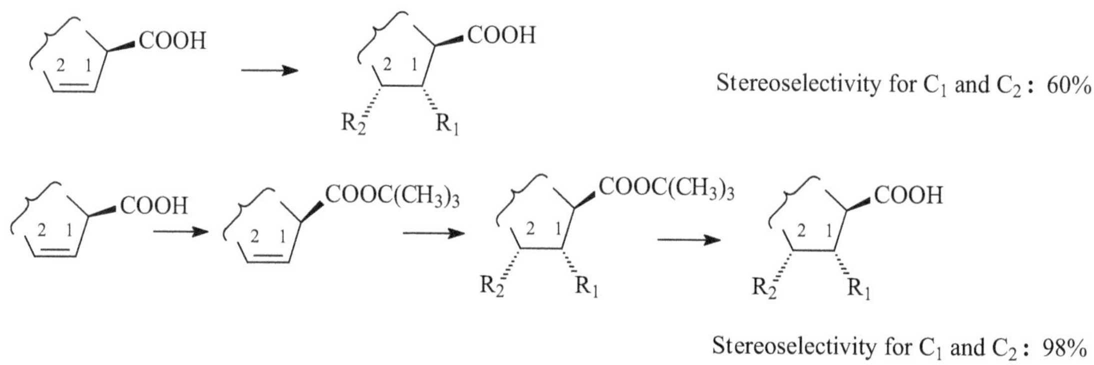

Fig. 1. The strategy to the synthesis: improving the stereoselectivity

In addition, the different reaction conditions such as temperature, pressure and the addition of special chiral catalysts may likely affect the stereoselectivity of the reaction, there are a lot of books and literature can be consulted, the test can be designed according to the actual situation and the literatures. It should be noted that the current use of some common chiral catalysts such as ruthenium, rhodium, etc have high toxicity, and so the strictly measurement should be adopted to control the residues of the mental catalysts. Identify of the limits can consult Guideline on the Specification Limits for Residues of Metal Catalysts or Metal Reagents issued by the EU EMEA[4].

2.2 Control of the starting materials

The chiral starting materials, besides some common chiral materials like L-amino acids, D-tartaric acid, other chiral starting materials purchased from other companies should be established the corresponding chiral purity control item, and should be provided the production techniques and detailed quality control about it, evaluated the rationality of the process. In the actual evaluation, a lot of applicants did not provide the production techniques and detailed quality control about the chiral starting materials purchased, and did not carry out the optical control on the chiral starting materials, directly impact on the quality control of starting materials and the evaluation on its quality. For example: a purchased key side-chain has two chiral centers that is used in the synthesis of antilipemic drug Atorvastatin calcium by some applicants (the structure described in Fig. 2), but the applicants don't accomplish the corresponding chiral purity control item, that will affect on the evaluation of the drug application, and the drug standard doesn't include the chiral quality index about the product, so that the application isn't approved.

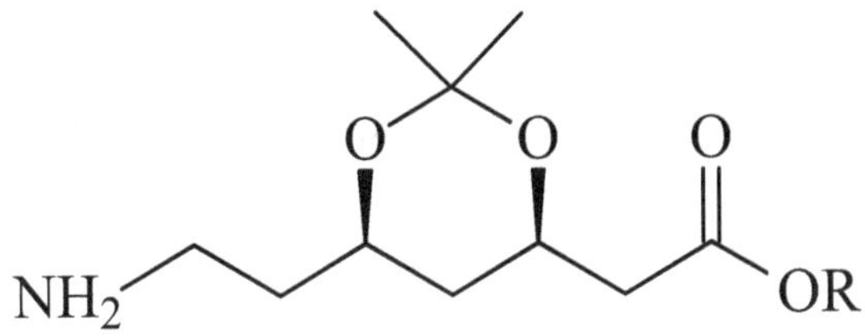

Fig. 2. The key side chains in the synthesis of Atorvastatin calcium

And some applicants have already accomplished a rough chiral purity control item, such as controlling the optical rotation of the starting materials. but the control of optical rotation is not enough to ensure the high content of the optical isomerism, especially when the starting material contains two or more chiral centers, and the different chiral center will contribute to the addition of optical rotation, it's not enough that only to utilize the optical rotation of the starting materials to afford a high content of steric isomerism. in addition, the range of the optical rotation is usually too rough, even if there is considerable quantity of of isomerism impurities, the optical rotation can still meet the requirement of the limit. For example, the optical rotation is usually controlled in the range ± 5° in the current specification, if a chiral drug contains one chiral center, even if there is only 5% enantiomers in the final product, the determination of the optical rotation traps in the range of the standard, and these should be limited more exacting than the limits. So if the optical rotation is used as a chiral purity control item, sufficient validation about its accuracy and precision should be made to ensure its confidence, and must be shown an accurate definition. There is a chiral drug with multiple chiral carbon atoms, because each chiral carbon atom contributes to the apparent optical rotation of the final product, then it will is more complex to calculate the optical rotation, here to control the optical purity through the optical rotation of the product will be more difficult. If a following chemistry reaction is achieved by the use of a low purity of the starting material, it will be more difficult to develop the sequent purification and quality control, and it will greatly increase the cost of the synthesis of final product.
Based on those reasons, we suggested that appropriate optical purity guideposts about the chiral starting material should be established, and the chiral HPLC method should be used if necessary. In addition, it should provide detailed production process of chiral starting material and detailed quality control process to evaluate the rationality of the craft.

2.3 Intermediates control

In addition to the introduction of chiral centers from chiral starting materials, it may also be introduced during the reaction. We should focus on steps that generate chiral centers. The intermediate, which will generate the new chiral center, should be controlled and internal quality control standard should be established. After introducing this chiral center, possible stereomeride should be focused on and monitored. In order to fully control the optical purity of products, we should understand the reaction mechanism of introducing chiral center, analysis isomer structure and different isomer proportion; establish effective isomers separation control method. It could not only depend on refining to improve the optical purity of final products. It needs to note that if this starting material used containing more than one chiral center, and this step reaction did not affected other chiral center, then this step reaction formed the diastereoisomer which could be separated by the ordinary HPLC methods. This requires adequate method validation. By those, we could control such key intermediates effectively intermediates.

2.4 Process control and process control index

Comparing with non-chiral drugs, in-process control is very important in synthesizing of chiral drugs, especially when the chiral drugs containing more than one chiral center. Each step stereoisomer impurities should be detected, analyzed and possibility of conformational changes be monitored, rather than using an ordinary HPLC monitoring method or TLC method.

Optimizing reaction parameters, monitoring the optical purity of reaction products could help us to determine this step reaction process condition and reaction products optical purity control item. After the introduction of chiral centers, follow-up reaction can make configuration changes. According to the difficulty of the final product quality control, different control methods were used to control the optical purity of the final product.

During the process research, the stereoisomers of impurities were detected after the introduction of chiral centers in each step, the possibility of conformational changes were analyzed and monitored. If there were no configuration changes, it should strictly control the process parametersits in the preparation process according to the results of process optimization and verification. If such changes may occur, indicators should also be targeted using the optical purity of the intermediate control, in addition to strictly control the process parameters.

With the reaction mechanism in each step and possible side effects, we should comprehensive analysis the stereoisomers structure of impurities, determine the scope of the possible structure of impurities, and to verify the method of structural confirmation. So to reduce the work load of the impurities structure confirmation. For example, an innovative chiral drug, the reaction generated 4 diastereoisomer in step; these isomers were isolated and determined by NMR spectra. Combined with the reaction principle and the theoretical values determined different isomers structure were confirmed, and the formation of these isomers ratio of process parameters were optimized, and also provides a strong proof to the confirmation of the final product structure.

3. Characterisation research of chiral drugs

3.1 The general principles to the structure identification of chiral drugs

During the study of structural confirmation of chiral drugs, it should not only be consistent with the general principles of structural confirmation, but also pay particular attention to the research and conclusive evidence of configuration according with the requirements of the guiding principles. For innovative chiral drugs, chiral centers on the absolute configuration should be confirmed clearly; for generic drugs absolute configuration should be confirmed with orignal drugs. Since enantiomers have the same general physical and chemical properties, chromatographic retention behavior (non-chiral packing column) and spectral characteristics (IR, Ultraviolet spectrum, nuclear magnetic resonance (NMR) spectroscopy, mass spectrometry), so the conventional method can not corroborate the configuration of chiral drugs, even if the conventional structure comparison with the configuration of standard product, still can't confirm their stereo configuration. In the actual evaluation about chiral drugs, we can often see that some drugs have multiple chiral carbons, but the applicants work over only by the four conventional spectrum analysis methods in the structure corroboration, not for chiral center,which causes the supplement rate of these drugs higher than the normal drugs in the structure corroboration.

It should be known that, the methods of structure corroboration about chiral drugs are classified, and the main method of configurational corroborating respectively is introduced, which are comprehensive. The methods concreted and their principles may refer to the guiding principle and relevant professional books, which are not mentioned in this no longer. In the following, only the questions found in the structure corroboration and the specific application of various methods will be stated.

3.2 The direct methods

Single-crystal X-ray diffraction method belongs to the direct methods, and is the preferred method of configuration corroboration about chiral drugs. The indirect methods need a lot of jobs to do, especially in corroborating innovative drug configuration or in the drugs of multiple chiral centers. but the single-crystal X-ray diffraction method can provide directly configuration information. So we should get the drug samples of single crystal determination of single crystal X-ray diffraction as far as possible through various measures. Of course, if the indirect method is simple, and can be relatively easy to identify the absolute configuration, there is no need to perform the single crystal determination. The point need stressed is that the object of single-crystal X-ray diffraction structure analysis only to be one crystal among the samples to be measured, which will not be representative. So it is necessary that the drug samples will be measured with powder X-ray diffraction, and gets the theoretical powder X-ray diffraction spectrum of chiral drugs through the calculation of single crystal structure data., and then is compared with that of sample drugs powder. The single-crystal sample will be proved to be representative when two crystal diffraction spectrums are consistent, and then corroborate configuration of the chiral drugs. Although the point is stressed in this guiding principle, but the declaring enterprises all do not have a research about this, which can cause evaluation personnel some questions, ever if some samples have a detection of the single-crystal X-ray diffraction. So attention must be brought to the applicants.

3.3 The indirect methods

When it is difficult to raise single crystal, more indirect combined application methods should be made. Usually, an indirect method to identify the absolute stereo configuration is limited, should as far as possible use more than one indirect methods to mutual self-evident. In the following, the application of indirect methods will be introduced though some examples in the evaluation.

3.3.1 The specific rotation

For the chiral drug only containing a chiral center, such as Levocarnitine, (S)-Amlodipine, its stereo configuration can be determined by rotation detection and enantiomer control. If the result of rotation detection is consistent with literature value, and the enantiomer can be generally effective controlled in the quality standards, the chiral drugs' stereo configuration may be identify in according to the conventional method. But if the chiral drugs are innovative drugs, their absolute configuration should still be corroborated.

3.3.2 Chiral HPLC positioning method and specific rotation

For the chiral drug containing two chiral centers, such as Sertraline Hydrochloride, it has a enantiomer and two diastereomers. These isomers can be separated and positioned through chiral HPLC conditions in the reference when their configuration are corroborated. According to the result of specific rotation detection, we affirm that its configuration would be consistent with the marketed drug if they have the same chromatograms. If marketed standard substance to be available, we affirm that its configuration would be consistent with the marketed drug through the way combining chiral HPLC method with NMR spectroscopy.

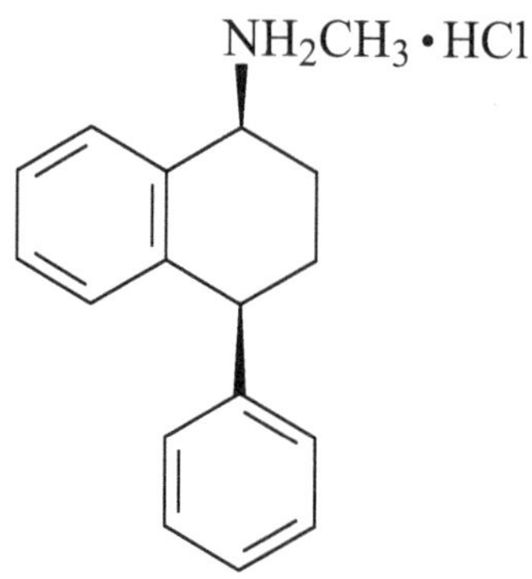

Fig. 3. Sertraline Hydrochloride

3.3.3 Literature comparative method

For the chiral drug containing multiple chiral centers, the determination of other items must be detected in order to corroborate three-dimensional structure of every chiral center besides specific rotation detection. For these compounds, the literature data obtained outside is also very important, except for the methods mentioned in this guiding principle of direct or indirect method. Because of multiple chiral centers, the presence of the final product including enantiomers are less, rather than non-enantiomers in the NMR spectrum are obvious differences, through the literature data by comparison with the measured data confirm the stereochemistry. Such as the muscle relaxant Vecuronium Bromide (Figure 4),

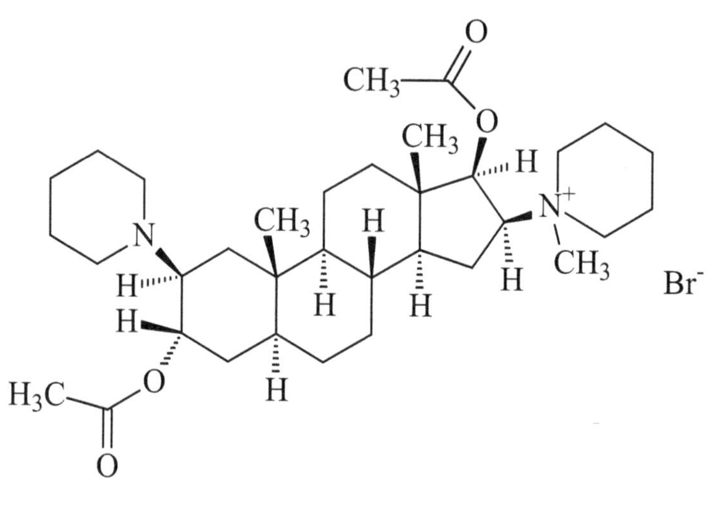

Fig. 4. Vecuronium Bromide

the structure contains ten chiral carbon, but one of the six chiral carbon in a rigid steroid ring, in the subsequent reaction of steroid body chiral carbon on the ring flip is unlikely occurrence, follow-up of non-response is only possible non-enantiomers. The literature clearly shows the various possible non-enantiomers of the NMR data and maps, which compare the sample through the NMR measured values with the literature, combined with other evidence of testing to confirm the relatively easy three-dimensional product configuration.

3.3.4 The inverse method of intermediate configuration

The determination of the intermediate single crystal X-diffraction is significant to the determination of the structure of the final product. Sometimes, the end product of the single crystal can not be obtained. At the same time, they can study and explore the availability of the last step reaction of the intermediate 1,2-crystal. When the intermediates of single crystal can be obtained, and chiral center does not changes or changes in control centers in the subsequent reaction, these intermediate configuration of the confirmation of the final product configuration is the very useful evidence for confirmation. such as the Chiral drug A, its single crystal is not available. But the intermediate steps before a chiral drug L-Menthylacetat single crystal is available, through its configuration can be anti-speculation chiral drug A by the conclusive evidence, shown in Figure 5.

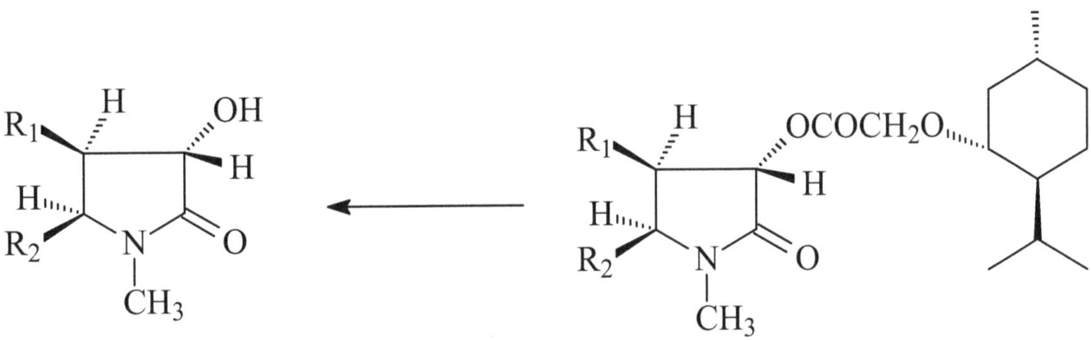

Chiral drug A　　　　Chiral drug A-3-L-Menthylacetat

Fig. 5. Anti-speculation process

3.3.5 NMR

NMR is useful to the confirmed of general structure of the drug. But he confirmed of the structure of chiral drugs has serious limitations, because the isotropic probe in the NMR determination is connatural. It makes the map of measured isomer NMR spectrum is identical. If distinguished by NMR mapping isomers, enantiomers shoud be changed into diastereoisomers, and then receive the appropriate tests. The methods of Common detection include: adding chiral shift reagent, add chiral solvent and chiral derivatization method and so on. After adding chiral derivatization reagent, it can make the formation of chiral drugs covalent bond. Then though the determination of NMR spectra, it can effectively distinguish different enantiomers with the configuration of the end product. This method is in common, and the different structure of chiral drugs can have a variety of derivatization reagent for selection. Referring to the specific relevant professional books, the guidelines are an increase Mosher Law adding chiral derivatization method.

3.3.6 Theoretical analysis & NMR

Reasonable theoretical analysis for the validation of the configuration of the final product is important. When a chiral drug in the chiral center from the starting material or reagent introduced, and the chiral centers in the subsequent reaction is not affected, or the configuration of chiral center of the quantitative impact is clearly occurring At this point, if the starting materials or reagents of three-dimensional structure is known, by classical chemical correlation method can be confirmed in the API configuration of chiral centers. Such as cisatracurium besylate (structure shown in Figure 6) confirmed the structure of the drug exists in four chiral centers, configuration is 1R, 1'R, 2R, 2'R type, and its structure confirmed by theoretical analysis and nuclear magnetic resonance methods: the synthesis of this product to R-Tetrahydropapaverine synthesized R-Tetrahydropapaverine does not involve the chiral carbon papaverine chiral reversal, the basic validation of 1,1 '-bit conformation; 2,2 '-bit configuration determined using NOESY spectra, NOESY spectra of C1-bit display connected to the methylene on the benzyl hydrogen and N2 connected propionate methylene hydrogen are related, but and N2-methyl hydrogen does not exist on the relationship, indicating that the connection C1 and N2 connected benzyl propionate in the cis part of the basic goods can confirm the stereochemistry.

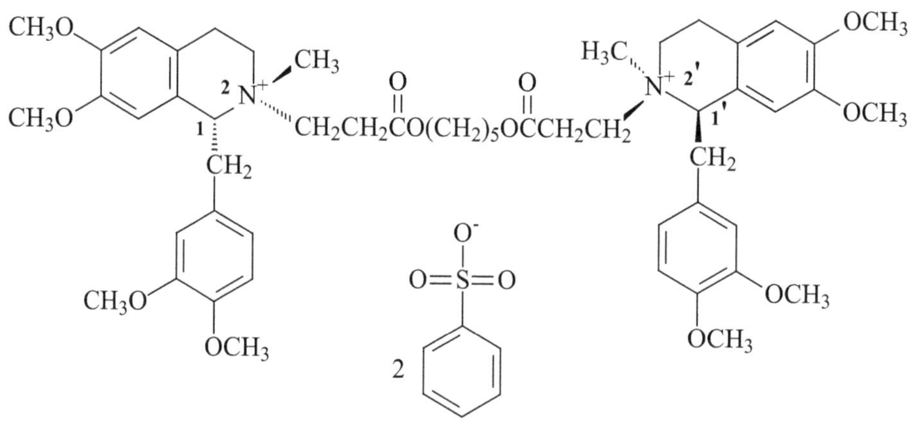

Fig. 6. Cisatracurium besylate

In addition, impurities can be combined with process research and study results to determine the configuration of end products, such as some examples in the Technology Application Unit of which the results of theoretical synthesis of the four possible isomers were separated and identified, but also for configuration of the main components of the quality of the establishment and follow-up study provides strong evidence.

4. References

[1] FDA CDER Guideline: Development of New Stereoisomeric Drugs. [S]. 1992- 05-01.

[2] SFDA Guideline: Guidance for industry. 16 Technical Guidelines for the research of the Chemical Drugs. [S]. 2005-03-18.

[3] SFDA Guideline: Guidance for industry. The Quality Control of Chiral Drugs. [S]. 2006-12-19.

[4] EMEA/CHMP: Guideline on the Specification Limits for Residues of Metal Catalysts or Metal Reagents. [S]. 2008-02-21.

6

Quality Control of *Cordyceps sinensis* Teleomorph, Anamorph, and its Products

Chih-Sheng Chen, Ruey-Shyang Hseu and Ching-Tsan Huang
National Taiwan University, Taipei
Taiwan,
Republic of China

1. Introduction

1.1 *Cordyceps sinensis* general description and habitat

Cordyceps sinensis (Berk.) Sacc. is a caterpillar fungus of the genus *Cordyceps* (Clavicipitaceae, Hypocreales, Pyrenomycetes, Ascomycota, Eukaryota) (Fig. 1).

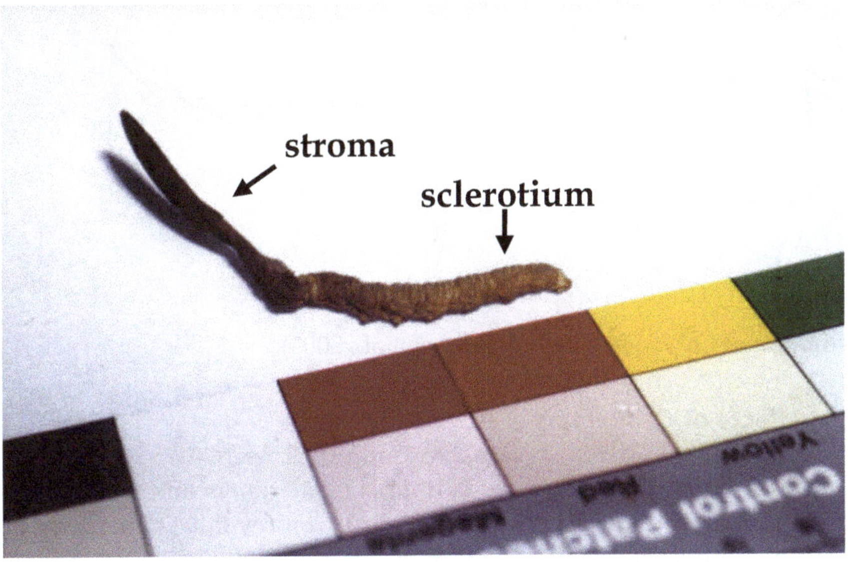

Fig. 1. The stroma and sclerotium of a *Cordyceps sinensis* specimen (image with back shadow)

The fungus is endemic mostly to the alpine shrub-meadow zone of high mountains (3000–5000 m altitude) or highlands of the south western of China (the Tibet Autonomous Region and the Qinghai, Sichuan, Yunnan and Gansu provinces) and to some countries of the Himalayan south slope (Nepal, Bhutan, and North East India) (Fig. 2). It grows parasitically on Lepidoptera larvae, particularly those belonging to the genus *Hepialus* (bat moths), which are found in cool weather conditions (Kinjo & Zang, 2001; Pegler et al., 1994).

After host larval infection with either meiotic or mitotic spores, the fungus multiplies in the host by yeast-like budding, eventually killing the host. The fungus then grows in the form of thread-like hyphae. Following overwintering, the fungus ruptures the host body, forming a sexual sporulating structure (a perithecial stroma) that is connected to the dead larva below ground and grows upward to emerge above the soil surface. It is this stroma, either with or without the host larva, that is traditionally used for medicinal purposes (Buenz et al., 2005).

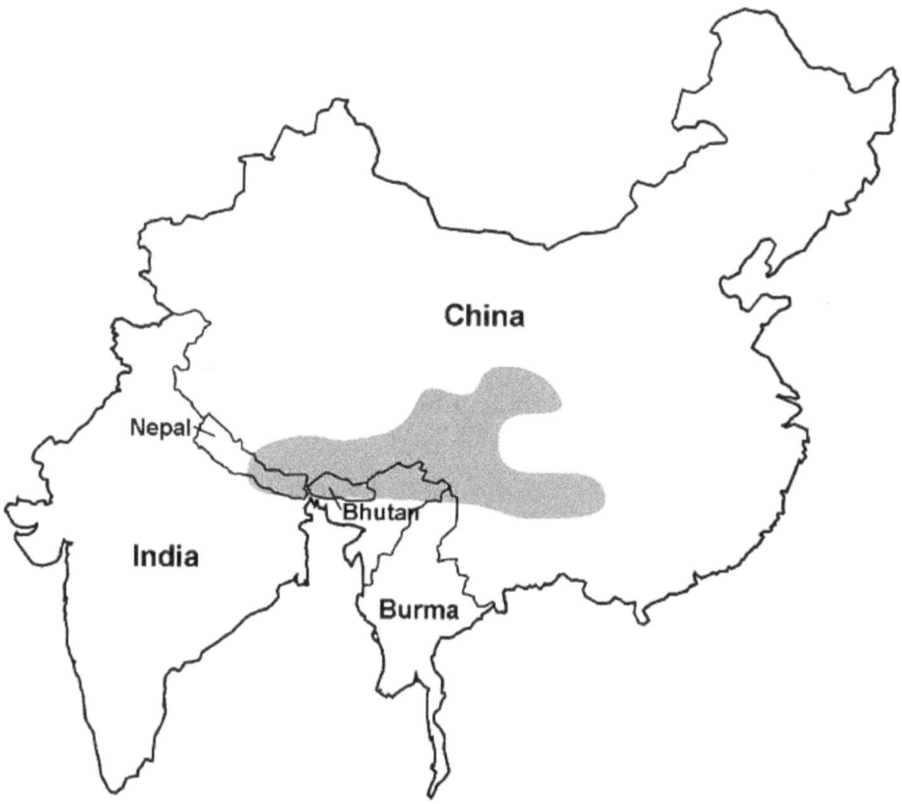

Fig. 2. Distribution of *Cordyceps sinensis* (Buenz et al., 2005)

1.2 Medicinal effects of *C. sinensis*

In Asia, *C. sinensis* is considered a valuable traditional herb that has several medicinal effects. It has been reported that *C. sinensis* nourishes the lungs and kidneys (Pegler et al., 1994), strengthens the immune system (Kuo et al., 1996), revitalizes the body after serious illness, acts as an aphrodisiac (Bhattarai, 1993), is a free-radical scavenger (Yamaguchi et al., 2000), exerts an anti-tumour effect (Chen et al., 1997b), and possesses the ability to alter apoptotic homeostasis (Buenz et al., 2005).

1.3 Morphology of the *C. sinensis* teleomorph

C. sinensis has a sexual stage (teleomorph) and an asexual stage (anamorph). It is generally seen in the sexual stage with a stalked fruit body. Recently, an inadequate teleomorph supply has raised its price to around 30,000–50,000 USD per kilogram (depending on size and quality). This high price results in many fake products on the market, e.g. other *Cordyceps* spp. (e.g. *C. cicadicola*, *C. liangshanensis*, *C. hawkesii*, *C. militaris*, *C. ophioglossoides*, *C. shanxiensis*, *C. sobolifera*, etc.) or some plant root and stem products; therefore, accurate *C. sinensis* teleomorph identification is very important (Chen et al., 2009).

Fungus identification is traditionally via morphological observation. The fungus holotype (K. H0221) kept in the Herbarium of the Royal Botanic Gardens, Kew, was labelled as *Sphaeria sinensis* Berk., Stroma, China. Morphological characteristics according to holotype were described as 'the stroma single, cylindrical 1.7 - 2.2 cm, 2.4 - 4 mm diameter, with sterile acuminate apex. Ascogenous portion glabrous or punctate with ostioles of the perithecia. Stipes 2–2.6 cm, 2–2.6 mm diameter with silky surface. Perithecia globoid or vase-shaped, 150–380 (-550) × 110–240 µm. The cortex usually consisting of one layer of closely interwoven hyphae, pseudoparenchymatous 80–170-µm thick. Asci cylindrical, narrowing below, 160–240 (-400) × 5.2–6.5 (-12) µm with a hemispherical thickening of the wall at the apex, asci not fully mature and hence thinner. Ascospores hyaline, filiform, smooth, mutiseptate, 120–190 × 0.6–1.3 µm, never breaking up into secondary spores; faintly tapered to both ends' (Zang & Kinjo, 1996).

All of these characteristics should be observed using mature and complete tissues (stroma, ascus, ascospore, etc.), but most *C. sinensis* teleomorphs are collected before maturation and sold as desiccated specimens. Nothing about the powdered products has been said. Therefore, it is important that molecular methods to accurately identify *C. sinensis* be developed.

1.4 *C. sinensis* anamorph

Due to the serious decline of teleomorph resources, cultured *C. sinensis* anamorph mycelia have been used as a substitute. However, anamorph culture did not produce a uniform mycelium, and several species have subsequently been reported as possible *C. sinensis* anamorphs, including *Stachybotrys* sp. (Kobayasi, 1982), *Paecilomyces sinensis* (Chen et al., 1984), *Scytalidium hepiali* (Li & Sun, 1988), *Tolypocladium sinensis* (Li, 1988), *Chrysosporium sinensis* (Liang, 1991a), *Hirsutella sinensis* (Liu et al., 1989), *Synnematium sinensis* (Yin & Shen, 1990), *Cephalosporium* sp. (Shen, 1983), *Paecilomyces hepiali*, *Mortierella hepiali*, and *Scytalidium hepiali* (Chen et al., 2009). Many mycelia products made by these species are marketed as '*C. sinensis* mycelia products', which confuses consumers.

H. sinensis has been confirmed as a *C. sinensis* anamorph based on microcyclic conidiation (short life cycle) observation (Liang, 1991b; Liu et al., 2001). However, the short life cycle is difficult to observe, and its use is very limited for other species. Similar problems have been encountered with regard to the morphological identification of the desiccated and powdered mycelia products. Thus, development of molecular biological techniques is important in order to extract and analyse fungal DNA even from dead fungi and to infer simple, rapid, and reliable anamorph-teleomorph connections (Egger & Sigler, 1992).

1.5 *C. sinensis* identification using molecular biology methods

Although *C. sinensis* has different phenotypes during its life cycle, its genotype during the different stages is unique. Genetic analyses of *C. sinensis* examined the patterns of genetic variability exhibited by randomly amplified polymorphic DNA (RAPD) markers and nuclear ribosomal DNA (nrDNA) sequence diversity. However, most DNA-based studies have examined genetic differentiation at the population rather than the species level (Buenz et al., 2005).

RAPD-polymerase chain reaction (RAPD-PCR) techniques have been used to study the relationship between *H. sinensis* and *C. sinensis* (Chen et al., 1999; Li et al., 2000) and those among the geographical populations of *C. sinensis* (Chen et al., 1999; Chen et al., 1997a). Twenty-nine *C. sinensis* samples were divided into 3 clusters, i.e. the north population (NP), middle population (MP), and south population (SP) and were considered as different subspecies rather than as different species (Chen et al., 1999; Chen et al., 1997a). The unstable RAPD patterns and large time commitment restricted the application of RAPD-PCR.

Using phylogenetic trees and probes based on ITS-region nrDNA sequences (ITS 1, 5.8S, and ITS 2 nrDNA sequences), Chen et al. (2001b) designed 2 *C. sinensis*-specific probes for species-level identification. A PCR single-stranded conformation polymorphism (PCR-SSCP)-based method was developed in Taiwan to identify *C. sinensis* and its fermented products (Kuo et al., 2006; Kuo et al., 2005).

Kinjo and Zang (2001) suggest that the 17 collections of *C. sinensis* isolates from 11 southwestern localities in China could be divided into 2 subgroups based on their ITS region sequences. Stensrud et al. (2007) analysed ITS-region nrDNA variations among 71 sequences of *C. sinensis* made available by the EMBL/GenBank databases. These authors suggested that *C. sinensis* isolates can be divided into 3 sub-species groups; however, the 2 *C. sinensis*-specific probes (Chen et al., 2001b), as well as the PCR-SSCP-based method (Kuo et al., 2006; Kuo et al., 2005), could only detect group 2 of Kinjo and Zang (2001) and group A of Stensrud et al. (2007).

The objective of this study was to develop an innovative and direct method that can detect all 3 subspecies groups of *C. sinensis* teleomorph, anamorph, and its derivative products.

2. Materials and methods

2.1 Fungal specimens and strains

The specimens and strains used in this study are listed in Table 1. The specimens were washed with sterile water and divided into 3 parts: the stroma (fruiting body), upper part of the sclerotium (head, h), and lower part of the sclerotium (tail, t). Some of the smaller sclerotia (body, b) were used for subsequent experiments.

The strains were cultured in 250 mL of potato dextrose broth (PDB; DIFCO, Detroit, MI, USA) in 500-mL flasks and agitated at 100 rpm at 14 °C. The mycelia were harvested after 8 weeks and washed with sterile water. All the specimens and mycelia were then lyophilized and stored at -20°C for subsequent analysis.

2.2 DNA preparation

DNA was isolated as described by Moncalvo et al. (1995). In brief, the ground sample (60 mg) was transferred to a 1.5-mL microcentrifuge tube containing 600 μL of lysis buffer (50 mM Tris-HCl, 50 mM EDTA, 3% SDS, and 1% 2-mercaptoethanol; pH 7.2). The tube was incubated in a water bath at 65 °C for 1 h, and the aqueous phase was then extracted twice using 600 μL of PCI (phenol:chloroform:isoamyl alcohol = 25:24:1; Sigma Co., St. Louis, MO, USA). After extraction, the aqueous phase was transferred to a new tube and the precipitated DNA was mixed with 0.1 volumes of 3 M sodium acetate and 0.6 volumes of isopropanol. The DNA was pelleted by centrifugation at 15,000 × *g* for 5 min, washed twice with cold 70% ethanol, and dried for 30 min in a vacuum oven at 37 °C.

The DNA was resuspended in 100 μL of TE buffer (10 mM Tris-HCl and 1 mM EDTA; pH 8.0) containing 2 μL of RNase (500 μg/mL; Roche Applied Science Co., Mannheim, Germany) and incubated in a water bath at 37 °C for 1 h. After addition of 100 μL of chloroform, the aqueous phase was transferred directly into a new tube. DNA was precipitated with 0.1 volumes of 3 M sodium acetate and 0.6 volumes of isopropanol and then pelleted by centrifugation at 15,000 × *g* for 5 min. The DNA was resuspended in 100 μL of sterile water and stored at -20°C.

2.3 PCR amplification

Partial 18S nrDNA were amplified using the primer pairs NS5 (5′-AACTTAAAGGAATTGACGGAAG-3′)/NS6 (5′-GCATCACAGACCTGTTATTGCCTC-3′). The 18S (partial), ITS 1, 5.8S, ITS 2, and 28S (partial) regions were amplified using the following primer pairs (Fig. 3) (White et al., 1990):
ITS1 (5′-TCCGTAGGTGAACCTGCGG-3′)/ITS4, (5′-TCCTCCGCTTATTGATATGC-3′) and
ITS5 (5′-GGAAGTAAAAGTCGTAACAAGG-3′)/ITS4
The amplifications were carried out in a Perkin-Elmer Thermocycler 480 (Applied Biosystems, Foster City, CA, USA) in 25 μL of the reaction mixture containing 50 ng template DNA, 2.5 μL of 10× PCR buffer (ProTech Professional Technical Services, Inc., Pittsburgh, PA, USA), 0.2 mM of each dNTP, 0.5 μM of each primer, and 0.625 U of Super *Taq* DNA polymerase (ProTech Professional Technical Services, Inc.).

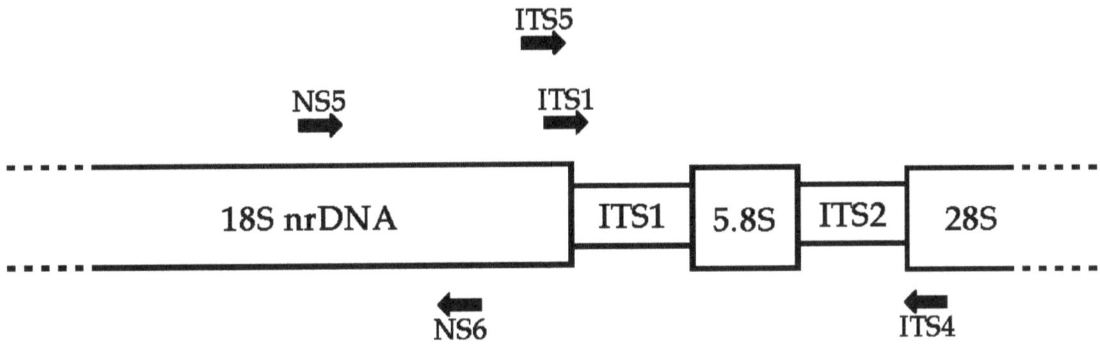

Fig. 3. PCR primer locations on the nrDNA. The arrowheads represent the 3′ end of each primer (White et al., 1990)

Amplifications were performed using the following PCR program: initial denaturation at 96 °C for 2 min followed by 35 cycles at 96 °C for 45 s, 52 °C for 45 s, 72 °C for 2 min, and a final extension step at 72 °C for 10 min. A negative control (dsH_2O) was included. Gel electrophoresis of the PCR products was performed on a 1.2% agarose gel. The gels were photographed under a UV transilluminator.

2.4 DNA sequencing and analyses

The PCR-amplified products were sequenced by the Mission Biotech Company (Taipei, Taiwan) (Chen & Hseu, 2002). The sequences were analyzed by an autosequencer (Applied Biosystems) using a Terminator Cycler Sequencing Ready Reaction Kit (Applied Biosystems). The sequences were imported into the BioEdit Sequence Alignment Editor version 7.0.9.0 (Hall, 1999) and aligned using the CLUSTAL W (Thompson et al., 1994) option.

2.5 Restriction fragment length polymorphisms (RFLPs)

For RFLP analysis, 20 μL of the PCR products was digested with 1 μL each of the restriction enzyme *Cfo*I (GCG↓C; 10 U/μl; Roche Applied Science Co.) and *Rsa*I (GT↓AC; 10 U/μL;

Roche Applied Science Co.), 5 μL of 10× SuRE/Cut buffer L (Roche Applied Science Co.), and distilled water to a final volume of 50 μL. Tubes were incubated at 37 °C for at least 4 h before separation on a 2.0% agarose gel and visualization by staining in ethidium bromide and UV transillumination (Chen & Hseu, 1999).

Species	Isolate No.	Tissue	Locality/Source	**Collection date**	ITS	18S
Cordyceps sinensis	Cs824a	Stroma	Sichuan, China	Oct. 1995	AJ488272	-
		Sclerotium (body)	Sichuan, China	Oct. 1995	-	AJ274527
	Cs824b	Sclerotium (body)	Sichuan, China	Oct. 1995	AJ488267	AJ274528
	W1023	Stroma	Sichuan, China	Sep. 1996	AJ488260	AJ274531
		Sclerotium (tail)	Sichuan, China	Sep. 1996	AJ488259	-
	Cs1014C	Sclerotium (body)	Tibet, China	May 1997	AJ488268	-
	Cs7528A	Stroma	Tibet, China	May 1997	AJ488253	AJ007567
		Sclerotium	Tibet, China	May 1997	AJ488252	AJ007566
	Cs7528J	Stroma	China	May 1997	AJ488278	AJ007568
		Sclerotium (tail)	China	May 1997	AJ488239	AJ007569
	Cs7528H	Stroma	China	May 1997	AJ488245	-
		Sclerotium (head)	China	May 1997	AJ488251	-
		Sclerotium (tail)	China	May 1997	AJ488250	AJ274529
	RSCsI	Stroma	-	May 1997	AJ488236	-
		Sclerotium (head)	-	May 1997	AJ488237	-
		Sclerotium (tail)	-	May 1997	AJ488238	-
	RSCsK	Stroma	-	May 1997	AJ488249	-
		Sclerotium (head)	-	May 1997	AJ488248	-
		Sclerotium (tail)	-	May 1997	AJ488247	-
	RSCsL	Stroma	-	May 1997	AJ488240	-
		Sclerotium (head)	-	May 1997	AJ488246	-
		Sclerotium (tail)	-	May 1997	AJ488241	-
	RSCsM	Stroma	-	May 1997	AJ488242	-

Species	Isolate No.	Tissue	Locality/Source	Collection date	ITS	18S
		Sclerotium (head)	-	May 1997	AJ488243	-
		Sclerotium (tail)	-	May 1997	AJ488244	-
	Csd	Stroma	-	May 1997	AJ488269	-
		Sclerotium (body)	-	May 1997	AJ488270	-
	Cs824d	Stroma	-	May 1997	AJ488271	-
	S1023	Stroma	Tibet, China	Oct. 1998	AJ488257	AJ274534
		Sclerotium (head)	Tibet, China	Oct. 1998	AJ488256	-
		Sclerotium (tail)	Tibet, China	Oct. 1998	AJ488258	-
	T1023	Stroma	Qinghai, China	Oct. 1998	AJ488263	AJ274532
		Sclerotium (head)	Qinghai, China	Oct. 1998	AJ488261	-
		Sclerotium (tail)	Qinghai, China	Oct. 1998	AJ488262	-
	H1023	Stroma	Qinghai, China	Oct. 1998	AJ488254	AJ274535
		Sclerotium (tail)	Qinghai, China	Oct. 1998	AJ488255	-
	K1023	Stroma	-	Oct. 1998	AJ488264	AJ274536
		Sclerotium (head)	-	Oct. 1998	AJ488265	-
		Sclerotium (tail)	-	Oct. 1998	AJ488266	-
Hirsutella sinensis	RS2	Mycelium	Tibet, China	May 1997	AJ488275	AJ274540
	RS3	Mycelium	Tibet, China	May 1997	AJ488274	AJ274537
C. liangshanensis	CC1014a	Stroma	China	–	–	AJ239070
Cordyceps sp.	ATCC 36337	Mycelium	ATCC	–	–	AJ239076
C. memorabilis	ATCC 36743	Mycelium	ATCC	–		AJ242432
C. militaris	ATCC 26848	Mycelium	ATCC	–	–	AJ239074
	CMC2	Stroma	China	-	AJ488277	-
C. ophioglossoides	ATCC 36865	Mycelium	ATCC	–	–	AJ239075

Table 1. Examined species and isolates and their GenBank nrDNA sequences

3. Results

3.1 PCR amplification and DNA sequencing

We amplified and sequenced the NS5/NS6 region and ITS region nrDNA sequences of the *Cordyceps* species collected in our laboratory. Their GenBank Accession Numbers (http://www.ncbi.nlm.nih.gov/) are provided in Table 1. The ITS region yielded products of approximately 550 bp, while those of the NS5/NS6 region were approximately 310 bp.

In the present study, the 18S or ITS nrDNA sequences of the stroma and sclerotium (head, tail, and whole body) from each isolate were identical [Cs7528A(b) vs. Cs7528A(f); W1023(f) vs. W1023(t); Cs824a(f) vs. Cs824a(b); Cs7528H(f) vs. Cs7528H(h) vs. Cs7528H(t); Cs7528J(f) vs. Cs7528J(t); K1023(f) vs. K1023(h) vs. K1023(t); H1023(f) vs. H1023(t); T1023(f) vs. T1023(h) vs. T1023(t); S1023(f) vs. S1023(h) vs. S1023(t); Csd(f) vs. Csd(b); RSCsM(f) vs. RSCsM(h) vs. RSCsM(t); RSCsL(f) vs. RSCsL(h) vs. RSCsL(t); RSCsK(f) vs. RSCsK(h) vs. RSCsK(t); and RSCsI(f) vs. RSCsI(h) vs. RSCsI(t)] (Table 1). This result suggested that the stroma and sclerotium from each isolate originated from the same species.

3.2 Phylogenetic analysis

The phylogenetic tree based on the ITS region sequences is illustrated in Fig. 4. It was constructed using the sequencing data collected in this study as well as from GenBank. The *C. memorabilis* strain ATCC 36743 was set as the out-group. The 3 *C. militaris* sequences—GenBank Accession Nos. AJ242923, AJ243774, and CMC2—were grouped.

The *C. sinensis* specimens could be divided into 5 subgroups. Group A included the following isolates: (1) Tibet isolates Cs824d(f), K1023(f), RS2, Csd(b), and Cs7528A(f) as well as those with GenBank Accession Nos. AJ243775, AJ243776, AJ243778, AJ243979, AJ243980, AJ245559, AJ413178, AJ413179, AJ413180, AJ507399, AJ507400, AJ507401, AJ507402, and AB067713; (2) Sichuan isolates Cs824a(f) and Cs824b(b) as well as those with GenBank Accession Nos. AJ413183, AJ413184, AB067715, and AB067717; (3) Qinghai isolates T1023(t) and those with GenBank Accession Nos. AJ413181, AJ413182, and AJ507404; (4) Yunnan isolates with GenBank Accession Nos. AJ309354, AJ309361, and AJ507403; (5) Gansu isolates with GenBank Accession Nos. AJ507405 and AB067716; and (6) uncertain locality isolates with GenBank Accession Nos. AB067718, AB067721, and AJ309357. This group is similar to subgroup 2 of Kinjo and Zang (2001), and the bootstrap level was 994.

Group B included the following isolates: (1) Tibet isolates with GenBank Accession Nos. AB067739 (isolate Nyaramu-1), AB067740 (isolate Nyaramu-2), AB067743 (isolate Yagyusan), and AB067744 (isolate Satoku); (2) Sichuan isolates with GenBank Accession Nos. AB067742 (isolate Ritan), AB067745 (isolate Kandin Clone A1), AB067746 (isolate Kandin Clone A2), AB067747 (isolate Kandin Clone A4), AB067748 (isolate Kandin Clone B3), and AB067749 (isolate Kandin Clone B6); and (3) Qinghai isolate with GenBank Accession No. AB067741 (isolate Rusyasya). This group is close to subgroup 1 of Kinjo and Zang (2001), and the bootstrap level was 1000.

Group C, which we discovered earlier (Chen et al., 2004), included the following: (1) Tibet isolate Cs1014C(b) and (2) Sichuan isolate W1023(f). The bootstrap level of Group C was 1000. Although this group was remote from *C. sinensis* Groups A and B, the 2 isolates were identified to be *C. sinensis* based on morphological observations.

Group D included the following isolates/strains: GenBank Accession Nos. AF122030 (strain BCRC 36421), AF291749 (strain MPNU 8002), and AB067720 (isolate SHANGHAI). The bootstrap level of Group D was 1000. Although these isolates were scientifically named C.

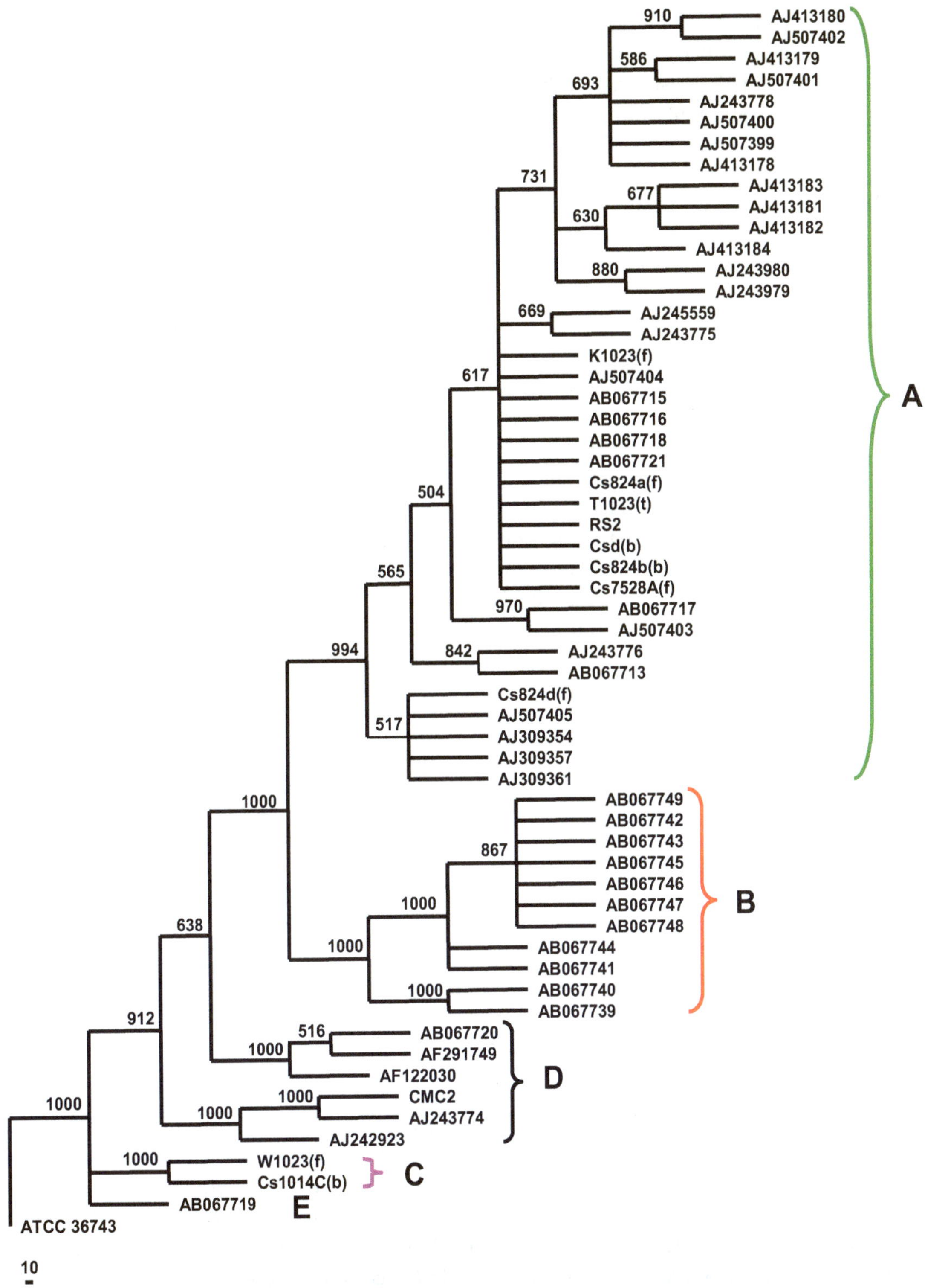

Fig. 4. Phylogenetic tree resulting from the Neighbour-Joining Method (NJ) of the nrDNA ITS1, 5.8S, and ITS2 region sequences of *Cordyceps sinensis* and other related fungi. NJ bootstrap percentage values are shown at each branch

sinensis, the 3 strains shall not be considered *C. sinensis*. They might belong to the anamorphic species *Tolypocladium*, a relative of *C. subsessilis* (Hodge et al., 1996). Another possibility was that the 3 strains might be contaminants or associated fungi of *C. sinensis* because many contaminant anamorphic fungi were associated with *Cordyceps* species (Kinjo & Zang, 2001).

Group E included only 1 isolate that had the GenBank Accession No. AB067719 (isolate SANMEI). It was not accurately represented in the GenBank format by Kinjo. The isolate was not considered a *C. sinensis* anamorph strain because of the large identity difference in its 18S nrDNA sequences and those of *C. sinensis* specimens (discussed below).

According to the above-mentioned findings, Groups A, B, and C were considered the real *C. sinensis*. Group A included *C. sinensis* isolates from 5 sources (Tibet, Sichuan, Qinghai, Yunnan, and Gansu); Group B, 3 sources (Tibet, Sichuan, and Qinghai); and Group C, 2 sources (Tibet and Sichuan). This indicated that the intra-group isolates from different geographic regions were identical subspecies. However, the inter-group isolates were different subspecies. The identity between Groups A and B was 86.0%–89.4% as compared to 63.2%–66.0% between Groups A and C and 56.6%–57.8% between Groups B and C. Only Group A members could be detected using the 2 probes developed by Chen et al. (2001a).

The ITS region and NS5/NS6 region sequences of *C. sinensis* in the present study and GenBank (Table 1) were aligned and analysed. The identity between each ITS region sequence was 56.6%–100%; however, the NS5/NS6 region sequences of the isolates were almost completely identical. Therefore, the NS5/NS6 region sequence of *C. sinensis* was compared to those of other *Cordyceps* spp. to determine the diversity therein.

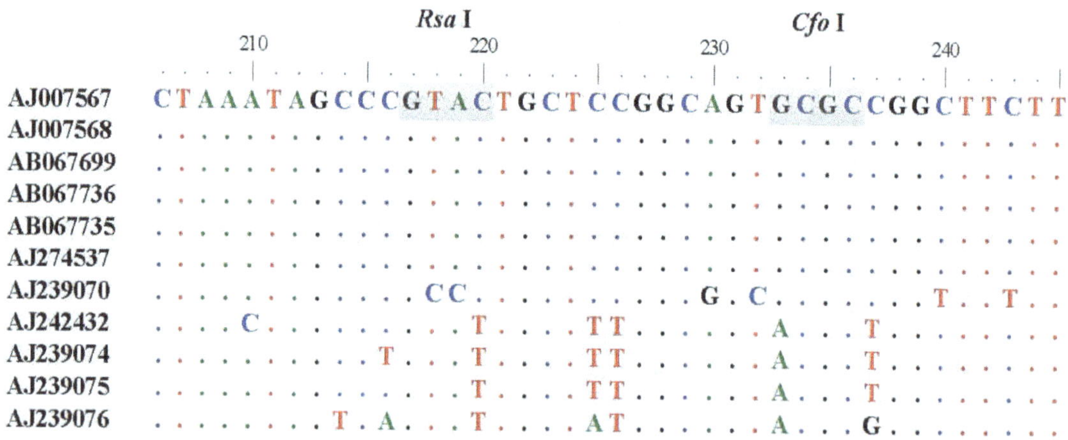

Fig. 5. Sequence alignment of 18S nrDNA NS5/NS6 region sequences of *C. sinensis* Cs7528A(f) (Accession No. AJ007567), *C. sinensis* Cs7528J(f) (Accession No. AJ007568), *C. sinensis* MARCH (Accession No. AB067699), *C. sinensis* Kandin (Accession No. AB067736), *C. sinensis* Nyaramu-1 (Accession No. AB067735), *H. sinensis* (Accession No. AJ274537), other *C. liangshanensis* CC1014a (Accession No. AJ239070), *C. memorabilis* ATCC 36743 (Accession No. AJ242432), *C. militaris* ATCC 26848 (Accession No. AJ239074), *C. ophioglossoides* ATCC 36865 (Accession No. AJ239075), and *Cordyceps* sp. ATCC 36337 (Accession No. AJ239076) in the present study. The shades are the restriction sites of *Cfo*I (GCG↓C) and *Rsa*I (GT↓AC)

Obviously, *C. sinensis* had 2 restriction sites—*Cfo*I and *Rsa*I (the signature sequence)—that could be used to differentiate *C. sinensis* from other *Cordyceps* spp. (Fig. 5). To ensure specificity of the signature sequence, the GenBank database was searched using the search phrase '*Cordyceps* 18S rRNA gene'. Simultaneously, the NS5/NS6 region sequence was uploaded to GenBank and the database was searched for the sequences that were mostly closely related using the Basic Local Alignment Search Tool (BLAST) program (Altschul et al., 1990). None of the sequences contained both restriction sites (data not shown); thus, *C. sinensis* could be definitively identified based on the 2 restriction sites.

The PCR-RFLP method based on the signature sequence was developed and used to characterize *C. sinensis* fermented products in Taiwan (Table 3).

Marketing Sample[a]	Sample Origin[b]	Collection Date
C. sinensis mycelium	A	June 2004
C. sinensis mycelium	AV	June 2004
C. sinensis mycelium	B	June 2004
C. sinensis mycelium	C	June 2004
C. sinensis and *Ganoderma lucidum* mycelia	DP	June 2004
C. sinensis mycelium	G1	June 2004
C. sinensis mycelium	Gen	June 2004
C. sinensis mycelium	L	June 2004
C. sinensis mycelium	NT	June 2004
C. sinensis mycelium	P	June 2004
C. sinensis mycelium	PH	June 2004
C. sinensis mycelium	4B	June 2004

[a]The marketing sample content descriptions were provided by the respective suppliers.
[b]Full company names related to the marketing samples are not shown here.

Table 3. *Cordyceps sinensis* mycelium fermented products collected in the present study

Among the 12 fermented products, only AV and L matched the signature sequence and were, therefore, considered genuine *C. sinensis* mycelium products (Fig. 6).

Another 8 products—A, B, C, G1, Gen, NT, PH, and 4B, none of which were digested by *Cfo*I and *Rsa*I—were considered fake products. The product DP, whose content was labeled *C. sinensis* and *Ganoderma lucidum* mycelia, had 2 corresponding polymorphism patterns; however, the product P, whose content was labeled only as *C. sinensis* mycelium, must not exclusively comprise pure *C. sinensis* mycelium.

4. Discussion

ITS-region nrDNA, which consists of the 2 variable non-coding regions ITS 1 and ITS 2, was more broadly used in phylogenetic analysis than 18S nrDNA. However, the 2 *C. sinensis*-

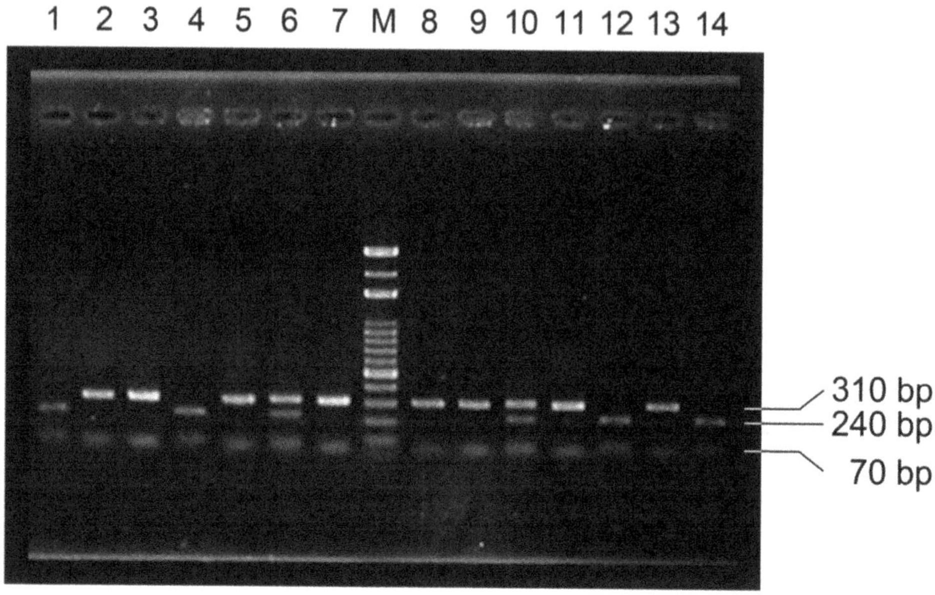

(a)

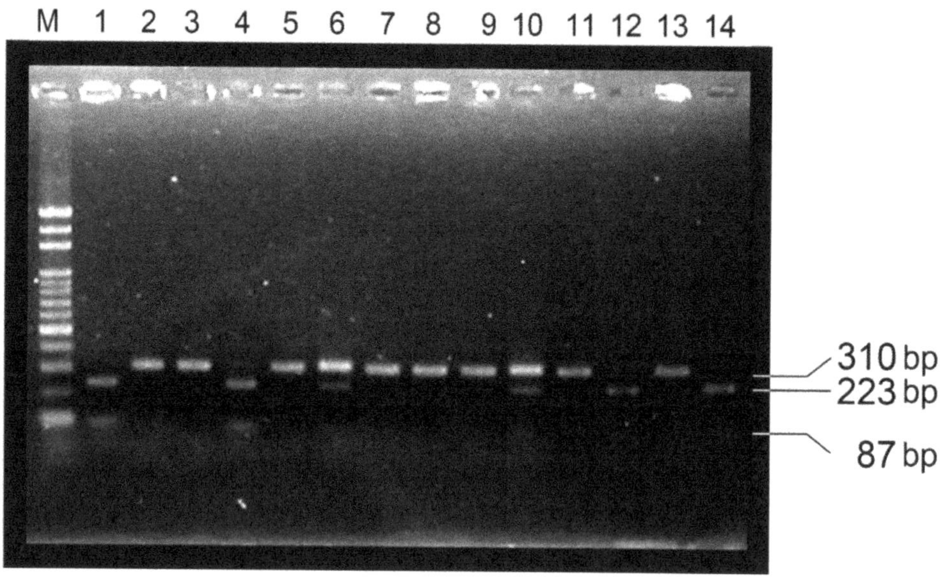

(b)

Fig. 6. Restriction maps of the 18S nrDNA PCR products of *C. sinensis* and various mycelium fermented products. Amplification of 18S nrDNA by PCR using primer pair NS5/NS6. The products were digested using restriction enzyme (A) *Cfo*I (GCG↓C) and (B) *Rsa*I (GT↓AC) and then visualized in 2.0% agarose gel stained with ethidium bromide. Lane M, 100-bp DNA marker; lane 1, *C. sinensis* Cs7528A; lane 2, product A; lane 3, product B; lane 4, product AV; lane 5, product C; lane 6, product DP; lane 7, product G1; lane 8, product Gen; lane 9, product NT; lane 10, product P; lane 11, product PH; lane 12, product L; lane 13, product 4B; and lane 14, *C. sinensis* Cs7528J

specific probes (Chen et al., 2001b) and the PCR-SSCP method (Kuo et al., 2006; Kuo et al., 2005) based on the ITS region nrDNA sequence could detect only group A in Fig. 4. Thus, the 18S nrDNA was used in the present study instead of the ITS region to develop a method by which to differentiate *C. sinensis*.

The signature sequence based on the *Cfo*I and *Rsa*I restriction sites of the NS5/NS6 region was an innovative and species-level genetic marker of *C. sinensis*. It could be broadly used to determine *C. sinensis* teleomorph, anamorph, and the identification and differentiation of derivative products. In addition, the *C. sinensis* was further divided into 3 intra-species groups, based on the ITS-region sequences. These molecular systematic indicators could serve as the foundation for further research and applications.

Many teleomorph and anamorph fermented products in the market do not comprise *C. sinensis* (i.e. fake products), and some of them are not made exclusively of pure *C. sinensis* (Fig. 6). They might be made of or mixed with other *Cordyceps* spp.—*C. sinensis*-related anamorph strains, plant powders, or other materials. Although many of these ingredients were reported as having various biological functions, the fake or impure products, labelled as '*C. sinensis* mycelium products', might cause serious problems with regards to food safety. Thus, the signature sequence will be a powerful tool in assaying *C. sinensis* fermented products and performing quality control measures.

On the basis of morphological observation and signature sequence confirmation, strain RS3 was identified as *C. sinensis* anamorph, i.e. *H. sinensis*. According to the ITS-region nrDNA sequence, it belongs to group A of Fig. 4. However, the genomic statuses of the anamorph strains of groups B and C remain unclear. Further work should be undertaken to collect live *C. sinensis* specimens for group B and group C anamorph strain isolation and for research into the morphological characteristics and medicinal effects of each group isolate.

5. Conclusion

In the present study, we successfully developed a molecular method that can detect all 3 sub-species groups of *C. sinensis*. This innovative method can be applied to *C. sinensis* teleomorph and anamorph identification and can be used to improve quality control.

6. Acknowledgment

This study was supported by a grant (Grant No. DOH-91-TD-1163) from the Department of Health, Executive Yuan, Taiwan, Republic of China.

7. References

Altschul, S.F., Gish, W., Miller, W., Myers, E.W., & Lipman, D.J. 1990. Basic local alignment search tool. *Journal of Molecular Biology*, 215, 403-410

Bhattarai, N.K. 1993. Folk herbal medicines of Dolakha District, Nepal. *Fitoterapia*, 66, 387-395

Buenz, E.J., Bauer, B.A., Osmundson, T.W., & Motley, T.J. 2005. The traditional Chinese medicine *Cordyceps sinensis* and its effects on apoptotic homeostasis. *Journal of Ethnopharmacology*, 96, 19-29

Chen, C.S. & Hseu, R.S. 1999. Differentiation of *Cordyceps sinensis* (Berk.) Sacc. specimen using restriction fragment length polymorphism of 18S rRNA gene. *Journal of The Chinese Agricultural Chemistry Society* 37: 533-545.

Chen, C.S. & Hseu, R.S. 2002. Differentiation of *Cordyceps sinensis* (Berk.) Sacc. with 18S rRNA Gene Sequences. *Taiwanese Journal of Agricultural Chemistry and Food Science* 40: 219-225.

Chen, C.S., Ling, C.H., & Hseu, R.S. 2004. Differentiation of *Cordyceps sinensis* (Berk.) Sacc. with Internal Transcribed Spacer1, 5.8S and Internal Transcribed Spacer 2 rRNA Gene Sequences. *Taiwanese Journal of Agricultural Chemistry and Food Science,* 42, 147-153

Chen, C.S., Huang, C.T., & Hseu, R.S. 2009. Identification of *Cordyceps sinensis* by 18S nrDNA Sequencing and Characterization of Fermented Products in Taiwan. *Food Biotechnology,* 23, 1-9

Chen, Q.-T., Xiao, S.R., & Shi, Z.-Y. 1984. *Paecilomyces sinensis* sp. nov. and its connection with *Cordceps sinensis*. *Acta Mycologica Sinica,* 3, 24-28

Chen, Y.-Q., Wang, N., Qu, L.-Q., Li, T.-H., & Zhang, W.-M. 2001a. Determination of the anamorph of *Cordyceps sinensis* inferred from the analysis of the ribosomal DNA internal transcribed spacers and 5.8S rDNA. *Biochemical Systematics and Ecology,* 29, 597-607

Chen, Y., Zhang, Y.P., Yang, Y., & Yang, D. 1999. Genetic diversity and taxonomic implication of *Cordyceps sinensis* as revealed by RAPD markers. *Biochemical Genetics,* 37, 201-213

Chen, Y., Wang, W., Yang, Y., Su, B., Zhang, Y., Xiong, L., He, Z., Shu, C., & Yang, D. 1997a. [Genetic divergence of *Cordyceps sinensis* as estimated by random amplified polymorphic DNA analysis]. *Yi Chuan Xue Bao,* 24, 410-416

Chen, Y.J., Shiao, M.S., Lee, S.S., & Wang, S.Y. 1997b. Effect of *Cordyceps sinensis* on the proliferation and differentiation of human leukemic U937 cells. *Life Sciences,* 60, 2349-2359

Chen, Y.Q., Wang, N., Qu, L., Li, T., & Zhang, W. 2001b. Determination of the anamorph of *Cordyceps sinensis* inferred from the analysis of the ribosomal DNA internal transcribed spacers and 5.8S rDNA. *Biochemical Systematics and Ecology,* 29, 597-607,

Egger, K.N. & Sigler, L. 1992. Using molecular data to infer anamorph-teleomorph connection: the case of *Scytalidium vaccinii* and *Hymenoscyphus aricae* in the fungal holomorph: mitotic, meiotic and pleomorphic speciation in fungal systematics CAB International, Wallingford. pp.

Hall, T.A. 1999. BioEdit: a user-friendly biological sequence alignment editor and analysis program for Windows 95/98/NT. *Nucleic Acids Symposium Series,* 41, 95-98,

Hodge, K.T.; Krasnoff, S.B., & Humber, R.A. 1996. *Tolypocladium inflatum* is the anamorph of *Cordyceps subsessils*. *Mycologia,* 88, 715-719

Kinjo, N. & Zang, M. 2001. Morphological and phylogenetic studies on *Cordyceps sinensis* distributed in southwestern China. *Mycoscience,* 42, 567-574,

Kobayasi, Y. 1982. Key to the taxa of the genus *Cordyceps* and *Torrubiella*. *Transactions of the Mycological Society of Japan,* 23, 329-364

Kuo, H.-C., Su, Y.-L., Yang, H.-L., Huang, I.-C., & Chen, T.-Y. 2006. Differentiation of *Cordyceps sinensis* by a PCR-Single-Stranded Conformation Polymorphism Based Method and Characterization of the Fermented Products in Taiwan. *Food Biotechnology,* 20, 161-170

Kuo, H.C., Su, Y.L., Yang, H.L., & Chen, T.Y. 2005. Identification of Chinese medicinal fungus *Cordyceps sinensis* by PCR-single-stranded conformation polymorphism and phylogenetic relationship. *Taiwanese Journal of Agricultural Chemistry and Food Science,* 53, 3963-3968

Kuo, Y.C., Tsai, W.J., Shiao, M.S., Chen, C.F., & Lin, C.Y. 1996. *Cordyceps sinensis* as an immunomodulatory agent. *The American Journal of Chinese Medicine,* 24, 111-125,

Li, C.-L. 1988. A study of *Tolypocladium sinensis* Z. L. Li sp. nov and cyclosporin production. *Acta Mycologica Sinica,* 7, 93-98

Li, Z.-L. & Sun, Y.-H. 1988. A new species of *Scytalidium-Scytalidium helpiali. Acta Mycologica Sinica,* 7, 23-28

Li, Z.-Z., Huang, B., & Mei-Zhen, F. 2000. Molecular Evidence for Anamorph Determination of *Cordyceps sinensis* (Berk.) Sacc. *Mycosystema,* 19, 60-64

Liang, Z.-Q. 1991a. A new species of *Chrysosporium* from *Cordyceps sinensis* (Berk.) Sacc. *Acta Mycologica Sinica,* 10,

Liang, Z.Q. 1991b. Anamorphs of *Cordyceps* and determination of the relationship between anamorph and teleomorph. *Journal of Southwest Agriculture,* 4, 1-8

Liu, X.J., Guo, Y.L., Yu, Y.X., & Zeng, W. 1989. Isolation and identification of the anamorphic stage of *Cordyceps sinensis* (Berk.) Sacc. *Acta Mycologica Sinica,* 8, 35-40

Liu, Z.-Y., Yao, Y.-J., Liang, Z.Q., Pegler, D.N., & Chase, M.W. 2001. Molecular evidence for the anamorph-teleomorph connection in *Cordyceps sinensis. Mycological Research,* 105, 827-832

Moncalvo, J.M., Wang, H.H., & Hseu, R.S. 1995. Gene phylogeny of the *Ganoderma lucidum* complex based on ribosomal DNA sequences. Comparison with traditional taxonomic characters. *Mycological Research,* 99, 1489-1499

Pegler, D.N., Yao, Y.J., & Li, Y. 1994. The Chinese 'caterpillar fungus'. *The Mycologist,* 8, 3-5,

Shen, N.-Y. 1983. Brief account of research on *Cordyceps sinensis. Medicinal Fungi,* 1-2, 85, 88,

Stensrud, Ø., Schumacher, T., Shalchian-Tabrizi, K., Svegarden, I.B., & Kauserud, H. 2007. Accelerated nrDNA evolution and profound AT bias in the medicinal fungus *Cordyceps sinensis. Mycological Research,* 111, 409-415

Thompson, J.D., Higgins, D.G., & Gibson, T.J. 1994. CLUSTAL W: improving the sensitivity of progressive multiple sequence alignment through sequence weighting, position-specific gap penalties and weight matrix choice. *Nucleic Acids Research,* 22, 4673-4680

White, T.J., Bruns, T., Lee, S., & Taylor, J. 1990. Amplification and direct sequencing of fungal ribosomal DNA for phylogenetics. In: *PCR Protocols: a Guide to Methods and Applications.* M. A. Innis, D. H. Gelfand, J. J. Sninsky, & T. J. White (eds.), 315-322, Academic Press, Inc., San Diego, California.

Yamaguchi, Y., Kagota, S., Nakamura, K., Shinozuka, K., & Kunitomo, M. 2000. Antioxidant activity of the extracts from fruiting bodies of cultured *Cordyceps sinensis. Phytotherapy Research,* 14, 647-649

Yin, X.-C. & Shen, L.-Y. 1990. The conidial state of *Cordyceps sinensis* (Berk.) Sacc. *Synnematium sinense* Yin et Shen, sp. nov. *Acta Biologica Plateau Sinica,* 9, 1-5

Zang, M. & Kinjo, N. 1996. Type study on the *Cordyceps sinensis. Acta Botanica Yunnanica,* 17, 63-65

7

Method Development and Validation of Analytical Procedures

Kapil Kalra
Dev Bhoomi Institute of Pharmacy and Research, Dehradun, Uttarakhand, India

1. Introduction

Method validation is the process used to confirm that the analytical procedure employed for a specific test is suitable for its intended use. Results from method validation can be used to judge the quality, reliability and consistency of analytical results; it is an integral part of any good analytical practice. It is the process of defining an analytical requirement, and confirms that the method under consideration has performance capabilities consistent with what the application requires. Use of equipment that is within specification, working correctly and adequately calibrated is fundamental to the method validation process. Likewise the operator carrying out the studies must be competent in the analysis under study and have sufficient knowledge of the method/analysis to draw conclusions from the observations as the validation work proceeds. Quite often method validation evolves from method development and so the two activities are often closely tied, with the validation study employing the techniques and steps in the analysis as defined by the method development.

Analytical methods need to be validated or revalidated

- before their introduction into routine use;
- whenever the conditions change for which the method has been validated (e.g., an instrument with different characteristics or samples with a different matrix); and
- whenever the method is changed and the change is outside the original scope of the method.

Method validation has received considerable attention in the literature and from industrial committees and regulatory agencies.

- The U.S. FDA CGMP request in section 211.165 (e) methods to be validated: The accuracy, sensitivity, specificity, and reproducibility of test methods employed by the firm shall be established and documented. Such validation and documentation may be accomplished in accordance with Sec. 211.194(a). These requirements include a statement of each method used in testing the sample to meet proper standards of accuracy and reliability, as applied to the tested product. The U.S. FDA has also proposed industry guidance for Analytical Procedures and Methods Validation.
- ISO/IEC 17025 includes a chapter on the validation of methods with a list of nine validation parameters. The ICH has developed a consensus text on the validation of analytical procedures. The document includes definitions for eight validation characteristics. ICH also developed guidance with detailed methodology.

- The U.S. EPA prepared guidance for method's development and validation for the Resource Conservation and Recovery Act (RCRA). The AOAC, the EPA and other scientific organizations provide methods that are validated through multi-laboratory studies.

1.1 When should methods be validated?

A method should be validated when it is necessary to verify that its performance parameters are adequate for use for a particular analytical problem. For example:

- Method just developed
- Revised method or established method adapted to a new problem;
- When a review of quality control indicates an established method is changing with time;
- When an established method is used in a different laboratory, with different analysts or with mdifferent equipment
- Demonstration of the equivalence between two methods, e.g. a new method and a standard. Certain areas of analytical practices, such as in clinical chemistry will specify validation requirements relevant to the method. This ensures that particular validation terminology together with the statistics used is interpreted in a manner consistent within the relevant sector. Official recognition of a method may require characterisation using a collaborative study.

1.2 Strategy for the validation of methods

The validity of a specific method should be demonstrated in laboratory experiments using samples or standards that are similar to unknown samples analyzed routinely. The preparation and execution should follow a validation protocol, preferably written in a step-by-step instruction format. This proposed procedure assumes that the instrument has been selected and the method has been developed. It meets criteria such as ease of use; ability to be automated and to be controlled by computer systems; costs per analysis; sample throughput; turnaround time; and environmental, health and safety requirements.

1. Develop a validation protocol, an operating procedure or a validation master plan for the validation
2. For a specific validation project define owners and responsibilities
3. Develop a validation project plan
4. Define the application, purpose and scope of the method
5. Define the performance parameters and acceptance criteria
6. Define validation experiments
7. Verify relevant performance characteristics of equipment
8. Qualify materials, e.g. standards and reagents for purity, accurate amounts and sufficient stability
9. Perform pre-validation experiments
10. Adjust method parameters or/and acceptance criteria if necessary
11. Perform full internal (and external) validation experiments
12. Develop SOPs for executing the method in the routine
13. Define criteria for revalidation
14. Define type and frequency of system suitability tests and/or analytical quality control (AQC) checks for the routine
15. Document validation experiments and results in the validation report

2. Steps in method validation

Successful acceptance of the validation parameters and performance criteria, by all parties involved, requires the cooperative efforts of several departments, including analytical development, QC, regulatory affairs and the individuals requiring the analytical data. The operating procedure or the Validation Master Plan (VMP) should clearly define the roles and responsibilities of each department involved in the validation of analytical methods.

The scope of the method and its validation criteria should be defined early in the process. These include the following questions:

- What analytes should be detected?
- What are the expected concentration levels?
- What are the sample matrices?
- Are there interfering substances expected, and, if so, should they be detected and quantified?
- Are there any specific legislative or regulatory requirements?
- Should information be qualitative or quantitative?
- What are the required detection and quantitation limits?
- What is the expected concentration range?
- What precision and accuracy is expected?
- How robust should the method be?
- Which type of equipment should be used? Is the method for one specific instrument, or should it be used by all instruments of the same type?
- Will the method be used in one specific laboratory or should it be applicable in all laboratories at one side or around the globe?
- What skills do the anticipated users of the method have?

The method's performance characteristics should be based on the intended use of the method. It is not always necessary to validate all analytical parameters that are available for a specific technique. For example, if the method is to be used for qualitative trace level analysis, there is no need to test and validate the method's limit of quantitation, or the linearity, over the full dynamic range of the equipment. Initial parameters should be chosen according to the analyst's experience and best judgment. Final parameters should be agreed between the lab or analytical chemist performing the validation and the lab or individual applying the method and users of the data to be generated by the method.

2.1 Quality control plan and implementation for routine

For any method that will be used for routine analysis, a QC plan should be developed. This plan should ensure that the method, together with the equipment, delivers consistently accurate results. The plan may include recommendations for the following:

1. Selection, handling and testing of QC standards
2. Type and frequency of equipment checks and calibrations (for example, should the wavelength accuracy and the baseline noise of an HPLC UV detector be checked after each sample analysis, or on a daily or weekly basis?)
3. Type and frequency of system suitability testing (for example, at which point during the sequence system should suitability standards be analyzed?)
4. Type and frequency of QC samples (for example, should a QC sample be analyzed after 1, 5, 20 or 50 unknown samples, and should there be single or duplicate QC sample analysis, or should this be run at one or several concentrations?)

5. Acceptance criteria for equipment checks, system suitability tests and QC sample analysis
6. Action plan in case criteria 2, 3 and/or 4 are not met.

In many cases, methods are developed and validated in service laboratories that are specialized in this task. When the method is transferred to the routine analytical laboratory, care should be taken that the method and its critical parameters are well understood by the workers in the departments who apply the method. A detailed validation protocol, a documented procedure for method implementation and good communication between the development and operation departments are equally important. If the method is used by a number of departments, it is recommended to verify method validation parameters and to test the applicability and usability of the method in a couple of these departments before it is distributed to other departments. In this way, problems can be identified and corrected before the method is distributed to a larger audience. If the method is intended to be used by just one or two departments, an analyst from the development department should assist the users of the method during initial operation. Users of the method should be encouraged to give constant feedback on the applicability and usability of the method to the development department. The latter should correct problems if any arise.

2.2 Transferring validated routine methods

Validated routine methods are transferred between laboratories at the same or different sites when contract laboratories offer services for routine analysis in different areas or when products are manufactured in different areas. When validated routine methods are transferred between laboratories and sites, their validated state should be maintained to ensure the same reliable results in the receiving laboratory. This means the competence of the receiving laboratory to use the method should be demonstrated through tests, for example, repeat critical method validation experiments and run samples in parallel in the transferring and receiving laboratories. The transfer should be controlled by a procedure, The recommended steps are:

- Designate a project owner
- Develop a transfer plan
- Define transfer tests and acceptance criteria (validation experiments, sample analysis: sample type, #replicates)
- Describe rational for tests
- Train receiving lab operators in transferring lab on equipment, method, critical parameters and troubleshooting
- Repeat 2 critical method validation tests in routine lab
- Analyze at least three samples in transferring and receiving lab
- Document transfer results

2.3 Revalidation

Most likely some method parameters have to be changed or adjusted during the life of the method if the method performance criteria fall outside their acceptance criteria. The question is whether such change requires revalidation. In order to clarify this question upfront, operating ranges should be defined for each method, either based on experience with similar methods or else investigated during method development. These ranges should be verified during method validation in robustness studies and should be part of the method characteristics. Availability of such operating ranges makes it easier to decide when

a method should be revalidated. A revalidation is necessary whenever a method is changed, and the new parameter lies outside the operating range. If, for example, the operating range of the column temperature has been specified to be between 30 and 40°C, the method should be revalidated if, for whatever reason, the new operating parameter is 41°C.
Revalidation is also required if the scope of the method has been changed or extended, for example, if the sample matrix changes or if operating conditions change. Furthermore, revalidation is necessary if the intention is to use instruments with different characteristics, and these new characteristics have not been covered by the initial validation. For example, an HPLC method may have been developed and validated on a pump with a delay volume of 5 mL, but the new pump has a delay volume of only 0.5 mL.

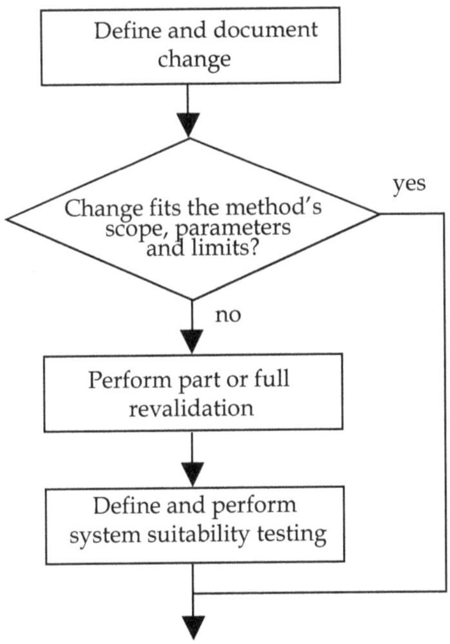

Fig. 1. Flow diagram for revalidation

Part or full revalidation may also be considered if system suitability tests, or the results of QC sample analysis, lie outside preset acceptance criteria and where the source of the error cannot be traced back to the instruments or any other cause.
Whenever there is a change that may require part or full revalidation, the change should follow a documented change control system. The change should be defined, authorized for implementation and documented. Possible changes may include

- new samples with new compounds or new matrices,
- new analysts with different skills,
- new instruments with different characteristics,
- new location with different environmental conditions,
- new chemicals and/or reference standards and
- modification of analytical parameters.

An evaluation should determine whether the change is within the scope of the method. If so, no revalidation is required. If the change lies outside the scope, the parameters for revalidation should be defined. After the validation experiments, the system suitability test parameters should be investigated and redefined, if necessary.

2.4 Bionalytical method development and validation

The process by which a specific bioanalytical method is developed, validated, and used in routine sample analysis can be divided into

1. Reference Standard preparation
2. Bioanalytical method develo`pment and establishment of assay procedure
3. Application of validated bioanalytical method to routine drug analysis and acceptance criteria for the analytical run and/or batch.

3. Parameters for method validation

The parameters for method validation have been defined in different working groups of national and international committees and are described in the literature. Unfortunately, some of the definitions vary between the different organizations. An attempt at harmonization was made for pharmaceutical applications through the ICH where representatives from the industry and regulatory agencies from the United States, Europe and Japan defined parameters, requirements and, to some extent, methodology for analytical methods validation.

3.1 Selectivity/specificity

The terms selectivity and specificity are often used interchangeably, the term specific generally refers to a method that produces a response for a single analyte only, while the term selective refers to a method that provides responses for a number of chemical entities that may or may not be distinguished from each other. If the response is distinguished from all other responses, the method is said to be selective. Since there are very few methods that respond to only one analyte, the term selectivity is usually more appropriate Selectivity and specificity are measures of the reliability of measurements in the presence of interferences. Where the measurement stage is non-specific, method development should indicate which analytes do not interfere. There will be cases where chemical interferences can be identified for a particular method but the chances of encountering them in real life may be improbable. The analyst has to decide at what point it is reasonable to stop looking for interferences. These parameters apply to both qualitative and quantitative analysis. The selectivity of a method is usually investigated by studying its ability to measure the analyte of interest in test portions to which specific interferences have been deliberately introduced (those thought likely to be present in samples). Where it is unclear whether or not interferences are already present, the selectivity of the method can be investigated by studying its ability to measure compared to other independent method/techniques. Another aspect of selectivity which must be considered is where an analyte may exist in the sample in more than one form such as: free or complexed; inorganic or organometallic; or the possibility of a component such as Chromium ion being present in different oxidation states such as Cr^{3+} or Cr^{6+}.

3.2 Precision and reproducibility

Precision is method and concentration specific, which in prac tice can be very varied. The two most common precision measures are 'repeatability' and reproducibility'. They represent the two extreme measures of precision, which can be obtained. Repeatability (the smallest expected precision) will give an idea of the sort of variability to be expected when a method is performed by a single analyst on one piece of equipment over a short timescale, i.e. the sort of variability to be expected between results when a sample is analysed in duplicate. If a sample is to be analysed by a number of laboratories for comparative purposes then a more meaningful precision measure is reproducibility (this is the largest

measure of precision normally encountered). It may be that some in-between measure is the most useful in particular cases; for example precision measured between different analysts, over extended timescales, within a single laboratory. This is sometimes known as 'intermediate precision', but the exact conditions should be stated. Precision is usually stated in terms of standard deviation or relative standard deviation. Both repeatability and reproducibility are generally dependent on analyte concentration, and so should be determined at a number of concentrations and if relevant, the relationship between precision and analyte concentration should be established. The Purpose of carrying out a determination is to obtain a valid estimate of a 'true' value. When one considers the criteria according to which an analytical procedure is selected, precision and accuracy are usually the first time to come to mind. Precision and accuracy together determine the error of an individual determination. They are among the most important criteria for judging analytical procedures by their results. Precision refers to the reproducibility of measurement within a set, that is, to the scatter of dispersion of a set about its central values. The term 'set' is defined as referring to a number (n) of independent replicate measurements of some property. One of the most common statistical terms employed is the standard deviation of a population of observation. Standard deviation is the square root of the sum of squares of a deviations of individual results for the mean, divided by one less than the number of results in the set.
The standard deviation S, is given by

$$S = \sigma = \sqrt{\frac{1}{N}\sum_{i=1}^{N}(x_i - \overline{x})^2},$$

Standard deviation has the same units as the property being measured.
The square of standard deviation is called variance (s^2). Relative standard deviation is the standard deviation as a fraction of the mean, i.e. S/x. It is some times multiplied by 100 and expressed as a percent relative standard deviation. It becomes a more reliable expression of precision.

$$\% \text{ Relative Standard Deviation (RSD)} = S * 100/x$$

3.3 Accuracy and recovery

The accuracy of an analytical method is the extent to which test results generated by the method and the true value agree. Accuracy can also be described as the closeness of agreement between the value that is adopted, either as a conventional, true or accepted reference value, and the value found. The true value for accuracy assessment can be obtained in several ways. One alternative is to compare the results of the method with results from an established reference method. This approach assumes that the uncertainty of the reference method is known. Secondly, accuracy can be assessed by analyzing a sample with known concentrations (e.g., a control sample or certified reference material) and comparing the measured value with the true value as supplied with the material. If certified reference materials or control samples are not available, a blank sample matrix of interest can be spiked with a known concentration by weight or volume. After extraction of the analyte from the matrix and injection into the analytical instrument, its recovery can be determined by comparing the response of the extract with the response of the reference material dissolved in a pure solvent. Because this accuracy assessment measures the effectiveness of sample preparation, care should be taken to mimic the actual sample preparation as closely as possible. If validated correctly, the recovery factor determined for different concentrations can be used to correct the final results.

3.3.1 Calibration

Calibration is the most important step in bioactive compound analysis. A good Precision and accuracy can only be obtained when a good calibration procedure is adopted. In the Spectrophotometric methods, the concentration of a sample cannot be measured directly, but is determined using physical measuring quantity 'y' (absorbance of a solution). An unambiguous empirical or theoretical relationship can be shown between this quanity and the concentration of an analyte. The calibration between y = g(x) the calibration function can be obtained by fitting an adequate mathematical model through the experimental data. The most convenient calibration function is linear, goes through the origin and is applicable over a wide dynamic range. In practice however, many deviations from the ideal calibration line may occur. For the majority of analytical techniques uses the calibration equation.

$$Y = a + bX$$

In calibration, univarate regression is applied, when means that all observations are dependent upon a single variable X.

3.3.2 Standard deviation of slope (Sb)

The standard deviation of slope is proportional to standard error of estimate and inversely proportional to the range and square root of the number of data points.

3.3.3 Standard deviation of intercept, (Sa)

Intercept values of least squares fits of data are often to evaluate additive errors between or among different methods.

3.3.4 Correlation coefficient, (r)

The correlation coefficient r (x,y) is more useful to express the relationship of the chosen scales. To obtain a correlation coefficient the covariance is divided by the product of the standard deviation of x and y.

$$r = \frac{\sum_{i=1}^{n}(x_i - \overline{x})(y_i - \overline{y})}{\sqrt{\sum_{i=1}^{n}(x_i - \overline{x})^2 \sum_{i=1}^{n}(y_i - \overline{y})^2}}$$

The absolute recovery of analytical method as the response of a processed spiked matrix expressed as a percentage of the response of pure standard. Which has not been subjected to sample pre-treatment and indicates whether the method provides a response for the entire amount of analyte that is present in the sample. It is best established by comparing the responses of extracted samples at low, medium and high concentrations in replicates at least 6 with those non- extracted standards, which represent 100% recovery.

$$\text{Absolute recovery} = \frac{\text{response of an spike into matrix (processed)}}{\text{response of an analyte of pure standard (unprocessed)}} \times 100$$

If an internal standard is used, its recovery should be determined independently at the concentration levels used in the method.

3.3.5 Linearity and sensitivity of the method

It may be demonstrated directly on the drug substance (by dilution of a standard stock solution) and/or separate weighings of synthetic mixtures of the drug product components, using the proposed procedure. The latter aspect can be studied during investigation of the range. Linearity should be evaluated by visual inspection of a plot of signals as a function of analyte concentration or content.The correlation coefficient, y-intercept, slope of the regression line, and residual sum of squares should be submitted. A plot of the data should be included. According to the Beers Lambert Law, Absorbance is the ratio of logarithm of Intensity of incident light and Intensity of transmitted light, or A = εCT. Knowledge of the sensitivity of the color is important and the following terms are commonly employed for expressing sensitivity. The absorbance (A) is proportional to the concentration (C) of the absorbing species, if absorptivity (ε) and thickness of the medium (t) are constant. When concentration is in moles per litre, the constant is called molar absorptivity. Beers Law limits and E_{max} values are expressed as µg/ml and moles/cm respectively. Sandell's Sensitivity refers to the number of µg of the drug to be determining, converted to the colored product, which in a column solution of cross section $1cm^2$ shows an absorbance of 0.001(expressed as µg/cm).

3.4 Stability

The term system stability has been defined as the stability of the samples being analyzed in a sample solution. System stability should be determined by replicate analysis of the sample solution. System stability is considered appropriate when the RSD, calculated on the assay results obtained at different time intervals, does not exceed more than 20 percent of the corresponding value of the system precision. If, on plotting the assay results as a function of time, the value is higher, the maximum duration of the usability of the sample solution can be calculated.

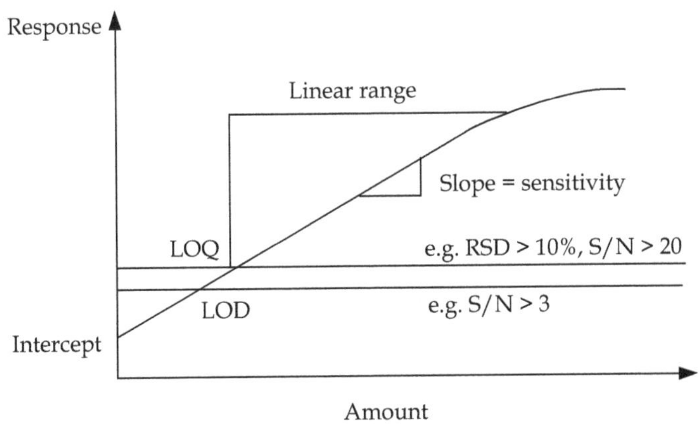

Fig. 2. Definitions for linearity, range, LOQ, LOD

3.5 Range

The range of an analytical method is the interval between the upper and lower levels (including these levels) that have been demonstrated to be determined with precision, accuracy and linearity using the method as written. The range is normally expressed in the same units as the test results (e.g., percentage, parts per million) obtained by the analytical method. For assay tests, the ICH (5) requires the minimum specified range to be 80 to 120 percent of the test concentration, and for the determination of an impurity, the range to extend from the limit of quantitation, or from 50 percent of the specification of each impurity, whichever is greater, to 120 percent of the specification.

3.6 Limit of detection

The limit of detection is the point at which a measured value is larger than the uncertainty associated with it. It is the lowest concentration of analyte in a sample that can be detected but not necessarily quantified. The limit of detection is frequently confused with the sensitivity of the method. The sensitivity of an analytical method is the capability of the method to discriminate small differences in concentration or mass of the test analyte. In practical terms, sensitivity is the slope of the calibration curve that is obtained by plotting the response against the analyte concentration or mass.

In chromatography, the detection limit is the injected amount that results in a peak with a height at least two or three times as high as the baseline noise level. Besides this signal/noise method, the ICH (4) describes three more methods:

1. Visual inspection: The detection limit is determined by the analysis of samples with known concentrations of analyte and by establishing the minimum level at which the analyte can be reliably detected.
2. Standard deviation of the response based on the standard deviation of the blank: Measurement of the magnitude of analytical background response is performed by analyzing an appropriate number of blank samples and calculating the standard deviation of these responses.
3. Standard deviation of the response based on the slope of the calibration curve: A specific calibration curve is studied using samples containing an analyte in the range of the limit of detection. The residual standard deviation of a regression line, or the standard deviation of y-intercepts of regression lines, may be used as the standard deviation.

3.7 Limit of quantitation

The limit of quantitation is the minimum injected amount that produces quantitative measurements in the target matrix with acceptable precision in chromatography, typically requiring peak heights 10 to 20 times higher than the baseline noise. If the required precision of the method at the limit of quantitation has been specified, the EURACHEM (22) approach can be used. A number of samples with decreasing amounts of the analyte are injected six times. The calculated RSD percent of the precision is plotted against the analyte amount. The amount that corresponds to the previously defined required precision is equal to the limit of quantitation. It is important to use not only pure standards for this test but also spiked matrices that closely represent the unknown samples. For the limit of detection, the ICH (5) recommends, in addition to the procedures as described above, the visual inspection and the standard deviation of the response and the slope of the calibration curve.

Any results of limits of detection and quantitation measurements must be verified by experimental tests with samples containing the analytes at levels across the two regions. It is equally important to assess other method validation parameters, such as precision, reproducibility and accuracy, close to the limits of detection and quantitation. Figure 6 illustrates the limit of quantitation (along with the limit of detection, range and linearity). Figure 7 illustrates both the limit of detection and the limit of quantitation.

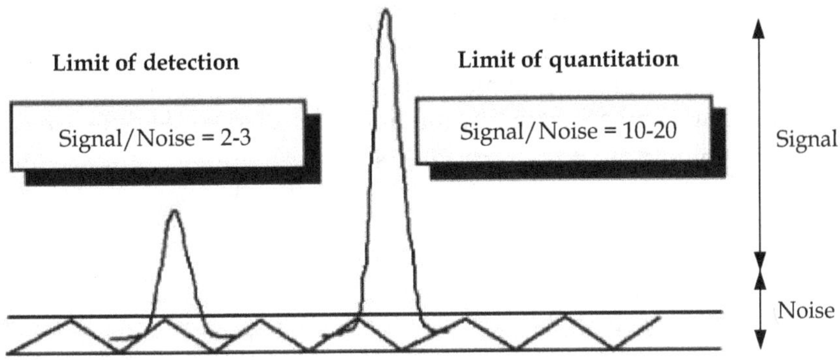

Fig. 3. Limit of detection and limit of quantitation via signal to noise

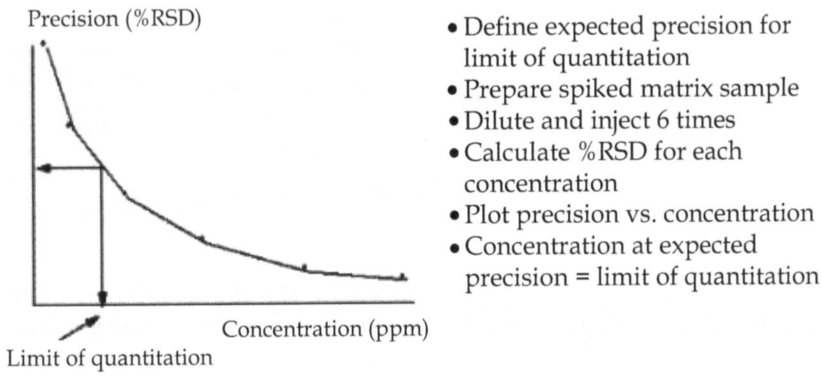

Fig. 4. Limit of quantitation with the EURACHEM (80) method

3.8 Repeatability

From the repeatability standard deviation or or sr it is useful to calculate the 'repeatability limit 'r'', which enables the analyst to decide whether the difference between duplicate analyses of a sample, determined under repeatability conditions, is significant.

3.9 Reproducibility

From the reproducibility standard deviation oR or sR it is useful to calculate the 'reproducibility limit 'R', 'which enables the analyst to decide wheth er the difference between duplicate analyses of a sample, determined under reproducibility conditions, is significant. These calculations can be performed directly with the built-in statistics function of the instrument, if available, or by using a pocket calculator or a PC (Personal Computer) with a suitable software pac kage (e.g. spreadsheet program).

3.10 Measurement uncertainty

Measurement uncertainty is a single parameter (usually a standard deviation with a coverage factor or confidence interval) expressing the range of values possible on the basis of the measurement result. A measurement uncertainty estimate takes account of all recognised effects operating on the result; the uncertainties associated with each effect are combined according to well-established procedures. An uncertainty estimate for analytical chemistry is often termed an 'uncertainty budget' and should take into account:

- The overall, long-term precision of the method;
- Bias and its uncertainty, including the statistical uncertainty involved in the bias measurements, and the reference material or method uncertainty. It may be necessary to increase the estimate where a significant bias is detected but left uncorrected.
- Calibration uncertainties. As most equipment calibration uncertainties will be negligibly small by comparison with overall precision and uncertainty in the bias; this needs only to be verified;
- Any significant effects operating in addition to the above. For example, temperature or time ranges permitted by the method may not be fully exercised in validation studies, and their effect may need to be added. Such effects can be usefully quantified by robustness studies (see 'Ruggedness' below) or related studies which establish the size of a given effect on the result. Where the contribution of individual effects is important, for example in calibration laboratories, it will be necessary to consider the individual contributions from all individual effects separately. Note that, subject to additional consideration of effects outside the scope of a collaborative trial, the reproducibility standard deviation forms a working estimate of a measurement uncertainty provided that the laboratory's bias, measured on relevant materials, is small with respect to the reproducibility standard deviation, the in-house repeatability precision is comparable to the standard method repeatability and the laboratory's intermediate precision is not large than the published reproducibility standard deviation.

3.11 Sensitivity

This is effectively the gradient of the response curve, i.e. the change in instrument response, which corresponds, to a change in analyte concentration. Where the response has been established as linear with respect to concentration, i.e. within the linear range of the method, and the intercept of the response curve has been determined, sensitivity is a useful parameter to calculate and use in formulae for quantitation. Sensitivity is sometimes used to refer to limit of detection but this use is not generally approved.

3.12 Ruggedness (or robustness)

Ruggedness is normally evaluated during method development, typically by the originating laboratory, before collaborating with other laboratories and is a measure how well a method stands up to less than perfect implementation. In any method there will be certain stages, which, if not carried out sufficiently carefully, will have a severe effect on method performance, and may even result in the method not working at all. These stages should be identified, usually as part of method development, and if possible, their influence on method performance evaluated using 'ruggedness tests', sometimes also called 'robustness tests'. This involves making deliberate variations to the method, and investigating the subsequent effect on performance. It is then possible to identify the variables in the method, which have the most significant effect and ensure that, when using the method, they are closely controlled. Where there is a need to improve the method further, improvements can probably be made by concentrating on those parts of the method known to be critical. Ruggedness tests are normally applied to investigate the effect on either precision or accuracy.

4. The validation tools

1. Reagent blanks: Reagents used during the analytical process (including solvents used for extraction or dissolution) are analysed in isolation in order to see whether they

contribute to the measurement signal. The measurement signal arising from the analyte can then be corrected accordingly.

2. Sample blanks: These are essentially matrices with no analyte. They are difficult to obtain but such materials are necessary to give a realistic estimate of interference that would be encountered in the analysis of test samples.
3. Samples / test materials: Test materials taken from real samples are useful because of the information they yield on interferences *etc.* which could be realistically encountered in day-to-day work. If the true analyte content of a test material is accurately know it can be used as a way of assessing the accuracy of the method. However the true analyte content is usually difficult to determine unless there is the possibility of using other methods which are known to show negligible bias.
4. Spiked material: These are material or solutions, which have been fortified with the analyte(s) of interest. These materials or solutions may already contain the analyte of interest so care is needed lest fortification inadvertently leads to levels outside of the range of applicability of the method. Fortification with a known amount of analyte enables the increase in response to the analyte to be measured and calculated in terms of the amount added (assuming 100% recovery), even though the absolute amounts of analyte present before and after the fortification are not know. Note that most methods of fortification add the analyte in such a way that it will not be as closely bound to the sample matrix as it would be if it was present naturally. Therefore, recovery determinations obtained by fortification can be expected to be over-optimistic. The nature of the spike obviously needs to be identified.
5. (Measurement) Standards: These are traditionally thought of as solutions of single substances but in practice can be anything in which a particular parameter or property has been characterized to a sufficient extent it can be used for reference or calibration purposes.
6. Reference materials: frequently confused with *certified reference materials*. Reference materials can be virtually any material used as a basis for reference, and could include laboratory reagents of known purity, industrial chemicals, or other artefacts. The property or analyte of interest needs to be stable and homogenous but the materials does not need to have the high degree of characterisation, traceability and certifi cation more properly associated with certified reference materials.
7. Certified reference materials: The characterisation of the parameter of interest in a *certified reference material* is generally more strictly controlled than for a *reference material,* and in addition the characterised value is certified with a stated uncertainty by a recognised institution. Characterisation is normally done using several different methods, so that as far as possible, any bias in the characterisation is reduced or even eliminated.

5. References

[1] Eric Reid, Ian D. Wilson, Methodological Survey in Biochemistry and Analysis Volume 20: Analysis for Drug and Metabolites, Including Anti-infective Agents, 1990,1-57

[2] U.S. Department of Health and Human Services, Food and Drug Administration., Guidance for Industry, Bioanalytical Method Validation, May2001

[3] Nowatzke W, Woolf E, Best Practices during Bioanalytical Method Validation for the Characterization of Assay Reagents and the Evaluation of Analyte Stability in Assay Standards, Quality Controls, and Study Samples, AAPS Journal. 9(2), 2007, E117-E122.

[4] Braggio S., Barnaby R. J., Grosi P, Cugola M., A strategy for validation of bioanalytical methods,Journal of Pharmaceutical and Biomedical Analysis 1996, 14, 375- 388

[5] Breda C.A., Breda M., Frigerio E.,Bioanalytical method validation: a risk-based approach?, Journal of Pharmaceutical and Biomedical Analysis,35, 2004, 887–89
[6] Nakashima Kenichiro, High-Performance Liquid Chromatography of drug of abuse in biological samples, Journal of Health Science, 51(3) 272-277 (2005)
[7] Boulanger B., Chiap P. Dewe W., Crommen J., Hubert Ph., An analysis of the SFSTP guide on validation of chromatographic bioanalytical methods: progresses and limitations Journal of Pharmaceutical and Biomedical Analysis,32, 2003,753-765
[8] Causon Roger, Validation of chromatographic methods in biomedical analysis viewpoint and discussion, Journal of Chromatography B, 689 (1997) 175-180
[9] Hartmann C., Smeyers-Verbeke J., Massart D. L., McDowall R.D., Validation of bioanalytical chromatographic methods, Journal of Pharmaceutical and Biomedical Analysis17, 1998,193–218
[10] G. C. Hokanson, A life cycle approach to the validation of analytical methods during pharmaceutical product development, Part II: Changes and the need for additional validation, Pharm.Tech., Oct. 1994, pp. 92–100.
[11] J. M. Green, A practical guide to analytical method validation, Anal. Chem. News & Features, 1 May 1996, pp. 305A–309A.
[12] B. Renger, H. Jehle, M. Fischer and W. Funk, Validation of analytical procedures in pharmaceutical analytical chemistry: HPTLC assay of theophylline in an effervescent tablet, J. Planar Chrom. 8:269–278 (July/August 1995).
[13] Wegscheider, Validation of analytical methods, in: Accreditation and quality assurance in analytical chemistry, edited by H. Guenzler, Springer Verlag, Berlin (1996).
[14] S. Seno, S. Ohtake and H. Kohno, Analytical validation in practice at a quality control laboratory in the Japanese pharmaceutical industry, Accred. Qual. Assur. 2:140–145 (1997).
[15] AOAC Peer-Verified Methods Program, Manual on policies and procedures, Arlington, Va., USA (1998). http://www.aoac.org/vmeth/PVM.pdf
[16] P. A. Winslow and R. F. Meyer, Defining a master plan for the validation of analytical methods, J. Validation Technology, pp. 361–367 (1997).
[17] Zhoua Shaolian, Songb Qi, Tangb Yong, Weng Naidonga, Critical Review of Development, Validation, and Transfer for High Throughput Bioanalytical LC-MS/MS Methods,Current Pharmaceutical Analysis, 2005, 1, 3-14 3
[18] Kelley M, DeSilva, B.,Key Elements of Bioanalytical Method Validation for Macromolecules., AAP Journal. 2007, 9(2), E156-E163.
[19] Findlay J.W.A., Smith W.C., Lee J.W.,Nordblom G.D., Das I., DeSilva B.S., Khan M.N., Bowsher R.R., Validation of immunoassays for bioanalysis: a pharmaceutical industry perspective Journal of Pharmaceutical and Biomedical Analysis, 2000, 21,1249–1273
[20] Shah Vinod P., Ph. D, History of Bioanalytical Validation and Regulation: Evolution of a Guidance Document on Bioanalytical Method Validation, AAPS 3rd Bioanalytical Workshop on Quantitative Bioanalytical Methods Validation and Implementation: Best Practices for Chromatographic and Ligand Binding Assays Crystal City, Arlington, VA, May 1-3, 2006
[21] Mohammad A.,Tabrizi-Fard, Ho-Leung, Fung, Reversed-phase high-performance liquid chromatography method for the analysis of nitro-arginine in rat plasma and urine, Journal of Chromatography B, 679, 1996, 7-12
[22] Bmscheck Torsten, Meyer Hartmut, Wellhrner Hans Herbert, a High-performance liquid chromatographic assay for the measurement of azathioprine in human serum samples, Journal of Chromatography B, 675, 1996,287-294

8

Quality Control Method for Herbal Medicine - Chemical Fingerprint Analysis

Zhang Yongyu, Sun Shujun, Dai Jianye,
Wang Wenyu, Cao Huijuan, Wu Jianbing and Gou Xiaojun
Shanghai University of Traditional Chinese P.R. China

1. Introduction

The herbal medicines (HMs) and their preparations have been widely used for thousands of years in many oriental countries, such as China, Korea, Japan, etc, (Liang Y.-Z. et al.,2004) and it is attracting more and more attention from all over the world. But the uncontrollable quality of HMs is the obstacle for internationalization and modernization. For HMs, both single and combinations contain a myriad of compounds, and multiple constituents of HMs represent their therapeutic effects. Moreover, the chemical constituents in herbs in the HM products may be diverse due to various harvest seasons, plant origins, origins, processing and other factors (Liang Y.-Z. et al.,2004).As to one kind of herbal medicine, any difference from above aspects can lead to variant efficacy. This point was illustrated in many literatures. (Pan Ruijing, et al., 2011;Qiu YQ, et al.,2007;Zeng Y.-X., et al., 2007;Zhang YY, et al., 2008) The content of bioactive components in the roots of *Salvia miltiorrhizae* (danshen) was closely related to germplasm and harvest time (He Chun'e, et al., 2010).As for HMs, the specific quality control of the tested samples usually was achieved through the identification and determination. Because of uncertainty and complexity, there is great difficulty in establishing a specific method of quality control of HMs. The techniques of authentication are not powerful enough to identify all the ingredients in a HM, target setting is too general to determine the active ingredient and the components that are regarded as markers are often not active. Hereby there are some problems in developing specific and objective quality standards of herb medicines. And just on based of this point, adulteration or inferior quality drugs appeared more and more in markets.

Subsequent evaluation revealed some products to be adulterated with other related plants from the same genus(Ma C.-H.,2011), for instance, in the U.S. market black cohosh products are adulterated widely with other species of *Actaea,* which are lower-priced and exert unknown effect on menopausal symptoms (Jiang B.,et al.,2006). At the same time also a large number of substitutes enjoy the same name but have different ingredients and efficiency, which causes confusion medicinal species and affects the safety and efficacy of HMs. In order to eliminate these quality problems, on one hand we must actively foster the concept of pharmaceutical production of good quality and the concept of legal system, and on the other hand, the scientific and technologically advanced quality control standards should be established as soon as possible.

The quality control standardization of HM contains standardization of herb medicinal substances, cut crude drug and preparations, and nowadays the emphasis is laid on that of HM substance. Without Quality control standardization of herb medicinal substances, there is not standardization of cut crude drug and preparations at all. The morphological identification and microscopic identification are utilized to determine the authenticity of HMs, and the physical and chemical characters are used to evaluate the quality of herbs in the existing quality standards. But by all above methods, the complexity of herbal medicines can not be elaborated, yet the chromatographic fingerprinting analysis was featured by the fundamental attributions of "integrity" and "fuzziness" or "sameness" and "difference", which can chemically represent the characteristics of the HM investigated(Xie P. S., 2001 as cited in Liang Y. Z. et al., 2004). Two key issues are involved in the development of a fingerprint method: (i) how to gain more effective and stable information and (ii) how to evaluate the similarity and difference with chemometric method(Liang X.-M. et al., 2009).
Mork and Chau grouped authentication and quality control of herbal medicines into the 'component-based' approach and 'pattern-based' approach (D.K.W. Mok & F.T. Chau,2006). In 2008, Zeng et.al (Zeng Z.D. et al., 2008) refined these two approaches into compound-oriented approach and pattern-oriented approach respectively. The compound-oriented approach includes the marker approach and the multi-compound approach. Generally, marker approach is utilized when the active ingredient was identified, such as paclitaxel and ephedrine. And multi-compound approach will be used when a single compound can not represent the efficacy of the HMs. Pattern-oriented approach namely fingerprint analysis is more popular now, because most HMs' chemical ingredients have been studied, but it is difficult to determine which compound is effective. In recent years, the combination of qualitative fingerprint profiles and quantitative multi-compounds detection was proposed and was applied into the quality control of HMs (Kong W. J. et al., 2009; Zhou F. Z. et al., 2008; Su J et al., 2008).
So far, during the production and circulation of HMs, there is no comprehensive and integrated quality control measure to reflect the variations of HM products, and to effectively control the quality in the whole process. The research and establishment of fingerprints contributed much to solving the problem. It can evaluate the integrative and holistic properties of herbal medicines by comparing the similarity and correlation of the analytes among the whole producing process, such as manufacture, processing and storage of raw materials for preparation, intermediate products, finished products and distribution products. The fingerprint analysis have been internationally accepted as one of the efficient methods to control the quality of herbal medicines (Liang Y.Z. et al.,2004). In this chapter we reviewed the quality control methods of HMs, especially fingerprint analysis methods. Moreover, a section named case study was given at the end of fingerprinting techniques. In this part, three carefully selected cases were described in details, aiming to demonstrate the whole process of fingerprint analysis.

2. Compound approach

On basis of the Chinese Pharmacopoeia, identification and quantification of chemical markers are crucial to the quality control of herbal medicines. Totally, 525 quantitative monographs by chemical markers were documented in the Chinese Pharmacopoeia (2005 edition) for control and evaluation of herbal medicinal materials, prepared slices, herbal extracts and preparations. For example, a HPLC method was used to identify and quantify the syringoside (content≥0.050%) in *radix acanthopanacis* and chrysophano (content≥0.20%) and aurantio-obtusin (content≥0.080%) in *semen cassiae* (CPh.2005,pp.288). Of course, additionally, the combination with morphological, phytochemical and physicochemical identification is essential. M.H. Jeon et al. developed a reversed-phase high-performance liquid chromatography-pulsed amperometric detection (RP-HPLC-PAD) method for the detection of albiflorin and paeoniflorin in *Paeoniae Radix* (Min-Hwan Jeon et al.,2009).As many herb medical substances contain the same compounds, thus just one or several markers approach fails to confirm the identity of a specific plant, let alone make any evaluation regarding its quality. This problem will appear when a specific class of compounds simultaneously exist in two substances (Xie P.S. et al., 2006). So the multi-compound approach and fingerprint approach are proposed, and the fingerprint approach will be discussed in the next section. Compared with marker approach, multi-compound approach study on more compounds, and does not necessarily require specific chemical markers. Chemometric deconvolution and resolution are the main methods in this approach (Zeng Z.D.,2008). Such as iterative OPA or non iterative EWOP (Guo F.Q., 2004), Artificial Neural Networks (ANNs), k-nearest neighbor (k-NN) (Tian R.T. et al., 2008.) et.al. Chemometric methods for evaluation of chromatographic separation quality from two-way data were reviewed in the literature (Xu L et al., 2008). For instance, total terpene lactones and total flavonol glycosides were detected for the quality control of ginkgo substances, ginkgo extraction and ginkgo tablet (CPh.2005, pp.292/322/663).A method, HPLC-DAD-ESI-MS, was established to qualitatively identify and quantitatively determine the 10 major active coumarins of Zushima (Su J. et al., 2009).And a HPLC-DAD method is firstly established for the simultaneous determination of 10 major components in different origins of *Carthamus tinctorius*, by L. Fan et al. (Fan L et al., 2009).

3. Fingerprint approach

By definition, a chromatographic fingerprint of a HM is, in practice, a chromatographic pattern of the extract of some common chemical components of pharmacologically active or chemically characteristics (Liang Y.Z.et al., 2004). Specifically, fingerprints of herbal medicine refer to the profiles which can illustrate the specific properties of the analyte including raw materials, slices, semi-finished products and finished products after appropriate processing, and be obtained by certain analysis techniques. The research of fingerprinting of herbal medicines is really an interdisciplinary and comprehensive research, which is based on the chemical composition of traditional Chinese medicine system. It needs crossover of herbal medicine, separation science, analytical science, and bioinformatics to provide a platform for the quality control of traditional herbal medicines. Those features make fingerprint analysis especially suitable for research on HMs which bearing characteristics of a complex mixture of chemical compounds.

Fingerprinting is now globally accepted as a quality evaluation model of herbal medicine. Due to different national conditions and traditions, the research thoughts and methods of fingerprinting are diverse in different countries. Japanese scientists accept the decoction of a prescription consisting of trueborn crude drug slices as standard extraction, and the fingerprint obtained from the standard extraction is taken for standard fingerprint. Food and Drug Administration has also started to accept fingerprint, because fingerprint method can be utilized to the quality control of the Botanical Drug Substances and Botanical Drug Products in application material named chemistry, manufacture and control (CMC) of

Investigation New Drug (IND). Furthermore, France, Germany, Britain, India and the WHO, adopted fingerprinting to evaluate the quality of medicinal plants. And Chinese manufacturers are required by the Chinese State Food and Drug Administration (SFDA) to standardize the injections and their corresponding raw materials made from Traditional Chinese Medicine, by using chromatographic fingerprinting method.

Just as in any single HM and its combinations, there are lots of unknown components and many of them are in low amount, researchers applied more and more techniques into this field. Fingerprinting, generally, was divided into chemical and biological fingerprint patterns. Chemical fingerprint is used to analyze the chemical constituents in HMs, consisting chromatographic fingerprint, such as thin layer chromatography (TLC), high-performance liquid chromatography (HPLC), gas chromatography (GC), capillary electrophoresis (CE) and spectral fingerprint, for instance, UV, IR, MS, X-ray and so on, and their hyphenated techniques. The biological fingerprints mainly refer to genomics fingerprints. Since genetic composition is unique for each individual, DNA methods for HMs' identification are less affected by age, physiological conditions, environmental factors, harvest, storage and processing methods. Genomic fingerprint has been used widely for the differentiation of plant individual, genus, homogeneity analysis, and detection of adulterants (Cheng KT et al., 1997; Huang Y et al., 2002; Wang C.Z. et al., 2007; Zhang X. et al., 2006). However, as for herbal instances processed or extractions of plants, DNA fingerprinting techniques usually can not do anything. Moreover, the efficiency of Chinese herbal medicines is based on the chemical components they contain, chemical analysis therefore better reflect the intrinsic quality of medicine. Consequently, DNA fingerprinting should be used as a complement tool of other quality control techniques.

In this part, the emphasis was put on chemical fingerprinting techniques, of which the classification and application were discussed in details, and at the end of this section, several carefully selected and systematical cases were presented to illustrate the methodology of fingerprints.

3.1 Chromatographic fingerprint analysis techniques and classification

3.1.1 Thin layer chromatography

TLC is the common fingerprint method for herbal analysis because of its simplicity, rapidity and economy. A major advantage of TLC is that it can provide the light images and fluorescence images, which is one more visual parameter than Chromatograms, and you can get different levels of profiles and corresponding integral data with chromatography scanning and digital processing, especially for routine analysis and on-site inspection test. But TLC analysis also has shortcomings: low resolution, low sensitivity and the difficulty of detection of trace components, etc.

Four species of herb medicines bailahuén-species Haplopappus remyanus, Haplopappus multifolius, and Haplopappus taedaare are all used in popular medicine for the same purpose, we supposed that chemical compounds would be very similar. But H. Vogel et al. identified them easily by TLC of the resins (Hermine Vogel et al., 2005). With this technique, authentication of various species of *Ginseng* and *Radix Puerariae* is possible, as well as the evaluation of stability and consistency of their preparations from different manufactures (Xie P.S et al., 2006). HPTLC fingerprint is mainly used to study the compounds with low or moderate polarities, but Di et al. established a fingerprint of fungal polysaccharide acid hydrolyzates by using automated multiple development (AMD) (Di X et al., 2003). Micro emulsion thin layer chromatography (ME-TLC) which differs significantly from conventional TLC, provides higher detection sensitivity and separation resolution and reproducibility (Cui S.F. et al.,2005). Researchers from Hong Kong Polytechnic University applied high performance thin layer chromatography (HPTLC) combining with digital imaging technology to compare the fingerprints of *Radix Puerariae Lobatae* and *Radix Puerariae Thomsonii.*, and directly revealed the chemical outline of two different species (Chen SB et al., 2006).

3.1.2 GC and its hyphenated techniques

Gas chromatography (GC) and GC-MS with high specificity, high sensitivity, stability and small amount of sample characteristics, are unanimously accepted as the method for the analysis of volatile constituents of HMs (Jiang Y, et al.). The combination of GC–MS fingerprinting analysis along with relative retention index (RRI) and related Chemometrics methods was developed to distinguish *Scutellaria Barbata D. Don* (SB) and its adulterants, simultaneously witness the consistent of SB from nine different origins (Pan R.J. et al.,2011). GC can detect almost all the volatile chemical compounds with high sensitivity, which is especially true for the usual FID detection and GC–MS. Moreover, the high selectivity of capillary columns enables separation of many volatile compounds simultaneously within very short time. However, it is not convenient for the analysis of samples of polar, non-volatile and heat-labile ingredients (Liang Y.Z. et al., 2004). The samples must be gasified by the tedious sample pretreatment such as derivatization, but the ingredients in most herbal instances are high polar compounds, which limits Gas chromatography's application in the chemical identification and authentication of HMs. To solve this problem, and expand the gas chromatography in the identification of herbal medicine, Chinese University of Hong Kong and Shanghai Innovative Research Center of Traditional Chinese Medicine combined to firstly set up off-line pyrolysis - gas chromatography - mass spectrometry fingerprint method to obtain the fingerprints of HMs (Chen W.D. et al., 2007).

3.1.3 HPLC and its hyphenated techniques

HPLC has been a popular and commonly used method in the research field of fingerprint analysis for Chinese medicines because it is easy to learn and use and is not limited by the volatility or stability of the sample compound (Liang Y.-Z. et al., 2004). Thus HPLC is utilized more widely than GC as the complement. One of the main advantages of HPLC is that many detectors can be connected to it, such as UV, DAD, ELSD, FLD, RID, MS, and NMR, etc, and even connect with two or more of them(Wang H.L. et al.,2010), which supplies much more possibilities for detecting different constituent types(Qi L.W. et al.,2008). HPLC fingerprinting technique is advisable for good quality control of Wuweizi (Lu Y. & Chen D.F., 2008). A method of HPLC–UV/MS was developed to determine the fiavonoid profile of S. *baicalensis* in (Liu G.Z.et al.,2009). Another method using liquid chromatography coupled to electrospray ionization mass spectrometry (LC–ESI-MS) has been optimized and established for the qualitative and quantitative analysis of ten active phenolic compounds originating from the pigeon pea leaves and a medicinal product (Tongluo Shenggu capsules)(Liu W et al.,2010). To investigate the possibility of using two non-official species of *Herba Cistanche* as alternatives to the official species, a high-performance liquid chromatography–diode array detection–mass spectrometry (HPLC–DAD–MS) fingerprint method was developed to comparatively analyze the crude herbs of these four species (Jiang Y. et al, 2008). C. Ma et al. used HPLC–ESI-TOF-MS/MS and chemometric analysis to identify marker compounds in the assessment of 4 species of Actaea. This method successfully distinguished different species of *Actaea* and made the black *cohosh* products high quality and unadulterated (Ma C.H. et al., 2011). And in recent years, coulometric electrode array detection (HPLC-CEAD) and charged aerosol detection (CAD) (Bai C.C.,et al., 2009) have also been used for the analysis of HMs. CAD is a quality detector (R.W. Dixon & D.S. Peterson,2002), and has similar properties with ELSD, suitable for detecting the compounds without or with weak UV absorption, but with higher sensitivity, wider test range and better reproducibility (Jiang Y. et al.,2010; Bai C.C.,et al., 2009). A binary chromatographic fingerprint analysis was developed using hydrophilic interaction chromatography (HILIC) and reversed-phase liquid chromatography (RPLC) to gain more chemical information about two parts of water-extracted fraction: the polar compounds and weakly polar compounds. The fingerprint of the polar compounds was analyzed with HILIC, whereas the fingerprint of the weakly polar compounds was analyzed with RPLC (Jin Y et al., 2008).

Except availability of more sensible detectors for HPLC, the appearance of capillary HPLC and ultra-performance (UPLC) have increased the analysis efficiency, so that shorter analytical time and better separation have been achieved (Zheng X.T. et al., 2008; Chen J.H. et al., 2008).UPLC also can be connected with different detectors, for instance, UV, TOF/MS, Q/TOF/MS, PAD and even two or more of them combined together. Those hyphenated techniques with the virtue of the high resolution, high speed of UPLC and the accurate mass measurement of TOF-MS, can get more information about the complex characteristics of herb medicine and can identify and quantify multi-components in HMs. Thus in recent years, UPLC technique, especially the hyphenated techniques are usually utilized in this field (Li S.-L. et al., 2009; Cheng J et al., 2010; H. Liu et al., 2009; Kong W.J. et al, 2009). Moreover, the UPLC-PDA-Q-TOF-MS was used to evaluate decocting-induced chemical transformations (S.-L. Li et al., 2010a)and chemical consistency between traditional and dispensing granule decoctions(S.-L. Li et al., 2010b).

3.1.4 Capillary electrophoresis and its Hyphenation

Capillary electrophoresis is the combination of a classic electrophoresis and modern micro-column separation technology, and in recent years it presents a rapid development and has been widely used in the medicine field. Capillary electrophoresis (CE), with high resolution, minimal sample and solvents consumption, short analysis time and high separation efficiency, is an effective tool for drug quality control. The methodology of CE was established to evaluate one herb drug in terms of specificity, sensitivity and precision, and the results were in agreement with those obtained by the HPLC method. Furthermore, the analysis time of the CE method was two times shorter than that in HPLC and solvent consumption was more than 100-fold less (Sombra L.L., et al., 2004). A characteristic fingerprint of *Flos Carthami* established using CE, simultaneously contributed to several objects in a study: identifying the raw herb, helping distinguish the substitute or adulterant and further assessing the differences of *Flos Carthami* grown in various areas of China (Sun Y et al., 2003). In addition, CE has a wide range of applications such as for use of organic, inorganic, neutral molecules, biological macromolecules, and so on. The hyphenated CE instruments, such as CE-DAD, CE-MS and CE-NMR, have been utilized in the past decades. However, Overlapping peaks in complex samples and irreproducible migration times are unintelligible defects of CE and hyphenations (Christophe Tistaert et al., 2011). Comparison of the CE and HPLC fingerprints of *radix Scutellariae* showed a decrease in analysis time from 40 to 12min for CE, but also a decrease in detected peaks from14 to 11(Wang L.C.,et al., 2005).

3.2 Evaluation of chemical fingerprint of herbal medicine

The whole process of evaluation of chemical fingerprint of herbal medicine was showed in fig.1. Evaluation of fingerprinting is important and critical for the quality assessment and quality control of herbal medicine. Due to experimental variations and column aging, shifts in retention time between fingerprints occur. However, data handling techniques require the same variable to contain synchronous information in every fingerprint. So when the fingerprints were obtained, peak-alignment or warping techniques are commonly applied to compensate for minor shifts in retention times. Many techniques in peak alignment have been proposed including target peak alignment (TPA), dynamic time warping (DTW), fuzzy warping (FW), parametric time warping (PTW), semi-parametric time warping (STW)and correlation optimized warping (COW) (Christophe Tistaert et al.,2011). And then, data information of fingerprint profiles should be normalized by being organized in a data matrix.

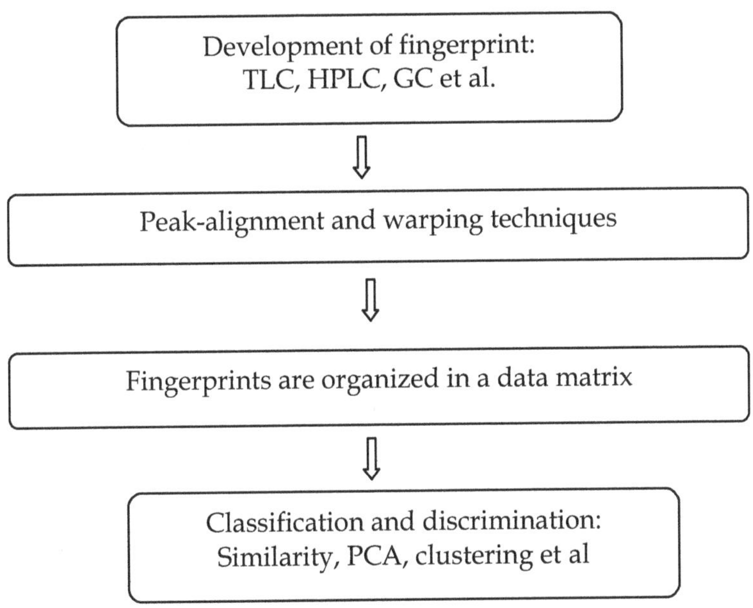

Fig. 1. The whole process of evaluation of chemical fingerprint of herbal medicine

The objective of this step is to achieve the relative proportions of the data (either peak height or peak area can be selected to express peak intensity) obtained from fingerprints. A chromatographic peak inheres in each profile is addressed as reference, and the ratio of peak height/area between other peaks and reference peak should be calculated in every sample. On the basis of the normalization processing, peaks whose peak height/area ratios change slightly in the same species but vary seriously between different species, could be picked out as candidate feature peaks using Stepwise Discriminant Analysis. The selected candidate feature peaks would be developed into characteristic spectrums that are used to evaluate the similarity and difference of fingerprints of analytes by some chemometric techniques such as Similarity Analysis, Principal Component Analysis, Clustering Analysis, etc.

Because of complexity and multiplicity of information from the fingerprints, pulsing minor differences in concentrations of some detected samples, more and more chemometric methods were applied to quality control and evaluation of HMs. Similarity comparison as one of the most common and earliest tools representing the equivalence of fingerprints of herbs, consists of both the point-point approach and the peak-peak approach. And the relationship within a set of fingerprints could be analyzed by (dis)similarity comparison of the substances with a certain standard fingerprint. So a reasonable standard (reference) should firstly be achieved. Popularly, the reference may be derived from not only standard extract or proportioned mixture of HMs (e.g. EGb761) but also computation by some mathematical methods (e.g. Principle Component Analysis) (Liang, Y.-Z., et al., 2004). Similarity evaluation could be achieved by many methods including congruence coefficient, correlation coefficient, distance coefficient, Nei coefficient, improved Nei coefficient, etc. These methods have their own characteristics and scope of application, which has be discussed in the reference (Nie L et al., 2005). Generally, congruence coefficient and correlation coefficient (Jin Y. et al., 2008)was the workhorse of chemometrics in the similarity analysis of data sets. However, it has been aware that the (dis)similarities of the herbal objects have shortcomings (Liang, Y.-Z., et al., 2004; Christophe Tistaert et al., 2011): a reference fingerprint is necessary, but in many instances, the herbal medicines, selected for producing reference fingerprints, often do not have the best efficacy, which might influence the outcome. And a second concern is the subjective threshold consideration for quality control and discrimination. Different thresholds may be used in different studies (Li Y. et al., 2010; Fan X.H. et al., 2005; Wei H. et al., 2010). And sometimes masking and swamping effects might occur, explicitly and implicitly.

In order to overcome the drawbacks of similarity evaluation, more methods appeared. Principal component analysis (PCA) and hierarchical cluster analysis (HCA) were used to discern HPLC fingerprints of 30 *Cortex cinnamomi* samples from different species and regions (Yang, J. et al., 2007). Ni et al. using pattern recognition models, PCA and HCA, successfully distinguished the fingerprints of 46 *Eucommia bark* samples originating from different locations, produced by the combination of LC-DAD and LC-MS techniques (Ni, Y. et al., 2008). Both PCA and HCA are exploratory data analysis tools which might be able to represent a multivariate data table as a low-dimensional plane: original variables are transformed into latent variables (LV) summarizing the systemic patterns of variation between the samples. Robust PCA (rPCA) (M.Hubert et al., 2001), Projection Pursuit (PP) (Daszykowski M. et al., 2002) also were devoted to gain insight in the structure of a multivariate data table as exploratory data analysis besides PCA and CA. Clustering techniques are divided into two subtypes: hierarchical (HCA) and non-hierarchical (FC, Fuzzy Clustering). And Hierarchical Clustering Analysis (HCA) is one of the most popular clustering techniques applied on herbal fingerprints, because of its flexibility to alter the similarity measurement criterion and the applied linkage method to suit different applications (Massart D.L. et al., 1997, as cited in Christophe Tistaert et al., 2011).

Another approach commonly used is Pattern Recognition that diverges from all above methods, as it makes use of discrete information on the samples in the calibration set. This information is described in a response vector Y. Recently, Pattern Recognition has been intensively used for the classification of data sets, including numerous linear and non-linear classification techniques. The most popular methods for the classification of herbal products include Linear Discriminant Analysis (LDA) (Lerma-García M.J et al., 2009; Ni Y. et al., 2008), K-nearest neighbors (k-NN) ,Artificial Neural Networks (ANN)(Tian R.T. et al.,2008),

Soft Independent Modelling of Class Analogy (SIMCA) (Chen Y. et al., 2008), Partial Least Squares–Discriminant Analysis (PLS-DA) (Toh D.F. et al., 2009) and Orthogonal Projections to Latent Structures–Discriminant Analysis (OPLS-DA) (Li S.L. et al., 2010). Advantage and disadvantage of each technique were reviewed in the literature (Christophe Tistaert et al., 2011).

3.3 Case study

The details of 3 carefully selected cases were discussed in this section, presenting establishment and evaluation of fingerprints.

Case I: Development, optimization and validation of a fingerprint of *Ginkgo biloba* extracts by high-performance liquid chromatography (Ji Y.B. et al., 2005)

This case presented four-step strategy for method development, optimization and validation of an HPLC fingerprint of *Ginkgo biloba* extracts (GBE 20030106): 1) Selection of a suitable chromatographic system including separation mode, stationary phase and mobile phase; 2) Screening design of some controllable parameters and the range of the factors; 3) Gradient optimization using a uniform design; 4) Methodology validation identical with that discussed in other cases. The theory of Screening design and uniform design could be discovered in the reference (Ji Y.B. et al.,2005,2006).

1) Selection of a suitable chromatographic system

Most compounds of interest are high polar components consisting of glycoside derivatives of quercetin, kaempferol and isorhamnetin, so reversed-phase liquid chromatography methods with ODS columns and acetonitrile–water mobile phases are recommended. Three columns were screened with a 30min-linear gradient elution, where acetonitrile/0.1% phosphoric acid (B/A; B%: 15%-30%) as mobile phase. And the Alltima C18 column (C) was selected according to selectivity and resolution. Then several mobile phases were investigated: methanol/ 0.1% phosphoric acid, acetonitrile/0.1% phosphoric acid and isopropanol and tetrahydrofuran added in mobile phase as organic modifier. Finally it was decided to use the chromatographic system consisting of the Alltima C18 column and an acetonitrile–0.1%phosphoric acid mobile phase combination.

Factor	Units	Level (-1)	Level (+1)
X1: concentration of phosphoric acid	%	0.1	0.5
X2: detector wavelength	nm	350	370
X3: column temperature	°C	30	50
X4: initial concentration of acetonitrile (B%)	%	12	18
X5: gradient time	min	30	50
X6: injection volume	μl	5	10
X7: concentration of isopropanol in mobile phase	%	0	10

Table 1. Factors and levels investigated in the screening design

2) Screening design

A fractional factorial design was utilized as screening design to identify significant main effects. The peak number was used as response and seven factors were examined (table 1). And the main effect plot determining the important factors and the best factor setting was shown in fig. 2. The main effect plots (Fig. 3) illustrated that detection wave-length and column temperature have main effects on the peak capacity (the total number of peaks observed). And it is reasonable that more information can be obtained using a higher injection volume.

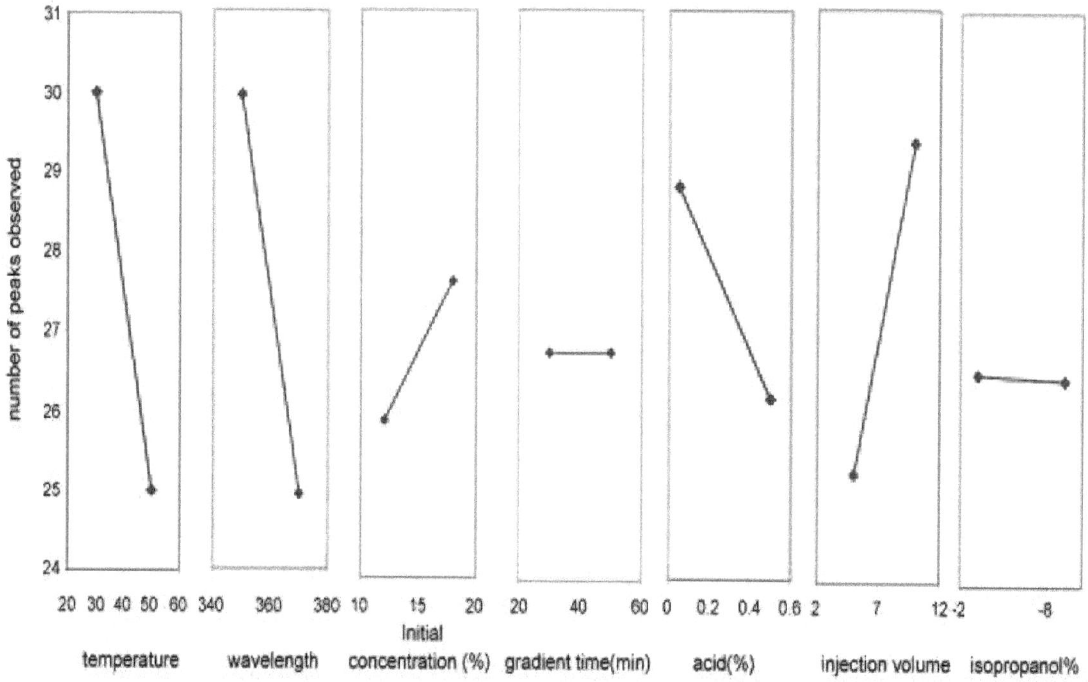

Fig. 2. Main effect plots from the screening design

From the results of the screening experiments, the values of some important controllable parameters can be selected and determined: detection wavelength (350nm), column temperature (30°C), acid concentration (0.1%) and injection volume (10μl), while no isopropanol was needed in the mobile phase. Another two factors, the initial concentration of organic solvent and the gradient time did not seem very important as presented in fig.2. However, the gradient optimization always be considered as a point of a general strategy to improve the HPLC separation. Hereby, it was selected for the next step.

3) Gradient optimization

Two parameters were chosen as optimization factors, the gradient time (t_G) and the concentration of organic solvent at the beginning of the gradient (B%). The optimization region selected was 28–52min for t_G and 11 to 17% for B%, according to the result of the screening experiment of step two. Uniform table U_7 (7^2) was given (table 2). And both the specific level investigated and the results including the values of hierarchical chromatographic response function (HCRF) were presented in table 3. HCRF can simultaneously assess the number of peaks that may be detected, the resolution and time of analysis.

No.	B_0(%)	t_G(min)	HCRF
1	14	40	43,068,057
2	13	52	41,068,045
3	15	28	39,056,069
4	12	32	39,034,066
5	11	44	40,067,053
6	17	36	41,080,057
7	16	48	46,068,049

Table 2. Uniform design table of $U_7(7^2)$

No.	Factor	
	X1	X2
1	4	4
2	3	7
3	5	1
4	2	2
5	1	5
6	7	3
7	6	6

Table 3. The result of the uniform design

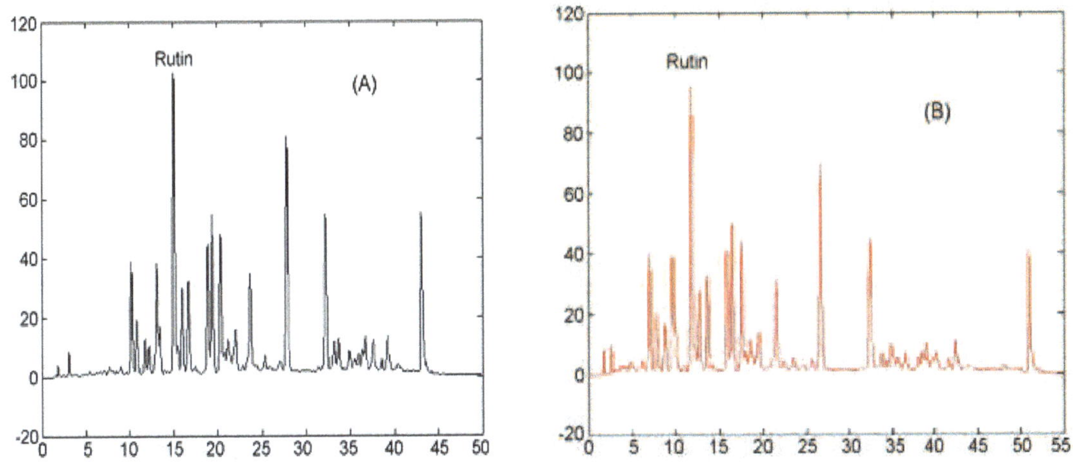

Fig. 3. HPLC fingerprints of *Ginkgo extract* in two different experiment conditions. (A) No. 1 (B) No. 7 experimental runs in a $U_7(7^2)$ design, HPLC conditions as in text

From the results of Table 3, the conditions of Experiment Nos.1 and 7 were selected (Fig. 3a and b). These two chromatograms are very similar, but shorter analysis time can be obtained in Fig. 3a, and the resolution of the peaks around 10min is better. So the conditions of Experiment No. 1 was chosen as optimized conditions: a linear gradient elution with acetonitrile/0.1% phosphoric acid (from 14/86 to 30/70 in 40min) as mobile phase, a column temperature of 30 °C, a detection wavelength of 350 nm, and an injection volume of 10 μl.

4) *Methodology validation*

The methodology of HPLC fingerprints from *Ginkgo biloba* extract was validated by identification and purity determination of chromatographic peaks, injection precision, repeatability and sample stability.

Conclusion and discussion

The process of development, optimization and validation of HPLC fingerprints of *Ginkgo biloba* extract was introduced in this case. The methods of development, optimization and validation of fingerprints are not limited to those discussed above, but all fingerprinting methods can be established imitating the process detailed in this part. A sequential procedure based on a uniform design approach was also applied in the development of CE fingerprints of *Ginkgo biloba* extract (Y.B. et al., 2006). Yet the authentic sample should be obtained or extracted from crude herbs before establishing the fingerprints, which is also very important for the final result. Recent developments in sample preparation techniques for the analysis, such as the extraction, clean-up, and concentration of analytes from HMs can be found in the references (Deng C.H et al., 2007). (Huie C.W., 2002).

Case II: Quantitative and chemical fingerprint analysis for quality control of *Rhizoma Coptidis chinensis* based on UPLC-PAD combined with chemometrics methods (Kong W.J. et al., 2009)

Rhizoma coptidis (Huanglian in Chinese), on one hand, as a traditional Chinese medicine, has been commonly used for the efficacy of suppressing fever, dispelling dampness, removing toxicosis and anti-microbes for many centuries, and on the other hand, phytochemical and modern pharmacological studies revealed that alkaloids therein it have the significant efficacy of anti-virus, anti-inflammatory, anti-cancer and anti-microbes (Huang et al. 2006; Enk et al. 2007; Hsu et al. 2007; Yan et al. 2008).

Since application of *Rhizoma Coptidis* is growing steadily, a quality control method using UPLC-PAD was developed to differentiate the *Rhizoma coptidis* from various sources by chemical fingerprints which were investigated by SA, HCA and PCA. Simultaneously, five markers were selected to carry out quantitative diagnosis. All the ten samples are dried and share the same origin: *Coptis chinensis Franch*. Sources and origins of raw herbs studied is presented in table 4.

Sample number	Sources	Harvesting time
S1	Shizhu, Sichuan	August, 2007
S2	Longchi, Sichuan	August, 2007
S3	Shuanghe, Hubei	September, 2007
S4	Huangshui,Chongqing	August, 2007
S5	Shizhu, Sichuan	December, 2007
S6	Huangshui,Chongqing	August, 2007
S7	Shizhu, Sichuan	February, 2007
S8	Wangsi, Sichuan	August, 2007
S9	Moudao, Hubei	September, 2007
S10	Xinchang, Sichuan	August, 2007

Table 4. Sources and origins of raw herbs

Development of fingerprint

In this study, the UPLC-PAD method was validated by linearity, detection limit and quantification limit, precision, reproducibility and stability after optimization. And then, ten fingerprints of *Rhizoma Coptidis* with reasonable heights and good resolutions were obtained.

Evaluation of fingerprints

There were 11 characteristic peaks (from peak 1 to peak 11) in the chromatogram, as shown in fig. 4B. Peaks purity was identified by comparison of retention time and PAD spectra. Peak 11 (berberine) with the biggest area peak, was chosen to calculate the relative retention time (RRT) and relative peak area (RPA) of all the other peaks.

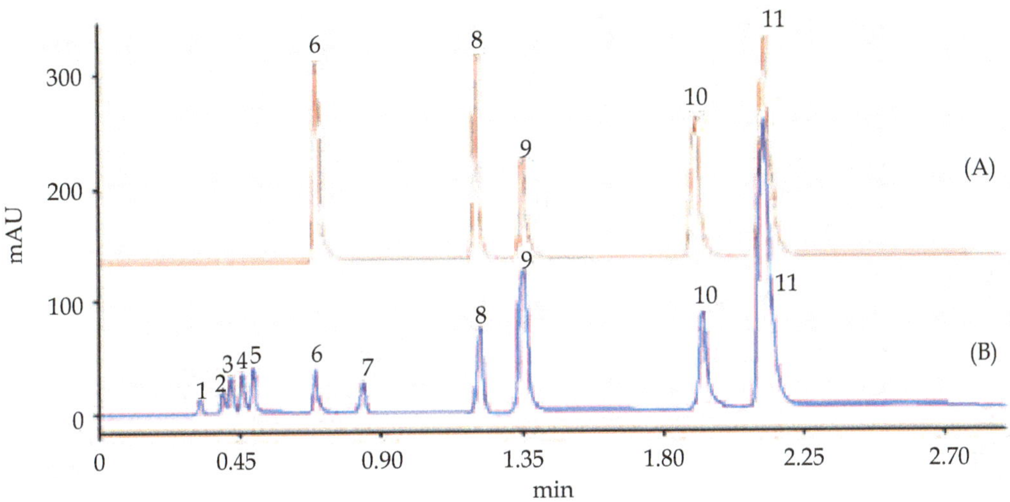

Fig. 4. Chromatogram of mixed standard compounds (A) and standardized chromatographic fingerprint of 10 batches *Rhizoma Coptidis* samples obtained by UPLC-PAD method at 350 nm(B)

Similarity analysis (SA)

The simulative mean chromatogram as reference fingerprint was derived from computation by Similarity Evaluation System for Chromatographic Fingerprint of Traditional Chinese Medicine. And the correlation coefficients between each fingerprint of *Rhizoma Coptidis* samples and the simulative mean chromatogram were 0.997, 0.981, 0.980, 0.983, 0.995, 0.971, 0.994, 0.981, 0.965 and 0.977, respectively. As we can see from the above results, different samples have different correlation coefficients and diverse internal quality. The correlation coefficients of the samples from the same source were similar, such as S1, S5 and S7, illustrating that productive origin is more influential than harvest time.

Hierarchical clustering analysis (HCA)

A hierarchical agglomerative clustering analysis was performed based on the relative peak areas of all the 11 common chromatographic peaks of *Rhizoma Coptidis* samples, using SPSS. The results of HCA as shown in Fig. 5, revealed the quality characteristics more clearly. Supposing an appropriate distance level (Level I) chosen, the samples could be classified into three quality clusters. Cluster-I including the samples collected from Shizhu city,

Sichuan province. The cluster II comprised the samples collected from other cities of Sichuan province and Chongqing city and cluster III was formed by samples collected from Hubei province. If a higher distance level (Level II) was adopted, the quality of samples was changed to two clusters, the first cluster comprised all samples collected from Sichuan province and Chongqing city, and the samples from Hubei province consisted in the second cluster.

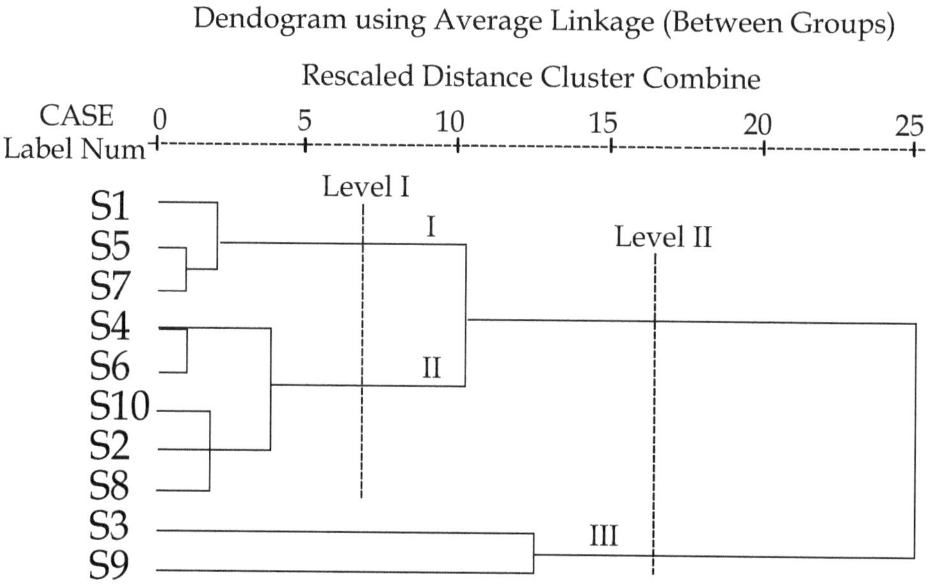

Fig. 5. Dendrogram of clustering of *Rhizoma coptidis* samples. This dendrogram was performed using SPSS 13.0 software (Chicago, USA). The Ward's method as the amalgamation rule and the squared Euclidean distance as metric were used to establish clusters

Principle component analysis (PCA)

PCA was employed to evaluate the discrimination ability of these common components used in SA and HCA, using the relative peak areas of common peaks as input data instead of the full fingerprints. The first two principal components PC1 and PC2 are used to present the inhomogeneity in the data sets. Fig. 6 showed the clear differentiation of samples in terms of cultivating locations, which is correspondence with the SA and same to HCA.

PCA analysis was also used to find the possible main chemical markers which have the most influence on the discrimination among different samples. For the log-centered data set with 81.26% of explained variance by the first two principal components, the loadings plot of the scores (Fig. 7) indicated that circled peaks 5, 8 (epiberberine), 9 (coptisine), 10 (palmatine), and 11 (berberine) may have more influence on the discrimination of the samples from different sources than other components. These peaks could be found in Fig. 4. The sequence of the total contents of the five alkaloids in different samples was S1 > S7 > S2 > S5 > S4 > S3 > S8 > S10 > S6 > S9. The higher content of five alkaloids, the better quality raw herbs have. This finding is also corresponding with the above results. So the five compounds may be used to qualitatively identify *Rhizoma coptidis* from various regions and harvest times.

Conclusion and discussion

A method with the combination of UPLC-PAD and chemometrics techniques in this study successfully classified ten samples of *Rhizoma Coptidis* from different regions, which is more effective than that in the official Chinese pharmacopoeia (China Pharmacopoeia Committee 2005). In Chinese pharmacopoeia berberine alone was detected for the quality evaluation of *Rhizoma Coptidis.*

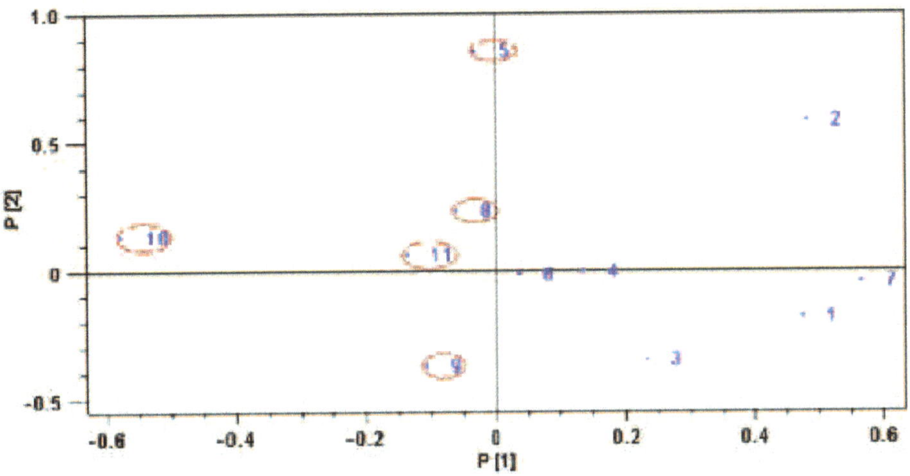

Fig. 6. The loadings plot from PCA for the common components. The loadings plot were performed with the original relative peak areas of the common compounds as input data using software of Unscrambler 9.7 from Camo AS (Trondheim, Norway); possible markers were marked with a circle

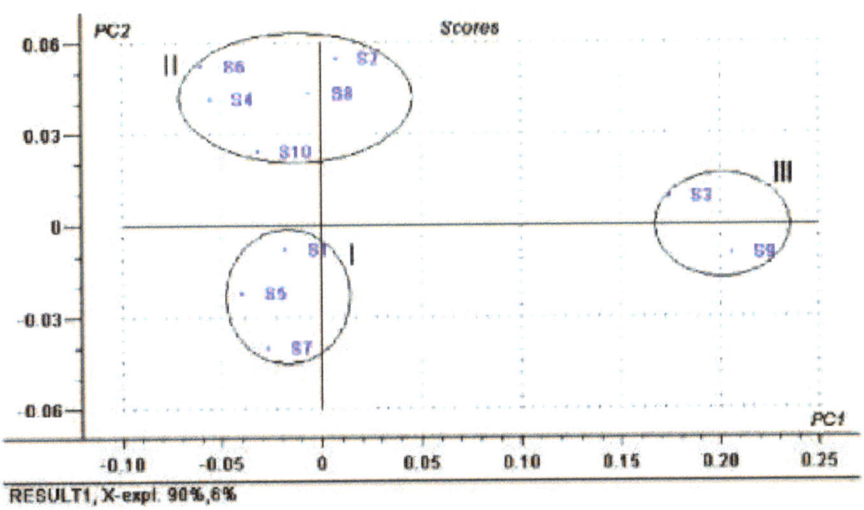

Fig. 7. Scores plot of PCA of *Rhizoma Coptidis* samples from various sources on the first two PCs. This plot of PCA on the first two PCs with the original peak areas of the 11 common compounds as input data was obtained using software of Unscrambler 9.7 from Camo AS (Trondheim, Norway). The labels of the sample refer to Table 4

The combination of fingerprint with multi-component quantification would be more powerful, because the qualitative and quantitative information of the analytes can be obtained at the same time. It has been proved to be a comprehensive method to assess the quality of herbs and herbal products. In this method, Zushima, Carthamus tinctorius and some preparations, such as ShuangHuang-lian oral liquid, xuesetong injection, etc. were successfully analyzed (Su J. et al., 2009; Fan L. et al., 2009; Cao Y.H. et al., 2006; Lai C.M. et al., 2005)

Case III: Combinative method using HPLC fingerprint and quantitative analyses for quality consistency evaluation of an herbal medicinal preparation produced by different manufacturers (Li Y, et al., 2010)

Yiqing is a medicinal preparation derived from the well-known traditional Chinese medicine (TCM) formula named San Huang Xie Xin (SHXX) decoction, composed of three herbs including *Rhizoma Coptidis* (*Coptis chinensis*), *Radix et Rhizoma Rhei* (*Rheum officinale*) and *Radix Scutellariae* (*Scutellaria baicalensis*). Fifteen samples (S1-15) of Yiqing preparations from twelve manufacturers were assessed using a combinative method of HPLC fingerprint and quantitative determination through analyzing nine bioactive compounds from Yiqing preparations. Meanwhile, four samples (S1-4) are different batches from one manufacture.

Development of fingerprint

Sample pretreatment conditions and HPLC chromatographic conditions were first optimized by investigating the effect of extraction solvents, extraction time and methods on the extraction efficiencies, and the effect of mobile phase and detection wavelength on the chromatographic separation efficiencies for marker compounds. And the optimal extraction and chromatographic conditions for Yiqing used in this study can be found in the literature (Li Y, et al., 2010). Consequently, a typical HPLC chromatogram fingerprint with satisfactory resolution of the nine chemical markers was shown in Fig. 8. Chromatographic fingerprints were achieved for 15 Yiqing samples from 12manufacturers, and about 40 peaks were found in each individual sample (Fig9. A). A simulative median fingerprint was generated by the professional software by analyzing all the 15 samples (Fig. 9B).

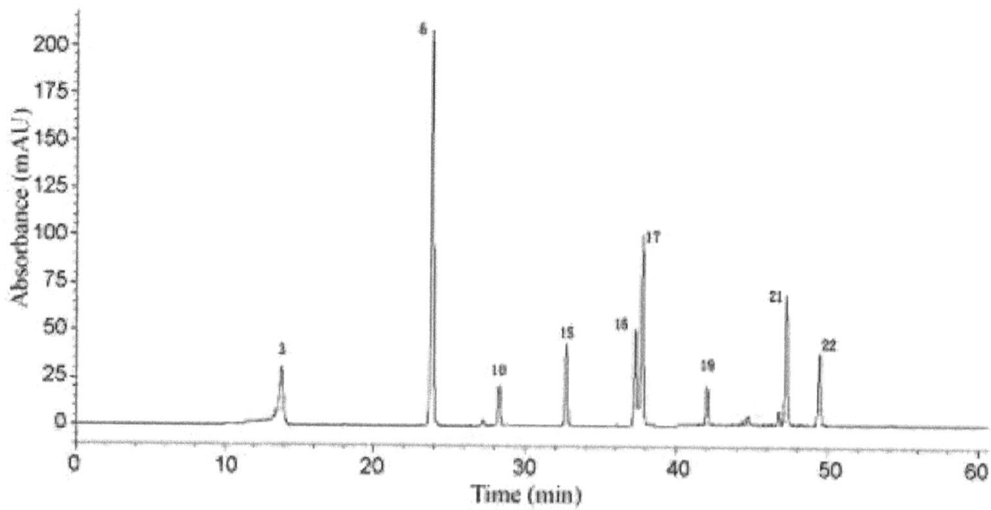

Fig. 8. The typical HPLC chromatographic profile of nine standards. The peaks marked with 3, 6, 10, 15, 16, 17, 19, 21 and 22 are berberine, baicalin, wogonoside, baicalein, wogonin, aloe-emodin, rhein, emodin and chrysophanol, respectively

Evaluation of fingerprints

15 samples' similarity values compared with simulative median fingerprint were 0.929, 0.982, 0.978, 0.978, 0.995, 0.997, 0.985, 0.987, 0.969, 0.781, 0.844, 0.980, 0.988, 0.780 and 0.978 respectively. Most of the similarity values were in the range of 0.992–0.997 for samples S1–S9, S12, S13, and S15, suggesting that similar chemical components were present in these samples regardless of manufacturer. But another three samples (S10, S11, and S14) demonstrated low similarity values of 0.871, 0.884 and 0.780, indicating that these three products were different from the other samples. Overall, the results from the chromatographic fingerprints illustrate that the principal components of Yiqing preparations were relatively stable.

Quantitative determination of the nine marker compounds

The Quantitative determination method was validated by the investigation of correlation coefficients, linear ranges, limit of detection (LOD) and limit of quantification (LOQ), intra-day and inter-day precision, repeatability and Recovery. The validation results indicated that the conditions used in the quantitative determination were acceptable. The contents of the nine marker compounds in 15 samples from 12 manufacturers were determined with above method. And the contents of each individual marker between manufacturers were different, and the RSD values are 118.20, 36.53, 115.20, 125.09, 116.31, 124.39, 128.05, 118.24, 100.92 respectively, almost of which beyond 100% except for baicalein (36.53%), indicating the large variations in their quality.

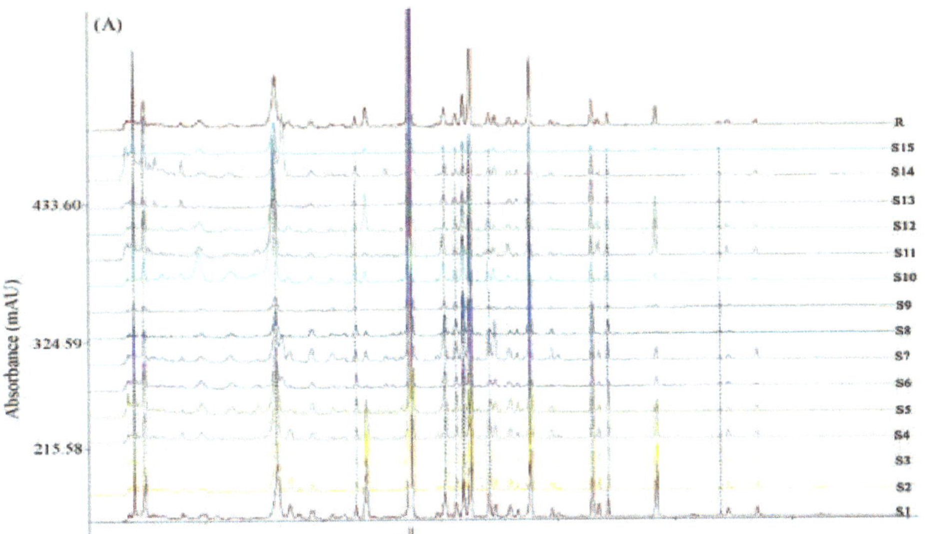

Fig. 9. HPLC chromatographic fingerprints of 15 Yiqing samples (A) and simulative median chromatogram obtained by Similarity Evaluation System for Chromatographic Fingerprint of Traditional Chinese Medicine software (B). The chromatograms marked with S1–S15, and R represents 15 Yiqing samples and the simulative median chromatogram, respectively. The peaks marked with 1–22 in the simulative median chromatogram represent 22 characteristic peaks

The HPLC fingerprint method combined with multi-component quantification utilized in this study is an efficient and comprehensive tool for quality control or consistency evaluations of herbal drugs and preparations. In terms of utilization of complex and large amount of information of fingerprints, chemometric techniques should be introduced into the study. It is believed that with chemometric techniques, much more principles could be found.

4. Conclusion

Due to long historical clinical use and reliable therapeutic efficiency, herbal medicines are attracting and increasing global attention. However, the herbal medicine's efficiency is based on their complex chemical constituents, so quality control of herbal medicine also raised the researchers' attention. Fingerprinting of herbal medicines is utilized on the authenticity and quality control of HMs and the total producing process of herbal preparation. The combination of qualitative fingerprinting and quantitive multi-component analysis is a novel and rational method to address the key issues of quality control of herbal medicine. This method is thought of more effective and rational than simple fingerprinting.

Generally speaking, fingerprinting technique concludes three phases: information acquisition, information processing and information excavation. Only if the specificity, reproducibility, stability of fingerprinting were guaranteed, a set of developed quality control standards could be established. However, to achieve good reproducibility and stability is not an easy task, because of the diversity of HMs' collection sources and time, processing methods, etc and the difference of experimental conditions (e.g. columns, solvents, equipment type, etc.) when analysis was undergoing. This is the main reason that fingerprinting technique is still hard to be generalized.

Fingerprinting analysis should be interdisciplinary collaborative researches involving the multi-dimensional fingerprint, efficacy testing and information processing. In fact, the fingerprint discussed in this chapter is the first step of quality control, because the discussed methods can only solve the problem of comparing the integrated sameness and difference of HMs, and controlling the stability of the available herbal products, the next step should combine the fingerprinting profiles with the therapeutic efficiency. In recent years, the fingerprint–efficacy study caused the scientists' interests, and many studies have been down or ongoing. For instance, for quality control of artificial Calculus bovis, an attempt on fingerprint–efficacy study of artificial C. bovis was developed in the literature (Kong W.J, et al., 2011). In this study, the chemical fingerprints of 10 batches of artificial C.bovis sample from various sources were established by UPLC–ELSD. Then, the antibacterial effects of these samples on E. coli growth were determined using microcalorimetry. The relationship between the fingerprints and efficacy of artificial C. bovis was elucidated. The fingerprint of most therapeutical HM should be determined as a reference for the quality control, and the result will be more convincing. Generally the fingerprint–efficacy study will provide a powerful way and feasible ideas for the quality control of HMs.

5. References

Bai C. C., Han S. Y., Chai X. Y., Jiang Y., Li P. & Tu P.F. (2009). Sensitive Determination of Saponins in Radix et Rhizoma Notoginseng by Charged Aerosol Detector Coupled with HPLC.*J. Liq. Chromatogr. Relat.Technol.* 32, (2009), pp.242-260, 1082-6076.

Cao Y. H., Wang L. C., Yu X. J. & Ye J. N. (2006). Development of the chromatographic fingerprint of herbal preparations Shuang–Huang–Lian oral liquid.*J. Pharm. Biomed. Anal.* 41, (June 2006), pp. 845-856, 0731-7085

Chen J.H., Wang F.M., Liu J., Lee F.S.C., Wang X.R. & Yang H.H. (2008). Analysis of alkaloids in *Coptis chinensis Franch* by accelerated solvent extraction combined with ultraperformance liquid chromatographic analysis with photodiode array and tandem mass spectrometry detections. *Anal. Chim. Acta.* 613, (2008), pp.184-195, 0003-2670

Chen S.B., Liu H.P., Tian R.T., Yang D.J., Chen S.L., Xu H.X, Albert S.C. Chana &Xie P.S.. (2006). High-performance thin-layer chromatographic fingerprints of isoflavonoids for distinguishing between *Radix Puerariae Lobate* and *Radix Puerariae Thomsonii. Chromatogr. A.* 1121, (July 2006), pp.114-119, 0021-9673

Chen Y., Zhu S.B., Xie M.Y., Nie S.P., Liu W., Li C., Gong X.F. & Wang Y.X. (2008). Quality control and original discrimination of *Ganoderma lucidum* based on high-performance liquid chromatographic fingerprints and combined chemometrics methods. *Anal. Chim. Acta.* 623, (August 2008), pp.146–156, 0003-2670

Chen W.D. , Zhan Q.F., Wu P, Ge X.W., Shu J.Z., Hui Y.Z., Wang J & Xu H.X. (2007). Study on Fingerprint of Herbal Material by Pyrolysis-GC/MS. *Journal of Chinese Mass Spectrometry Society*. 28, (2007), pp.267-274

Cheng K T, Chang H C, Su C H, & FL Hsu (1997). Identification of dried rhizomes of *coptis* species using random amplified polymorphic DNA. *Bot Bull Acad Sinica,* 38, (1997), p.241-244, 0006-8063

Christophe Tistaert, Bieke Dejaegher & Yvan Vander Heyden. (2011). Chromatographic separation techniques and data handling methods for herbal fingerprints: A review. *Analytica Chimica Acta.*690, (2011), pp.148–161, 0003-2670

Cui S.F., Fu B.Q., F.S.C. Lee & Wang X.R. (2005). Application of microemulsion thin layer chromatography for the fingerprinting of *licorice* (Glycyrrhiza spp.). *J. Chromatogr. B* 828 (December 2005), pp.33-40, 0378-4347

Di X, Kelvin K. C. Chan, Hei Wun Leung & Carmen W. Hui. (2003). Fingerprint profiling of acid hydrolyzates of polysaccharides extracted from the fruiting bodies and spores of Lingzhi by high-performance thin-layer chromatography. *J. Chromatogr. A.* 1018, (2003), pp.85-95, 0021-9673

Daszykowski M., Walczak B. & Massart D.L. (2002). Projection methods in chemistry. *Chemometr. Intell. Lab. Syst.* 65,(January 2003),pp. 97–112, 0169-7439

Deng C.H, Liu N., Gao M.X & Zhang X.M. (2007). Recent developments in sample preparation techniques for chromatography analysis of traditional Chinese medicines. *J. Chromatogr. A* .1153, (June 2007), pp. 90–96, 0021-9673

D.K.W. Mok & F.T. Chau (2006). Chemical information of Chinese medicines: A challenge to chemist. *J. Chemometrics and Intelligent Laboratory Systems* 82, (Sep. 2005), pp.210–217,0269–3879

Fan L, Zhao H.Y., Xu M., Zhou L., Guo H., Han J., Wang B.R. & Guo D.A. (2009). Qualitative evaluation and quantitative determination of 10 major active components in *Carthamus tinctorius L.* by high-performance liquid chromatography coupled with diode array detector. *J. Chromatogr. A.* 1216, (2009), pp.2063–2070, 0021-9673

Fan X.H., Y.Y. Cheng, Z.L. Ye, R.C. Lin & Z.Z. Qian (2005). Multiple chromatographic fingerprinting and its application to the quality control of herbal medicines. *Anal. Chim. Acta.* 555, (January 2006), pp.217–224, 0003-2670

Guo F.Q., Liang Y.Z., Xu C.J., Li X.N. & Huang L.F. (2004). Analyzing of the volatile chemical constituents in Artemisia *capillaris herba* by GC–MS and correlative chemometric resolution methods. *J. Journal of Pharmaceutical and Biomedical Analysis.* 35, (2004), pp.469–478, 0731-7085

He C.E, Wei J.-H., Jin Y & Chen S.-L. (2010). Bioactive components of the roots of *Salvia miltiorrhizae*: Changes related to harvest time and germplasm line Industrial *.Crops and Products* .32,(May 2010), pp.313–317, 0926-6690.

Huie C.W. (2002). A review of modern sample-preparation techniques for the extraction and analysis of medicinal plants. *J.Anal Bioanal Chem.* 373, (2002), pp.23–30, 1618-2642

Huang Y, Qin M. J., Yang G., Xu L.S. & Zhou K.Y., *Chinese Traditional and Herbal Drugs* Vol. 33, No.10,(2002)pp.935-937

Hermine Vogel, Mauricio González, Francesca Faini, Iván Razmilic, Jaime Rodríguez, José San Martín & Francisco Urbina. *Journal of Ethnopharmacology* 97 (2005), pp.97–100, 0378-8741

Ji Y.B., Xu Q.S., Hu Y.Z. & Yvan Vander Heyden (2005). Development, optimization and validation of a fingerprint of *Ginkgo biloba* extracts by high-performance liquid chromatography. *J. Chromatogr. A* 1066, (2005), pp. 97–104,0021-9673

Ji Y.B., Alaerts G., Xu C.J., Hu Y.Z. & Heyden Y.V. (2006). Sequential uniform designs for fingerprints development of *Ginkgo biloba* extracts by capillary electrophoresis. *J. Chromatogr. A.*1128, (2006), pp.273–281,0021-9673

Jiang B., F. Kronenberg, P. Nuntanakorn, Qiu M.H. & E.J. Kennelly (2006). Evaluation of the botanical authenticity and phytochemical profile of *black cohosh* products by high-performance liquid chromatography with selected ion monitoring liquid chromatography-mass spectrometry. *J. Agric. Food Chem.* 54, (May 2006), pp.3242-53, 0021-8561

Jiang Y, Li S.P., Wang Y.T., Chen X.J. & Tu P.F. (2008). Differentiation of *Herba Cistanches* by fingerprint with high-performance liquid chromatography–diode array detection–mass spectrometry. *J. Chromatogr. A* 1216 (March 2009) 2156–2162, 0021-9673

Jiang Y, Bruno David, Tu P.F. & Yves Barbin (2010). Recent analytical approaches in quality control of traditional Chinese medicines—A review. J. *Analytica Chimica Acta.* 657, (2010), pp.9–18, 0003-2670

Jin Y, Liang T, Fu Qi, Xiao Y.S., Feng X.T, Ke Y.X. & Liang X.M. (2008). Fingerprint analysis of Ligusticum chuanxiong using hydrophilic interaction chromatography and reversed-phase liquid chromatography. *J. Chromatogr. A.*1216, (March 2009), pp.2136–2141,0021-9673

Jin C, Kong W, Luo Y, Wang Jo, Wang H, Li Q & Xiao X. (2010). Development and validation of UPLC method for quality control of *Curcuma longaLinn.*: Fast simultaneous quantitation of three curcuminoids. *Journal of Pharmaceutical and Biomedical Analysis.* 53, (2010), pp.43–49 0731-7085

Kong W.J., Zhao Y.L., Xiao X.H., Jin C & Z L.L. (2009). Quantitative and chemical fingerprint analysis for quality control of *Rhizoma Coptidis chinensis* based on UPLC-PAD combined with chemometrics methods. *Phytomedicine* 16, (2009), pp.950–959, 0944-7113

Kong W.J, Wang J.B, Zang Q.C, Xing X.Y., Zhao Y.L., Liu W., Jin C., Li Z.L. & Xiao X.H. (2011). Fingerprint-efficacy study of artificial *Calculus bovis* in quality control of Chinese materia medica. *J.Food Chemistry*. 3, (2011), PP.1342-1347, 0308-8146

Lai CM, Li SP, Yu H Wan J.B., Kan K.W. & Wang Y.T. (2005). A rapid HPLC-ESI-MS/MS for qualitative and quantitative analysis of saponins in "XUESETONG" injection. *J Pharm and Biomed Anal*.40, (2006), pp.669-678,0731-7085.

Lerma-García M.J., Lantano C., Chiavaro E., Cerretani L., Herrero-Martínez J.M. & Simó-Alfonso E.F. (2009). Classification of extra virgin olive oils according to their geographical origin using phenolic compound profiles obtained by capillary electrochromatography. *Food Res. Int.* 42, (2009), pp.1446–1452, 0963-9969

Li S.L., Song J.Z., Qiao C.F., Zhou Y., Qian K.D., Kuo-Hsiung Leeb & Xu H.X. (2009). A novel strategy to rapidly explore potential chemical markers for the discrimination between raw and processed *Radix Rehmanniae* by UHPLC–TOFMS with multivariate statistical analysis. *Journal of Pharmaceutical and Biomedical Analysis*. 51, (2010), pp.812–823, 0731-7085

Li S.L., Shuk-Fan Lai, Song J.Z., Qiao C.F., Liu X, Zhou Y, Cai H, Cai B.C. & Xu H.X. (2010). Decocting-induced chemical transformations and global quality of Du–Shen–Tang, the decoction of ginseng evaluated by UPLC-Q-TOF-MS/MS based chemical profiling approach. *Journal of Pharmaceutical and Biomedical Analysis* 53 (2010) 946–957,0731-7085

Li S.L., Song J.Z., Qiao C.F., Zhou Y., Qian K.D. & Xu H.X. (2010). UPLC–PDA–TOFMS based chemical profiling approach to rapidly evaluate chemical consistency between traditional and dispensing granule decoctions of traditional medicine combinatorial formulae. *Journal of Pharmaceutical and Biomedical Analysis*. 52, (2010), pp.468–478, 0731-7085

Li Y., Wu T., Zhu J., Wan L., Yu Q., Li X., Cheng Z. & Guo C. (2010). Combinative method using HPLC fingerprint and quantitative analyses for quality consistency evaluation of an herbal medicinal preparation produced by different manufacturers .*J. Pharm. Biomed. Anal.* 52, (August 2010), pp.597–602,0731-7085

Liang, Y.-Z. Xie P.S. & Chan Kelvin. (2004). Quality control of herbal medicines. *Chromatogr. B* 812, (August 2004) pp.53–70,1570-0232.

Liang X.M., JinY, WangY.P, Jin G.W., Fu Q & Xiao Y.S. (2009). Qualitative and quantitative analysis in quality control of traditional Chinese medicines. *J. Chromatogr. A* .1216, (July 2008), pp.2033–2044, 0021-9673

Liu G.Z., Ma J.Y., Chen Y.Z., Tian Q.Q., Shen Y, Wang X.S., Bo C & Yao S.Z. (2009). Investigation of flavonoid profile of *Scutellaria bacalensis Georgi* by high performance liquid chromatography with diode array detection and electrospray ion trap mass spectrometry *J. Chromatogr. A* 1216 (June 2009) 4809–4814, 0021-9673

Liu W, Kong Y, Zu Y.G., Fu Y.J, Luo M, Zhang L & Li J. (2010). Determination and quantification of active phenolic compounds in *pigeon pea leaves* and its medicinal product using liquid chromatography–tandem mass spectrometry. *J. Chromatogr. A.* 1217, (July 2010), 4723–4731, 0021-9673

Liu H, Du Z.X. & Yuan Q.P. (2009). A novel rapid method for simultaneous determination of eight active compounds in silymarin using a reversed-phase UPLC-UV detector. *J. Chromatogr. B.* 877, (2009), pp.4159–4163, 1570-0232

Lu Y. & Chen D.F. (2008). Analysis of *Schisandra chinensis* and *Schisandra sphenanthera*. *J. Chromatogr. A* 1216, (2009), pp.1980–1990, 0021-9673

Ma C.-H., Adam R. Kavalier, Jiang B. & Edward J. Kennelly. Metabolic profiling of *Actaea* species extracts using high performance liquid chromatography coupled with electrospray ionization time-of-flight mass spectrometry. *Chromatogr. A* 1218, (2011), pp.1461–1476, 0021-9673

Min-Hwan Jeon, Ha-Jeong Kwon, Ji-Seon Jeong, Yong-Moon Lee & Seon-Pyo Hong (2009). Detection of albiflorin and paeoniflorin in Paeoniae Radix by reversed-phase high-performance liquid chromatography with pulsed amperometric detection. *J. Chromatogr. A* 1216, (March 2009), pp.4568–4573, 0021-9673

M.Hubert P. J. Rousseeuw & S.Verboven (2001). A fast method for robust principal components with applications to chemometrics. *Chemometr. Intell. Lab. Syst.* 60, (January 2002),pp.101–111, 0169-7439

Ni Y., Peng Y. & Kokot S. (2008). Fingerprinting of complex mixtures with the use of high performance liquid chromatography, inductively coupled plasma atomic emission spectroscopy and chemometrics. *Anal. Chim. Acta.* 616, (May 2008), pp.19–27, 0003-2670

Ni, Y., Peng, Y. & Koko, t S. (2008). Fingerprint analysis of *Eucommia bark* by LC-DAD and LC-MS with the aid of chemometrics. *Chromatographia* 67, (2008), pp.211−217, 0009-5893

Nie L, Cao J, Luo G.A. & Wang Y.M. (2005). Comparison of different methods for evaluating the similarity of the fingerprints of traditional Chinese medicines. *J. Chinese Traditional Patent Medicine.* 27,(2005),PP.249-252

Pan R.-J., Guo F.-Q., Lu H.-M., Feng W.-W. & Liang Y.-Z. (2011). Development of the chromatographic fingerprint of *Scutellaria barbata D.* Don by GC–MS combined with Chemometrics methods. *Journal of Pharmaceutical and Biomedical Analysis,* 55,(2011),pp.391–396, 0731-7085.

Qi L.W., Li P., Ren M.T., Yu Q.T., Wen X.D. & Wang Y.X. (2008). Application of high-performance liquid chromatography–electrospray ionization time-of-flight mass spectrometry for analysis and quality control of *Radix Astragali* and its preparations. *J. Chromatogr. A* 1216, (2009), 2087–2097,0021-9673

Qiu YQ, Lu X, Pang T, Zhu S.-H., Kong H.-W. & Xu G.W. (2007). Study of traditional Chinese medicine volatile oils from different geographical origins by comprehensive two-dimensional gas chromatography - time-of-flight mass spectrometry (GC×GC-TOFMS) in combination with multivariate analysis. *Journal of Pharmaceutical and Biomedical Analysis.*43, (January 2007) pp.1721–1727, 0731-7085.

R.W. Dixon & D.S. Peterson (2002). Development and Testing of a Detection Method for Liquid Chromatography Based on Aerosol Charging. *Anal. Chem.* 74, (2002), pp.2930-37, 0003-2700

Sombra L. L., Gómez M.R., Olsina R., Martínez L. D. & Silva M.F. (2004). Comparative study between capillary electrophoresis and high performance liquid chromatography in 'guarana' based phytopharmaceuticals. *Journal of Pharmaceutical and Biomedical Analysis.* 36, (2005), pp.989–994, 0731-7085

Su J, Zhang C, Zhang W, Shen Y.H., Li H.L., Liu R.H., Zhang X, Hu X.J. &Zhang W.D. (2008). Qualitative and quantitative determination of the major coumarins in

Zushima by high performance liquid chromatography with diode array detector and mass spectrometry. *J. Chromatogr. A* 1216 (2009) 2111–2117

Sun Y, Guo T, Sui Y & Li F. (2003). Fingerprint analysis of *Flos Carthami* by capillary electrophoresis. J. Chromatogr. B. 792, (2003), pp.147–152, 1570-0232

Tian R.T., Xie P.S. & Liu H.P. (2008). Evaluation of traditional Chinese herbal medicine: Chaihu (Bupleuri Radix) by both high-performance liquid chromatographic and high-performance thin-layer chromatographic fingerprint and chemometric analysis. *J.Chromatogr.A.* 1216, (2009), pp.2150–2155, 0021-9673

The State Pharmacopoeia Commission of People's Republic of China (2005). Pharmacopoeia of the People's Republic of China Beijing: Chemical Industry Press (2005), 7-117-06983-X/R·6984

Toh D.F., New L.S., Koh H.L. & Chan E.C.Y. (2009). Ultra-high performance liquid chromatography/time-of-flight mass spectrometry (UHPLC/TOFMS) for time-dependent profiling of raw and steamed Panax notoginseng. *J. Pharm. Biomed. Anal.*. 52,(May 2010),pp.43–50,0731-7085

Wang H.L., Yao W. F., Zhu D.N. & Hu Y.Z. (2010). Chemical Fingerprinting by HPLC-DAD-ELSD and Principal Component Analysis of Polygala japonica from Different Locations in China. *J.Chinese Journal of Natural Medicines.* 8, sep.2010), pp.343–348

Wei H., Sun L., Tai Z., Gao S., Xu W. & Chen W. (2010). A simple and sensitive HPLC method for the simultaneous determination of eight bioactive components and fingerprint analysis of Schisandra sphenanthera. *Anal. Chim. Acta* .662,(2010),pp.97–104, 0003-2670

Xie P.S., Chen S.B., Liang Y.Z., Wang X.H., Tian R.T. & Roy Upton (2006). Chromatographic fingerprint analysis—a rational approach for quality assessment of traditional Chinese herbal medicine *J. Chromatogr. A* 1112 (2006), pp.171–180,0021-9673

Xu L, Li-Juan Tang, Chen-Bo Cai, Hai-Long Wu, Guo-Li Shen, Ru-Qin Yu & Jian-Hui Jiang. (2008) Chemometric methods for evaluation of chromatographic separation quality from two-way data—A review. *analytica chimica acta.* 613, (2008), pp.121–134, 0003-2670

Yang, J., Chen, L.H., Zhang, Q., Lai M.X., & Wang Q. (2007). Quality assessment of Cortex cinnamomi by HPLC chemical fingerprint, principle component analysis and cluster analysis. *Journal of Separation Science* 30, (2007), pp.1276–1283, 1615-9306

Zeng Y.-X.,et al. (2007). Comparative analysis of volatile components from Clematis species growing in China. *Analytica Chimica Acta*, 595, (2007) pp.328–339, 0003-2670

Zhang YY, Dan M, Wu J.-B, Yang H.-Z, Huang H, Qi Y, Wei S.-D., Toru Okuyama,& Kaoru Nakajima. (2008). Study on the Chromatographic Fingerprinting of *Schisandra chinensis* (Turcz.) Baill. by LC Coupled with Principal Component Analysis. *Chromatographia* 68 (July 2008), pp.101-104, 0009-5893

Zeng Z.D., Foo-tim Chau, Hoi-yan Chan, Chui-yee Cheung, Tsui-yan Lau, Wei S.Y., Daniel Kam-wah Mok, Chi-on Chan & Liang Y.Z. (2008). Recent advances in the compound-oriented and pattern-oriented approaches to the quality control of herbal medicines. *Chinese medicine.* (August 2008), pp.3:9

Zhou F.R., Zhao M.B., Tu P.F. (2008). Qualitative evaluation and quantitative determination of 10 major active components in *Carthamus tinctorius L.* by high-performance liquid chromatography coupled with diode array detector. *J. Chromatogr. A* 1216, (2009), pp.2063–2070, 0021-9673

Wang C.Z., Li P., Ding J.Y., Peng X. & Yuan C.S. (2007). Simultaneous identification of Bulbus Fritillariae cirrhosae using PCR-RFLP analysis. *Phytomedicine.* 14, (2007), pp. 628-32, 0944-7113

Wang L.C., Cao Y.H., Xing X.P. & Ye J.N. (2005). Fingerprint Studies of Radix Scutellariae by Capillary Electrophoresis and High Performance Liquid Chromatography. *Chromatographia.* 62, (July 2005), pp.283–288, 0009-5893.

Zhang X., Xu Q., Xiao H., Liang X., Huang L. &Liu (2006). J. World Sci. Tech./Modern Trad. Chin. Med. Mat. Med. 8, (2006), pp.33.

Zheng X.T., Shi P.Y., Cheng Y.Y. & Qu H.B. (2008). Rapid analysis of a Chinese herbal prescription by liquid chromatography–time-of-flight tandem mass spectrometry. *J. Chromatogr. A.* 1206, (2008), pp.140-146,0026-9673

9

Validation of an Analytical Procedure

Ahmed Badr Eldin
Sigma Pharmaceutical Corp.,
Egypt

1. Introduction

Validation of an analytical procedure is performed in order to demonstrate that the procedure is suitable for its intended use. Validation is performed in order to show that the result(s) generated by a particular analytical procedure are reliable and accurate.
The principles and practices of validation of analytical procedures are covered by the International Conference on Harmonisation (ICH) and are published as guideline Q2 (R1), "Validation of Analytical Procedures: Text and Methodology". A full discussion of the terms and methodology applicable to validation of analytical procedures is provided in these documents.

2. Contents of the validation protocol for analytical method

- Statement of purpose and scope
- Responsibilities
- Documented test method
- List of materials and equipment
- Procedure for the experiments for each parameter
- Statistical analysis
- Acceptance criteria for each performance parameter

Full validation is necessary if;

- The method of synthesis changed from that of patented innovator's method
- Changes in the composition of the drug product (excipients, ...etc),
- Changes in the analytical procedure (critical change)
- Or if the method is not cited in the compendia (USP/BP/Eur. Ph)

Typical analytical performance characteristics that should be considered :
Accuracy - Precision - Specificity - Detection limit - Quantitation limit - Linearity - Range - Ruggedness[1]

3. Analytical performance characteristics

Specificity

Definition— The ICH documents define specificity as the ability to assess unequivocally the analyte in the presence of components that may be expected to be present, such as impurities, degradation products, and matrix components. Lack of specificity of an individual analytical procedure may be compensated for by other supporting analytical procedures. [NOTE— Other reputable international authorities (IUPAC, AOAC) have preferred the term "selectivity," reserving "specificity" for procedures that are completely selective.] For the test or assay methods below, the above definition has the following implications:

Identification tests— ensure the identity of the analyte.

Purity tests— ensure that all the analytical procedures performed allow an accurate statement of the content of impurities of an analyte (e.g., related substances test, heavy metals limit, organic volatile impurity limit).

Assays— provide an exact result, which allows an accurate statement on the content or potency of the analyte in a sample[1].

Determination— In qualitative analyses (identification tests), the ability to select between compounds of closely related structure that are likely to be present should be demonstrated. This ability should be confirmed by obtaining positive results (perhaps by comparison to a known reference material) from samples containing the analyte, coupled with negative results from samples that do not contain the analyte, and by confirming that a positive response is not obtained from materials structurally similar to or closely related to the analyte.

In an analytical procedure for impurities, specificity may be established by spiking the drug substance or product with appropriate levels of impurities and demonstrating that these impurities are determined with appropriate accuracy and precision. In an assay, demonstration of specificity requires that it can be shown that the procedure is unaffected by the presence of impurities or excipients. In practice, this can be done by spiking the drug substance or product with appropriate levels of impurities or excipients and demonstrating that the assay result is unaffected by the presence of these extraneous materials. If impurity or degradation product standards are unavailable, specificity may be demonstrated by comparing the test results of samples containing impurities or degradation products to a second well-characterized procedure (e.g., a pharmacopeial or other validated procedure). These comparisons should include samples stored under relevant stress conditions (e.g., light, heat, humidity, acid or base hydrolysis, oxidation). In an assay, the results should be compared; in chromatographic impurity tests, the impurity profiles should be compared. The ICH documents state that when[2] chromatographic procedures are used, representative chromatograms should be presented to demonstrate the degree of selectivity, and peaks should be appropriately labeled. Peak purity tests (e.g., using diode array or mass spectrometry) may be useful to show that the analyte chromatographic peak is not attributable to more than one component.

Linearity and range

Definition of Linearity— The linearity of an analytical method is its ability to elicit test results that are directly, or by a well-defined mathematical transformation, proportional to the concentration of analyte in samples within a given range.

Definition of Range— The range of an analytical method is the interval between the upper and lower levels of analyte (including these levels) that has been demonstrated to be determined with a suitable level of precision, accuracy, and linearity using the method as written. The range is normally expressed in the same units as test results (e.g., percent, parts per million) obtained by the analytical method. [1]

Determination of Linearity and Range— Linearity should be established across the range of the analytical procedure. It should be established initially by visual examination of a plot of signals as a function of analyte concentration of content. If there appears to be a linear relationship, test results should be established by appropriate statistical methods (e.g., by calculation of a regression line by the method of least squares). In some cases, to obtain linearity between the response of an analyte and its concentration, the test data may have to be subjected to a mathematical transformation. Data from the regression line itself may be helpful for providing mathematical estimates of the degree of linearity. The correlation coefficient, y-intercept, slope of the regression line, and residual sum of squares should be submitted. The range of the method is validated by verifying that the analytical method provides acceptable precision, accuracy, and linearity when applied to samples containing analyte at the extremes of the range as well as within the range.

ICH recommends that, for the establishment of linearity, a minimum of five concentrations normally be used. It is also recommended that the following minimum specified ranges should be considered:

Assay of a drug substance (or a finished product): from 80% to 120% of the test concentration.

Determination of an impurity: from 50% to 120% of the specification.

For content uniformity: a minimum of 70% to 130% of the test concentration, unless a wider or more appropriate range, based on the nature of the dosage form (e.g., metered-dose inhalers) is justified[1].

For dissolution testing: ±20% over the specified range (e.g., if the specifications for a controlled-release product cover a region from 20% after 1 hour, and up to 90% after 24 hours, the validated range would be 0% to 110% of the label claim).

Example:

The effect of varying the concentration of Misoprostol on its peak area is given in table 1

Peak area of Misoprostol	Concentration of Misoprostol (mcg / ml)	Concentration level (%)
355721.5	4.80	60
473319.5	6.40	80
591304.5	*8.00	100
702642	9.60	120
823837.5	11.20	140

* Concentration similar to that used in the test solution in the assay method.

Table 1. Effect of concentration of Misoprostol on its peak area

The regression equation is:

$$PA = C * 72847.15625 + 6587.75$$

Where:

PA: peak area

C: conc. (mcg / ml)

Note: Slope: 72847.156 - Intercept: 6587.75 - r: 0.9999, indicting good linear relationship

-A linear relationship exists between the peak area and the concentration of Misoprostol

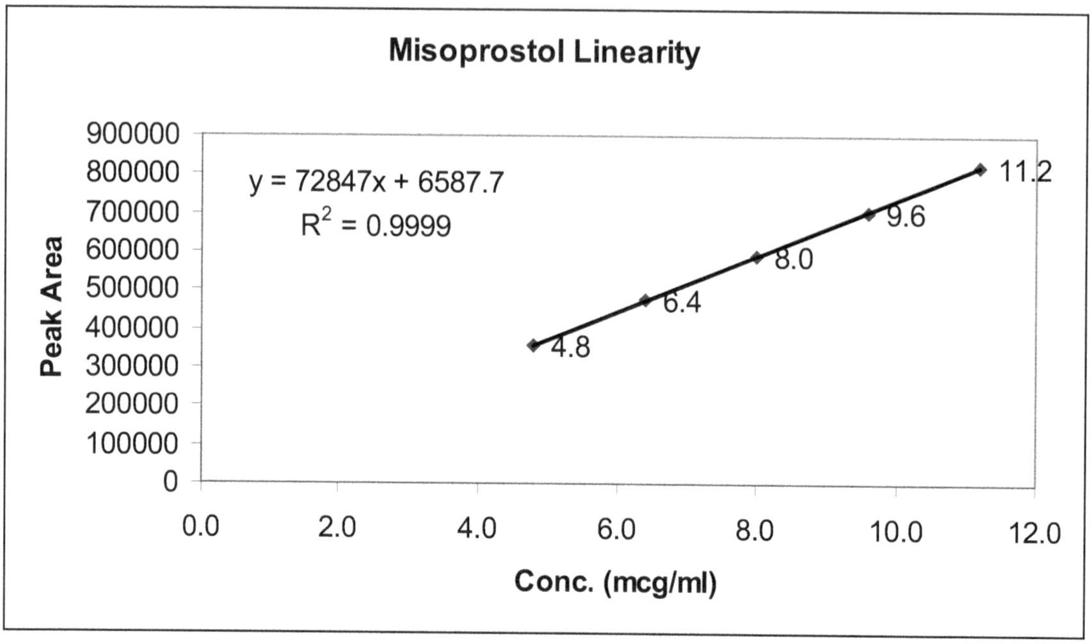

Fig. 1. A linear relationship exists between the peak area and the concentration of Misoprostol

[Example was taken from analytical method validation for Misotac 200 mcg tablets, produced by SIGMA pharmaceutical industries]

Accuracy

Definition— The accuracy of an analytical method is the closeness of test results obtained by that method to the true value. The accuracy of an analytical method should be established across its range. [2]

Determination— In assay of a drug substance, accuracy may be determined by application of the analytical method to an analyte of known purity (e.g., a Reference Standard) or by comparison of the results of the method with those of a second, well-characterized method, the accuracy of which has been stated or defined. In assay of a drug in a formulated product, accuracy may be determined by application of the analytical method to synthetic mixtures of the drug product components to which known amounts of analyte have been added within the range of the method. If it is not possible to obtain samples of all drug product components, it may be acceptable either to add known quantities of the analyte to the drug product (i.e., to "spike") or to compare results with those of a second, well-characterized method, the accuracy of which has been stated or defined. In quantitative analysis of impurities, accuracy should be assessed on samples (of drug substance or drug product) spiked with known amounts of impurities. Where it is not possible to obtain samples of certain impurities or degradation products, results should be compared with those obtained by an independent method. In the absence of other information, it may be necessary to calculate the amount of an impurity on the basis of comparison of its response to that of the drug substance; the ratio of the responses of equal amounts of the impurity and the drug substance (response factor) should be used if known.

Accuracy is calculated as the percentage of recovery by the assay of the known added amount of analyte in the sample, or as the difference between the mean and the accepted true value, together with confidence intervals.

The ICH documents recommend that accuracy be assessed using a minimum of nine determinations over a minimum of three concentration levels, covering the specified range (i.e., three concentrations and three replicates of each concentration) [3].

Precision

Definition— The precision of an analytical method is the degree of agreement among individual test results when the method is applied repeatedly to multiple samplings of a homogeneous sample. The precision of an analytical method is usually expressed as the standard deviation or relative standard deviation (coefficient of variation) of a series of measurements. Precision may be a measure of either the degree of reproducibility or repeatability of the analytical method under normal operating conditions. In this context, reproducibility refers to the use of the analytical procedure in different laboratories, as in a collaborative study. Intermediate precision expresses within-laboratory variation, as on different days, or with different analysts or equipment within the same laboratory. Repeatability refers to the use of the analytical procedure within a laboratory over a short period of time using the same analyst with the same equipment. For most purposes, repeatability is the criterion of concern in USP analytical procedures, although reproducibility between laboratories or intermediate precision may well be considered during the standardization of a procedure before it is submitted to the Pharmacopeia.

Determination— The precision of an analytical method is determined by assaying a sufficient number of aliquots of a homogeneous sample to be able to calculate statistically valid estimates of standard deviation or relative standard deviation (coefficient of variation). Assays in this context are independent analyses of samples that have been carried through the complete analytical procedure from sample preparation to final test result.

The ICH documents recommend that repeatability should be assessed using a minimum of nine determinations covering the specified range for the procedure (i.e., three concentrations and three replicates of each concentration, or a minimum of six determinations at 100% of the test concentration) [3].

Detection limit

Definition— The detection limit is a characteristic of limit tests. It is the lowest amount of analyte in a sample that can be detected, but not necessarily quantitated, under the stated experimental conditions. Thus, limit tests merely substantiate that the amount of analyte is above or below a certain level. The detection limit is usually expressed as the concentration of analyte (e.g., percentage, parts per billion) in the sample.

Determination— For noninstrumental methods, the detection limit is generally determined by the analysis of samples with known concentrations of analyte and by establishing the minimum level at which the analyte can be reliably detected[3].

For instrumental procedures, the same method may be used as for noninstrumental. In the case of methods submitted for consideration as official compendial methods, it is almost never necessary to determine the actual detection limit. Rather, the detection limit is shown to be sufficiently low by the analysis of samples with known concentrations of analyte above and below the required detection level. For example, if it is required to detect an impurity at the level of 0.1%, it should be demonstrated that the procedure will reliably detect the impurity at that level.

In the case of instrumental analytical procedures that exhibit background noise, the ICH documents describe a common approach, which is to compare measured signals from

samples with known low concentrations of analyte with those of blank samples. The minimum concentration at which the analyte can reliably be detected is established. Typically acceptable signal-to-noise ratios are 2:1 or 3:1. Other approaches depend on the determination of the slope of the calibration curve and the standard deviation of responses.
Where LOD = 3/Slope
S = slope of calibration curve
S may be carried out based on SD of blank or calibration curve
Whatever method is used, the detection limit should be subsequently validated by the analysis of a suitable number of samples known to be near, or prepared at, the detection limit. [3]

Quantitation limit

Definition— The quantitation limit is a characteristic of quantitative assays for low levels of compounds in sample matrices, such as impurities in bulk drug substances and degradation products in finished pharmaceuticals. It is the lowest amount of analyte in a sample that can be determined with acceptable precision and accuracy under the stated experimental conditions. The quantitation limit is expressed as the concentration of analyte (e.g., percentage, parts per billion) in the sample.
Determination— For noninstrumental methods, the quantitation limit is generally determined by the analysis of samples with known concentrations of analyte and by establishing the minimum level at which the analyte can be determined with acceptable accuracy and precision. For instrumental procedures, the same method may be used as for noninstrumental. In the case of methods submitted for consideration as official compendial methods, it is almost never necessary to determine the actual quantitation limit. Rather, the quantitation limit is shown to be sufficiently low by the analysis of samples with known concentrations of analyte above and below the quantitation level. For example, if it is required to assay an analyte at the level of 0.1 mg per tablet, it should be demonstrated that the method will reliably quantitate the analyte at that level. In the case of instrumental analytical methods that exhibit background noise, the ICH documents describe a common approach, which is to compare measured signals from samples with known low concentrations of analyte with those of blank samples. The minimum concentration at which the analyte can reliably be quantified is established. A typically acceptable signal-to-noise ratio is 10:1. Other approaches depend on the determination of the slope of the calibration curve and the standard deviation of responses. Whatever method is used, the quantitation limit should be subsequently validated by the analysis of a suitable number of samples known to be near, or prepared at, the quantitation limit[3].

Ruggedness

Definition— The ruggedness of an analytical method is the degree of reproducibility of test results obtained by the analysis of the same samples under a variety of conditions, such as different laboratories, analysts, instruments, lots of reagents, elapsed assay times, assay temperatures, or days. Ruggedness is normally expressed as the lack of influence on test results of operational and environmental variables of the analytical method. Ruggedness is a measure of reproducibility of test results under the variation in conditions normally expected from laboratory to laboratory and from analyst to analyst.
Determination— The ruggedness of an analytical method is determined by analysis of aliquots from homogeneous lots in different laboratories, by different analysts, using

operational and environmental conditions that may differ but are still within the specified parameters of the assay. The degree of reproducibility of test results is then determined as a function of the assay variables. This reproducibility may be compared to the precision of the assay under normal conditions to obtain a measure of the ruggedness of the analytical method[4].

Robustness

Definition— The robustness of an analytical method is a measure of its capacity to remain unaffected by small but deliberate variations in method parameters and provides an indication of its reliability during normal usage.

System suitability

If measurements are susceptible to variations in analytical conditions, these should be suitably controlled, or a precautionary statement should be included in the method. One consequence of the evaluation of ruggedness and robustness should be that a series of system suitability parameters is established to ensure that the validity of the analytical method is maintained whenever used. Typical variations are the stability of analytical solutions, equipment, and analysts. In liquid chromatography, typical variations are the pH of the mobile phase, the mobile phase composition, different lots or suppliers of columns, the temperature, and the flow rate. In the case of gas chromatography, typical variations are different lots or suppliers of columns, the temperature, and the flow rate. System suitability tests are based on the concept that the equipment, electronics, analytical operations, and samples to be analyzed constitute an integral system that can be evaluated as such. System suitability test parameters to be established for a particular method depend on the type of method being evaluated. They are especially important in the case of chromatographic methods, and submissions to the USP [1]

4. Data elements required for assay validation

Compendial assay procedures vary from highly exacting analytical determinations to subjective evaluation of attributes. Considering this variety of assays, it is only logical that different test methods require different schemes. This chapter covers only the most common categories of assays for which data should be required. These categories are as follows.

Category I: Analytical methods for quantitation of major components of bulk drug substances or active ingredients (including preservatives) in finished pharmaceutical products.

Category II: Analytical methods for determination of impurities in bulk drug substances or degradation compounds in finished pharmaceutical products. These methods include quantitative assays and limit tests.

Category III: Analytical methods for determination of performance characteristics (e.g., dissolution, drug release).

Category IV: Identification tests.

For each assay category, different analytical information is needed. Listed in Table 2 are data elements normally required for each of the categories of assays.

Already established general assays and tests (e.g., titrimetric method of water determination, bacterial endotoxins test) should be revalidated to verify their accuracy (and absence of possible interference) when used for a new product or raw material. The validity of an analytical method can be verified only by laboratory studies. Therefore, documentation of the successful completion of such studies is a basic requirement for determining whether a method is suitable for its intended applications. Appropriate documentation should accompany any proposal for new or revised compendial analytical procedures.

		Assay Category II			
		Limit Tests	Quantitative		
No	*	*	Yes	Yes	Accuracy
No	Yes	No	Yes	Yes	Precision
Yes	*	Yes	Yes	Yes	Specificity
No	*	Yes	No	No	Detection limit
No	*	No	Yes	No	Quantitation limit
No	*	No	Yes	Yes	Linearity
No	*	*	Yes	Yes	Range
* May be required, depending on the nature of the specific test.					

Table 2. Data elements required for assay validation[1]

5. References

[1] Pharmacopeia (USP-31) General Chapters: <1225> Validation of compendial methods.

[2] British Pharmacopeia 2008 SC III F. Validation of Analytical Procedures

[3] ICH Q2B, International Conference on Harmonisation, Validation of analytical procedures. Methodology, 2002.

[4] International Conference on Harmonisation Topic Q2B, Validation of Analytical Methods: Methodology. The Third International Conference on Harmonization of Technical Requirements for Registration of Pharmaceuticals for Human Use (ICH) Yokohama Japan

10

Improvement of Food Safety and Quality by Statistical Process Control (SPC) in Food Processing Systems: A Case Study of Traditional Sucuk (Sausage) Processing

A. Coşkun Dalgiç[1], Hasan Vardin[2] and K. Bülent Belibağli[1]
[1]*Department of Food Engineering, University of Gaziantep, Gaziantep,*
[2]*Department of Food Engineering, University of Harran, Şanlıurfa,*
Turkey

1. Introduction

Increasing costumer demand for safe food has lead food industry to build up food safety and quality systems. The food safety and quality are affected by insufficiency on administration, supplier, production technologies, working environment, human resources and control activities.

Hazard analyzes and critical control points (HACCP) is a system that identifies, evaluates and controls hazards which are significant for food safety. It is a structured, systematic approach for the control of food safety throughout the commodity system, from the farm to the plate. It requires a good understanding of the relationship between cause and effect in order to be more pro-active and it is a key element in Total Quality Management (TQM). The HACCP system has 7 elements called the HACCP principles and pre-requisite programs that must be in place for the system to operate effectively. HACCP is focused in two main steps, namely; (1) Hazard analysis and critical control points (CCPs) determination and (2) HACCP plan for the food processing. First step includes hazards identification, hazard assessment, preventive measure establishment, CCPs determination and their critical limits. The following step is to carry out HACCP plan preparation; monitoring system, corrective actions, verification system and related record system on each CCP.

Statistical tools are an effective way for improving process quality and safety. A large number of managers have achieved the benefits from statistical process control (SPC) implementation. SPC includes flow charts, pareto analysis, histograms, cause-and-effect or Ishikawa diagrams, scatter diagrams, and control charts. Control charts enable the monitoring of key variables during production and they give warning when the process is out-of-control. The best-known charts are the X and s charts that show the temporal variability of the average and standard deviation of the sample subgroups. SPC tools are, particularly control charts, for trend analysis, monitoring and evaluating the critical control points (CCPs) statistically, obtaining advance warning on the status of a critical control point and not just a "Pass/Fail" classification and measuring process outputs and identifying if they vary within statistically defined upper and lower control limits. Use of these tools is discussed by considering traditional sucuk (sausage) process. Sucuk, is a term used for a fermented dry meat product, is a very popular meat product in Turkey and countries located in Balkans, Middle East and Caucasus. Similar type products are also known in most Middle East countries and in European countries. This meat product has been chosen because of its liability to deteriorate easily.

Assuring HACCP effectiveness for food safety relies on application of many prerequisite programs. In addition, some processes (Documentation and record process, internal audit process, etc) applied with ISO 9000-Quality Management System (QMS) standard are used with the HACCP system. ISO 22000-Food Safety Management System (FSMS) standard is being introduced as organizing all of these requirements; moreover it is desired to be used as a single standard in the world. These management systems require statistical tools to have an effective implementation.

2. Food safety and quality systems

Food safety is a scientific discipline handling, preparation, and storage of food in ways that prevent food borne illness. HACCP is a management system in which food safety is addressed through the analysis and control of biological, chemical and physical hazards from raw material to the end product. ISO 22000 concentrates exclusively on food safety and will instruct food producers how they can build up the food safety system itself. Food quality is the quality characteristics of food that is acceptable to consumers. The ISO 9000:2000 includes all management, production, distribution, and product design and service activities.

2.1 TQM and ISO 9000-Quality management system standard

Total Quality Management (TQM) is a comprehensive and structured approach to organizational management that seeks to improve the quality of products and services through ongoing refinements in response to continuous feedback. TQM covers to meet customer requirements, to improve teams, to reduce product and service costs and to provide continuous improvement. TQM techniques have demonstrated an ability to significantly increase productivity and improve profitability. Total Quality Management (TQM) is a comprehensive philosophy of living and working in organizations that emphasizes the relentless pursuit of continuous improvement (Chase & Aquilano, 1995). The principles of TQM and other management systems are summarized in Table 1.

The basic principles for the Total Quality Management (TQM) philosophy of doing business are to satisfy the customer, satisfy the supplier, and continuously improve the business processes. Organizations depend on their customers and therefore should understand current and future customer needs, should met customer requirements and strive to exceed customer expectations. Nearly every organized activity can be looked upon as a process. This process is supported by on organization consisting of people and their relations, resources and tools. Continuous improvement is an integral part of a total quality management system. Common tool to achieve to continuous improvement could be the plan-do-check-act (PDCA) cycle, often called the Deming Wheel, which conveys the sequential and continual of the continuous improvement process.

ISO 9000:2000 is in fact families of standards developed to assist organizations implement and operate effective quality management systems (QMS). ISO 9000:2000 consisted of quality systems that focused on documenting all quality assurance and improvement processes in a company (ISO, 1999). Although the ISO 9000:2000 was originally developed for the manufacturing sector, it had been applied to many service organizations and was gaining some acceptance in the food industry.

TQM	ISO 9000:2000-QMS	HACCP	**ISO 22000-FSMS**
• Focus on customer • Leadership • Let everybody be committed • Approaching of process • Focus on system management • Continuous development • Reality approaching • Cooperation with suppliers	• Customer focus • Leadership • Involvement of people • Process approach • System approach to management • Continual improvement • Factual approach to decision making • Mutually beneficial supplier relationships	• Hazard analysis • Critical control points (CCPs) • Critical limits • Monitoring procedures • Corrective actions • Verification procedures • Documentation procedures	• Customer focus • Leadership and team work • Involvement of people • Process approach and food safety • System approach to management • Continual improvement • Factual approach to decision making • Mutually beneficial supplier relationships • Legislation, regulations • Science and experience • Interactive communication

Table 1. The Principles of TQM, ISO 9000:2000-QMS, ISO 22000-FSMS and HACCP

The ISO 9000:2000 standard describes a basic set of 8 elements by which quality management system can be developed and implemented. Table 2. represents the structure of ISO 9000:2000-QMS Standard.

2.2 HACCP and ISO 22000-Food safety management system standard

For the food industry, the HACCP program is currently recognized as the best approach to control food safety. Although concerns such as quality and economic adulteration are not included in the HACCP system, the implementation of an HACCP system means greater control over production process, which results in improvements in both the quality and safety of food. The HACCP system has 7 elements called the HACCP principles (Table 1.) and pre-requisite programs (Table 2.) that must be in place for the system to operate effectively (FAO, 1998; Codex, 2003).

The food processing industry has long used HACCP programs to make their products safer. Application of HACCP systems in many different manufacturing processes has led to more efficient prevention of adverse health effects associated with the consumption or use of the products. In addition, HACCP focused on the elimination of food-related health hazards. Companies involved in HACCP attempted to identify all critical points at which health hazards could be introduced into food and control those points to eliminate the associate risk (Mortimore & Wallace, 1998).

	Strategic	**Operational**	**Support**
ISO 9000:2000-QMS	QP.1 Market Research and Customer Relation QP.2 Internal Communications QP.3 Document and record Control QP.4 Planning QP.5 Resources Management	QP.6 Product Design QP.7 Food Manufacturing	QP.8 Purchasing QP.9 Internal Audit QP.10 Data Analysis QP.11 Maintenance of measurement's and process equipments QP.12 Calibration of measurement's equipment
ISO 22000:2005-FSMS	PR.1 Construction and lay-out of buildings and associated utilities PR.2 Lay-out of premises, including workspace and employee facilities PR.3 The suitability of equipment and its accessibility for cleaning, maintenance and preventative maintenance	PR.4 Supplies of air, water, energy and other utilities PR.5 Supporting services, including waste and sewage disposal PR.6 Cleaning and sanitizing PR.7 Pest control PR.8 Personnel hygiene PR.9 Measures for the prevention of cross contamination	PR.10 Management of purchased materials (e.g. raw materials, ingredients, chemicals and packaging), and supplies

QP: Quality Process, PR: Pre-requisite

Table 2. Some quality processes and prerequisite programs

HACCP is a system that identifies, evaluates and controls hazards which are significant for food safety (FAO, 1998). It is a structured, systematic approach for the control of food safety throughout the commodity system, from the farm to the plate.

ISO 22000-2005 FSMS aims to harmonize the requirements for food safety management in food and food related business (ISO, 2005). ISO 22000-2005 FSMS assists the food manufacturers in the use of HACCP principles. Main elements in ISO 22000:2005 FSMS are compatible with ISO 9000:2000 QMS. Both models consist of 5 major elements. For the proposed-integrated models, the principle aim is to provide simplicity and applicability. A common documentation system is provided by the integration (Figure 1.).

HACCP system had been required operational applications such as GMP, GHP, and SSOP before ISO 22000-FSMS Standard had been published. ISO 22000-FSMS Standard has included and organized the definition and detailed contents of these applications. Prerequisite programs, in this study, are classified as strategic, operational, and supportive programs (Table 2). ISO 22000-FSMS and ISO 9000-QMS have the same framework properties. The standards have built on customer focus, continuous improvement, and process approach. Figure 3 shows the properties and similarities of the standards. ISO 22000-FSMS standard includes HACCP principles with prerequisite programs (ISO, 2005). The prerequisite programs and processes that are required both ISO 9000-QMS and ISO 22000-FSMS are shown in Table 2. For example; the followings are in both standards; documentation and record process (QP 3), which are the fundamental items in both standards are in the article number 4. The planning (QP 4), and internal communication (QP 2) are in the article number 5, resource management process (QP 5) are in the article number 6.

2.3 Continuous improvement

Continuous improvement is a management philosophy that approaches the challenge of product and process improvement. Specifically, continuous improvement seeks continual improvement of machinery, materials, labor utilization, product quality and safety, and production methods through application of suggestions and ideas of team members (Chase & Aquilano, 1995).

ISO 9000:2000 Quality Management System and ISO 22000:2005 Food Safety Management System are based on the process model which includes the continuous improvements from suppliers to the customer chain. In both models the influence of Deming's cycle can be seen (Table 3.). In ISO 9000:2000-QMS and ISO 22000:2005 a far greater emphasis is placed on the use of measurement and analysis of results, feeding into the review and improvement process. The continued auditing and verification of HACCP system demand more attention than the initial development of a HACCP plan. Food companies sometimes focus on the process control portion of HACCP without documenting the product design. Important process in HACCP system verification includes the initial validation of HACCP plan and its periodic revalidation. HACCP is brought to a standard structure with ISO 22000:2005 which has similarities with ISO 9000:2000 QMS. Moreover, integration of standards will provide simplicity in practicing of them.

Figure 1 represents the continuous improvement of process models in product quality with ISO 9000:2000 QMS and product safety with ISO 22000:2005 FSMS. Continuous improvement can be well designed by applying the following steps;

2.3.1 Management responsibility

In both models top managements make/decide quality and safety policies. After this step, objectives to reach quality and safety policies should be determined. The customer requirements have to be included in this determination. Food quality and food safety management system planning is then followed. Planning will include strategies, resources and cost estimation.

2.3.2 Resource management

The required resources such as human resources, infrastructures, equipments, and work environment have to be organized. Infrastructure covers the hygienic and sanitary design of equipment and buildings. Required continuing education for employees has to be planned and supplied.

Deming Wheel (PDCA Cycle)	Quality and safety improvement steps	ISO 9000-QMS	ISO 22000-FSMS
Plan (P): The plan phase of the cycle is an improvement area and a specific problem with it to be identified. In this phase, objectives and strategies are developed and necessary sources are determined.	1. Theme Selection	5.3. Quality Policy	5.2. Food Safety Policy
	2. Current situation review and analysis	5.4. Quality planning	5.3. FSMS planning
	3. Preventive action planning	5.4. Quality planning	5.3. FSMS planning
Do (D): The do phase of the cycle deals with implementing the changes according to the plan.	4. Action	7. Product/Service Realization 7.5. Production & Service Provision	7. Realization of safe product 7.9. Operation of FSMS
Check (C): The check phase deals with evaluating data collected during implementation.	5. Analysis	8. Measurement, Analysis, and Improvement	8.2. Monitoring and measuring
Act (A): During the act phase, the improvement is codified as the new standard procedure; necessary revisions are applied and replicated in similar processes throughout the organization.	6. Standardization of the countermeasures	7.5. Production and Service Provision	8.4. Validation of control measure combinations
	7. Identification of remaining problems	8.3. Control of Nonconforming product	8.3. FSMS verification
	8. Evaluation of whole plans and procedures	8.5. Improvement 5.6. Management review	8.5. Improvement 5.6. Management review

Table 3. PDCA cycle with ISO 9000-QMS and ISO 22000-FSMS

2.3.3 Product/service realization

Following steps have to be studied in safe product and service realization;

- Planning of safe product and service
- Implementation of pre requisite programs
- Hazard and risk analysis
- Design (Safe product and/or service, HACCP plan, Operational procedures)
- Realization of purchasing after evaluating of supplier
- Realization of safe products and service by customer requirements

2.3.4 Measurement, verification, validation and improvement

Data obtained from suppliers, customer satisfaction, product quality and safety, process trends, critical control points, pre-requisite programs and quality-safety system have to be

analyzed. Quality and safety systems are usually analyzed and verified through internal audits (Sperber, 1998). After that, outputs coming from auditing are validated. In both systems, the control of non confirmative products (in terms of quality and safety aspects) is required. Preventive and corrective actions provide us to get improvements.
Management starts the review the data obtained through the former stages. Then, re-planning and validation are conducted.

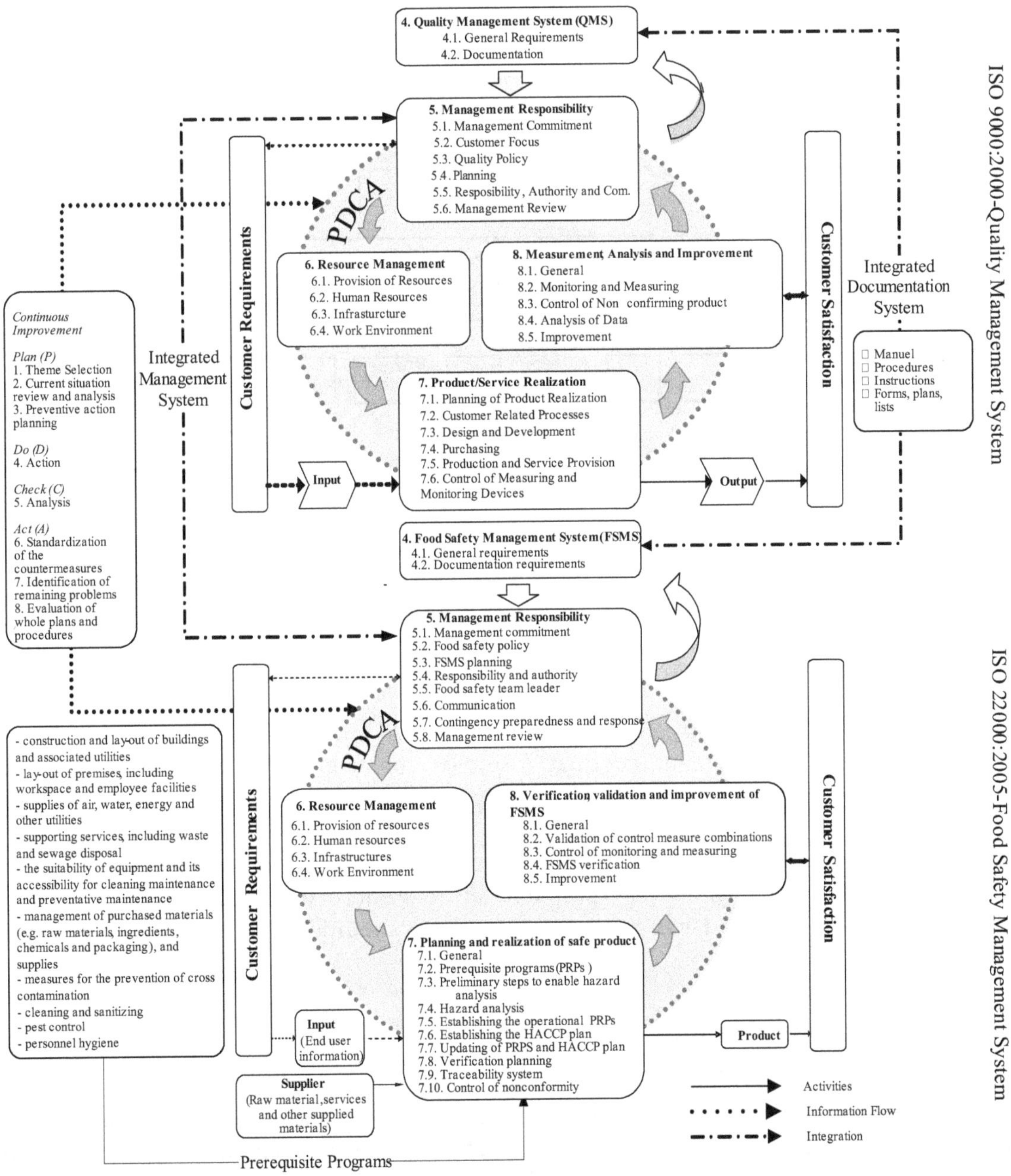

Fig. 1. Continuous Improvement Models in ISO 22000-Food Safety Management System and ISO 9000-Quality Management System (ISO, 1999; ISO, 2005)

2.4 Process management

Process is a collection of related, structured activities that produce a specific service or product from inputs given for particular customers. All of these activities are connected to each other with logic relations of processes. They provide the results by using sources of a organization to attain the goals. Process management between functional units of the institution within the hierarchical structure of production is a simple management system that provides work flows. In addition it is an effective management system in which responsibilities of employees are considered, inputs and outputs are clearly stated, performance criteria and the size of success are being measured, and continuous improvements are provided (Juran & Gryna, 1998).

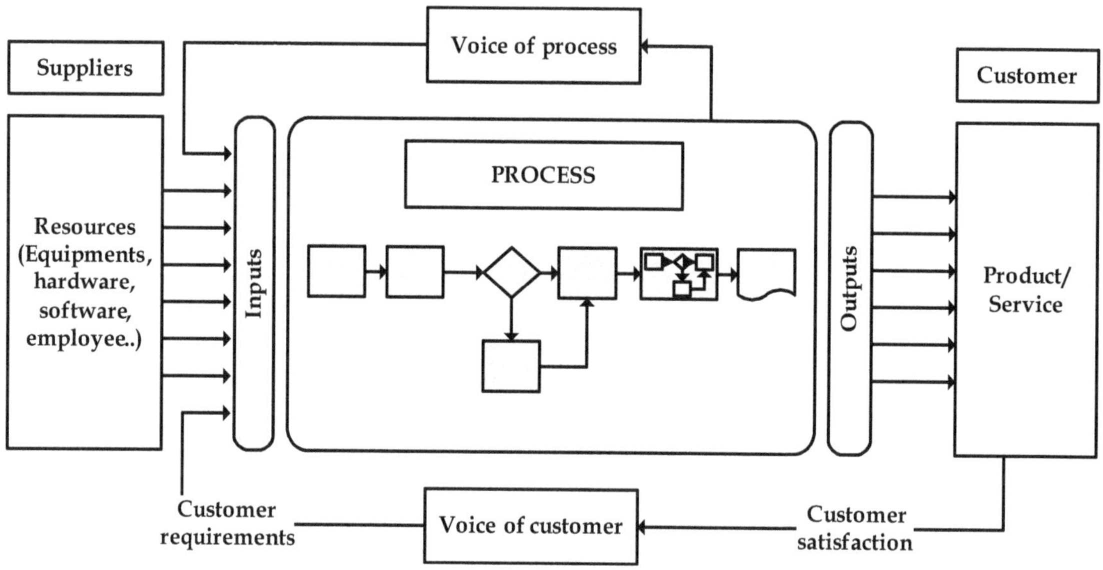

Fig. 2. Process model

ISO 9000:2000-Quality Management System standard requires process management activities, resource management, product / service implementation and identification of processes during monitoring. Within this scope, the processes specified in Table 2 can be prepared.

Documentation required by these processes vary according to the organizational structure, however, the documents should be prepared in accordance with ISO 9000:2000-Quality Management System standard, the necessity, their validities must be approved and implemented.

3. Statistical process control

Statistical process control (SPC) is defined as the application of statistical techniques to control a process. SPC is concerned with quality of conformance. There are a number of tools available to the quality engineer that is effective for problem-solving process. The seven quality tools are relatively simple but very powerful tools which every quality engineer. The tools are: flow chart, run chart, process control chart, check sheet, pareto diagram, cause and effect diagram, and scatter diagram (Juran & Gryna, 1998).

3.1 Flow charts

Flow charts are defined as the graphical representation of the steps of in a process. Flow charts facilitate an analysis of the steps in a process to determine relationships between the steps.

3.2 Check sheets

Check sheets are useful during data collection. They provide a simple means for recording data by categories and enable the analyst to determine the relative frequency of occurrence of the various categories of the data.

3.3 Cause and effect diagrams

Cause and effect diagrams (CED) are simple techniques for dissecting a problem or a process. CED identifies all possible relationships among input and output variables, that is, the five categories on the following skeleton (materials, machines, man, methods, and environment).

3.4 Histograms and pareto charts

A histogram is a bar chart showing the variation or distribution of the observations from a set of data. The pareto chart is a form of bar chart with each bar representing a cause of a problem and always arranged so that the most influential cause of a problem can be easily recognized, that is, arranging the problems in descending order. This information is helpful in focusing attention on the highest-priority category (Srikaeo & Hourigan, 2002).

3.5 Scatter diagrams

Scatter diagramming is a tool to study how different variables relate to each other or how they correlate. A scatter diagram demonstrates the results of a series of experiments which is conducted to document the relationship between the variables. Table 4. represents the mathematical models.

3.6 Process control charts

The primary function of a control chart is to determine which type of variation is present and whether adjustments need to be made to the process.

Variables data are those data which can be measured on a continuous scale. Variable data are plotted on a combination of two charts- usually an x-bar ($\overline{x}$) chart and a range (R) chart. The x-bar chart plots sample means. It is a measure of between-sample variation and is used to asses the centering and long term variation of the process. The range chart measure the within sample variation and asses the short term variation of the process (Juran & Gryna, 1998; Grigg, 1998).

Attribute charting is used for various types of defects, primarily by counting the number of nonconforming units or the nonconformities per units. The most commonly used attribute control chart is p-chart or the percentage of defective unit with variable sample size. The np-chart is used to monitor the percentage defective unit for constant sample size. The c-chart is used to monitor the number of defects on an item for constant sample size. The u-chart is fro number of unlimited defects in variable sample size.

Expression	Mathematical models	Geometric shape	Applications
Sigmoidal (Gompertz)	$y = y_0 + ae^{-e^{-(\frac{x-x_0}{b})}}$	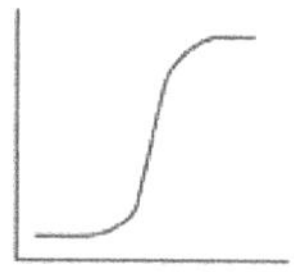	Growth curve Inactivation of microorganisms (Banani et al., 2007)Ray
Sigmoidal (Lojistic)	$y = y_0 + \frac{a}{1+(\frac{x}{x_0})^b}$		
Sigmoidal (Sigmoid)	$y = y_0 + \frac{a}{1+e^{-(\frac{x-x_0}{b})}}$		
Sigma (GAB)	$y = \frac{abcx}{(1-ax)(1-ax+abx)}$	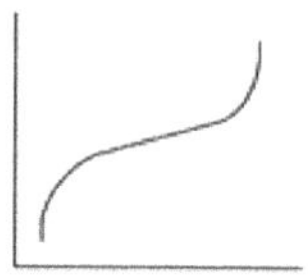	Moisture sorption isotherms (Ayranci & Dalgic, 1992)
Polynomial (linear)	$y = y_0 + ax$	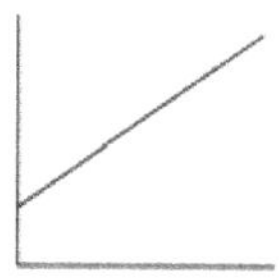	Linear relationships (Wu et al., 2007)
Polynomial (Quadratic)	$y = y_0 + ax + bx^2$	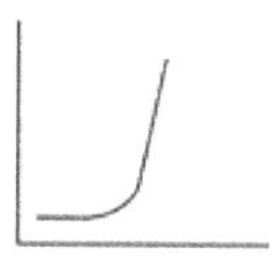	(Gao et al., 2007)
Polynomial (inverse first order)	$y = y_0 + \frac{a}{x}$	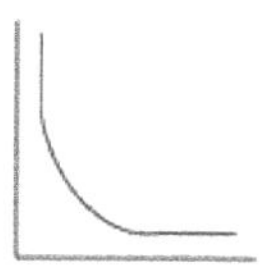	
Peak (Guassian)	$y = y_0 + ae^{\left[-0.5(\frac{x-x_0}{b})^2\right]}$	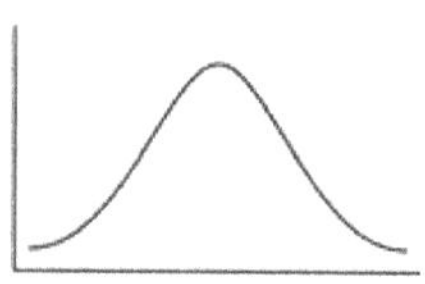	Distrubition (Peng & Lu, 2007).
Peak (Lorentzian)	$y = y_0 + \frac{a}{1+(\frac{x-x_0}{b})^2}$		
Exponential decay	$y = y_0 + ae^{-bx} + ce^{-dx}$	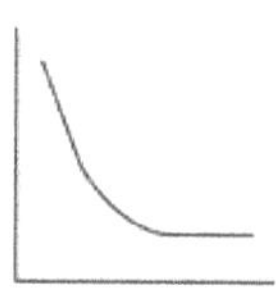	Drying Destruction curve for microorganisms (Bruce et al. 2009)
Exponential growth	$y = y_0 + ae^{bx} + ce^{dx}$	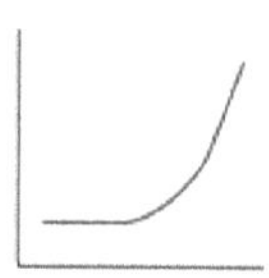	Growth curve (Daniela et al., 2009)

Table 4. Some mathematical models'formulas and their geometric shapes

	UCL & LCL	Mean	n*	A_2	D_3	D_4
X-Chart	$UCL_{\bar{X}} = \bar{\bar{X}} + A_2\bar{R}$ $LCL_{\bar{X}} = \bar{\bar{X}} - A_2\bar{R}$	$\bar{\bar{X}} = \frac{\sum_{i=1}^{n} \bar{x}_i}{n}$	2	1.88	0	3.27
			3	1.02	0	2.57
			4	0.73	0	2.28
			5	0.58	0	2.11
			6	0.48	0	2.00
R-Chart	$UCL_R = D_4\bar{R}$ $LCL_R = D_3\bar{R}$	$\bar{R} = \frac{\sum_{i=1}^{n} R_i}{n}$	7	0.42	0.08	1.92
			8	0.37	0.14	1.86
			9	0.34	0.18	1.82
			10	0.31	0.22	1.78

* Number of observations in each sample, UCL: upper control limit, LCL: lower control limit, A_2, D_3, and D_4 are constants

Table 5. The control diagrams for variable data and control chart factors (Juran & Gryna, 1998)

Chart	UCL and LCL	Center line
p	$UCL \alpha LCL = \bar{p} \pm 3\frac{\sqrt{\bar{p}(1-\bar{p})}}{\sqrt{n}}$	$\bar{p} = \frac{\sum np}{\sum n}$
np	$UCL \alpha LCL = n\bar{p} \pm 3\sqrt{n\bar{p}(1-\bar{p})}$	$n\bar{p} = \frac{\sum np}{k}$
c	$UCL \alpha LCL = \bar{c} \pm 3\sqrt{\bar{c}}$	$\bar{c} = \frac{\sum c}{k}$
u	$UCL \alpha LCL = \bar{u} \pm 3\frac{\sqrt{\bar{u}}}{\sqrt{n}}$	$\bar{u} = \frac{\sum c}{\sum n}$

n: the number of observations in each sample, k: number of samples

Table 6. Control diagrams for attributes

3.7 Failure mode and effect analysis

A failure modes and effects analysis (FMEA) is a procedure in product development and operations management for analysis of potential failure modes within a system for classification by the severity and likelihood of the failures. Failure modes are any errors or defects in a process, design, or item, especially those that affect the customer, and can be potential or actual. Effects analysis refers to studying the consequences of those failures.

Failure mode and effect analysis is a tool that examines potential product or process failures, evaluates risk priorities, and helps determine remedial actions to avoid identified problems. The spreadsheet format allows easy review of the analysis (Arvanitoyannis & Varzakas, 2007 and 2008).

4. A case study: Some applications of SPC in traditional sucuk processing

A traditional sucuk processing was partly investigated by SPC. The process data were retrieved from an industry and analyzed by SPC techniques. Data were obtained over a period of 3 months. The process variables considered were and moisture content, pH change during ripening. In addition to these, some and product variables (flavor, texture, saltiness etc.) were determined from a survey conducted in Gaziantep, Turkey. The SPC techniques included Check sheets, Cause and effect diagrams, Histograms and pareto charts, Scatter diagrams, Process control charts, Failure mode and effect analysis

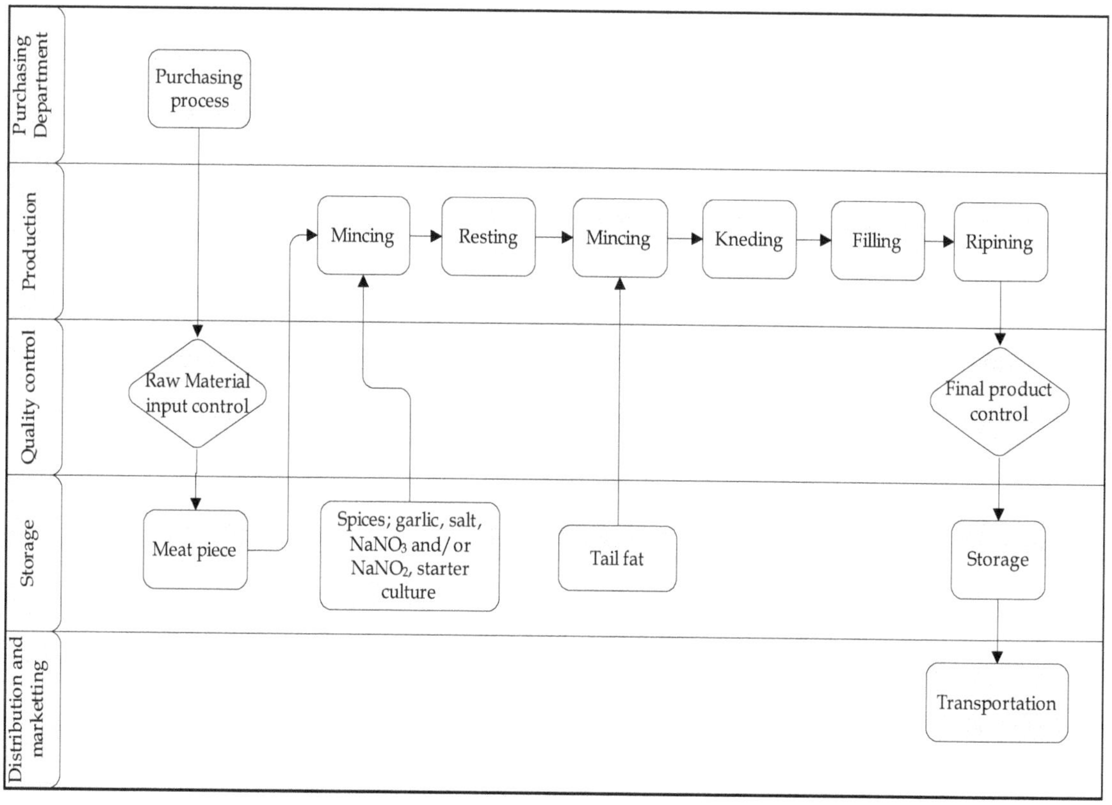

Fig. 3. Sucuk manufacturing process flow chart by various departments

4.1 Traditional sucuk processing and properties

Sucuk dough is prepared from meat (about 18% fat) mixed with tail fat, salt, sugar, clean dry garlic, spices, NaNO2, NaNO3, vegetable oil (generally olive oil), antioxidants and antimicrobial. Meat, fat and spices are added into sucuk dough according to the following recipe; 900 g sheep red meat (about 18% fat), 200 g tail fat, 5.5 g cumin, 1.1 g cinnamon, 11.42 g allspice, 0.48 g cloves, 5.5 g red pepper, 11 g black pepper, 20.76 g garlic, 4.4 g sugar, 18 g salt and 2.1 g olive oil are used to prepare sausage dough. A flow-chart of sucuk preparation is given in Figure 3. The meat is minced in a meat mincer to about 1.3–2.5 cm. After that spices and starter culture are added and mixed with minced meat. Starter culture mixture (*P. acidilactici*, *L. plantarum* and *S. carnosus*) is used as a 20 g commercial culture mixture per 100 kg meat. After that nitrate/nitrite, potassium pyrophosphate, dipotassium hydrogen phosphate, ascorbic acid and potassium sorbate which are dissolved in 25 ml of distilled water, are added into the prepared of sucuk dough. The sucuk dough is conditioned at 0-4 °C for 12 hours. The minced refrigerated tail fat is added and mixed into the sucuk dough. After that, the dough is filled into artificial collagen casings, of 38 mm diameter, under aseptic conditions, using a filling machine. Sucuks are fermented and matured from 95% to 60% RH and from 22 to 18 °C during 15 days. Sucuk samples are then stored at 50% RH and 30 °C (Bozkurt & Erkmen, 2007).

4.2 Application of pareto analysis in traditional sucuk processing

A survey study was done to collect customer complaints about the properties of sucuk products. According to Pareto analysis; the percentage of complaints are listed by the descending order and cumulative percentages are obtained by adding each other to previous ones. The priority problems are being identified by this order.

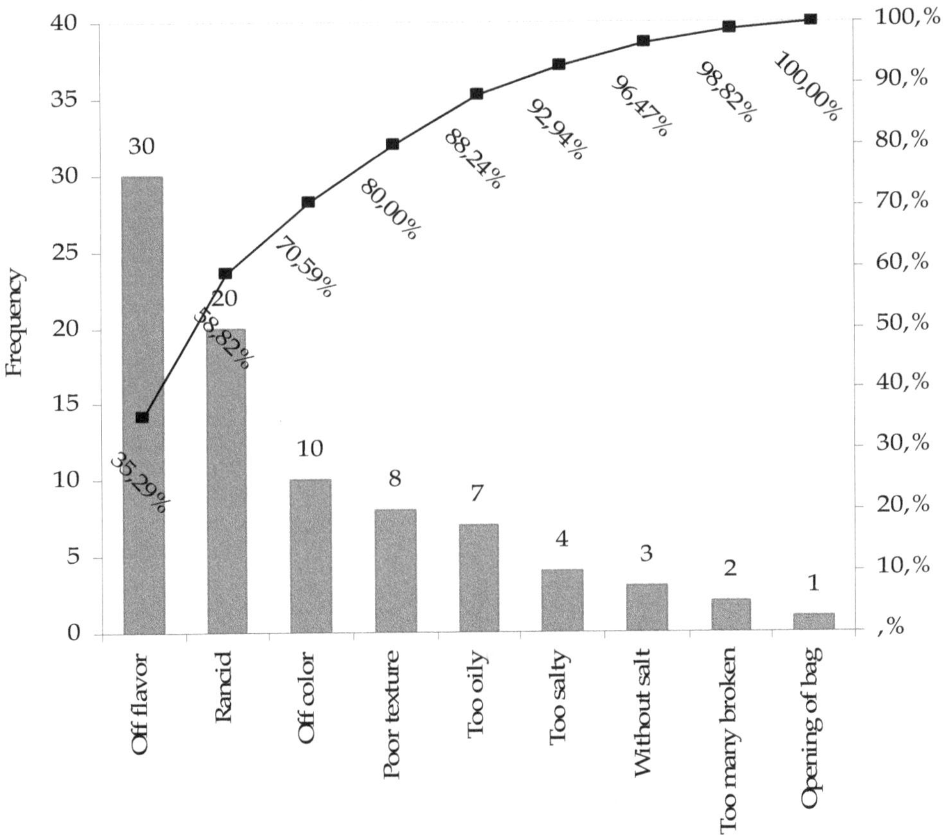

Fig. 4. Pareto analysis of customer complaints for sucuk product

4.3 Application of control charts in traditional sucuk processing

The amount of moisture in the production of sucuk is one of the quality parameters. Moisture content should be around 40%. The X-bar (x) and R-chart graphics in Table 7 are created from the moisture contents of 5 samples of 10 runs. The control limits drawn in both plots were obtained by using equations given in Table 5.

n	Final moisture content for each run (kg water/100 kg total sucuk)									
	1	2	3	4	5	6	7	8	9	10
1	43,36	43,54	42,38	41,17	40,15	43,25	41,15	40,97	40,75	39,98
2	42,45	44,05	43,56	43,78	42,38	42,97	43,54	41,43	43,35	42,75
3	43,38	42,48	42,15	43,56	43,75	44,06	41,91	44,38	44,09	44,75
4	42,96	43,54	43,75	44,17	44,51	43,65	42,54	43,76	42,75	43,75
5	43,78	44,15	42,96	41,24	43,75	43,54	43,89	42,54	41,76	42,75
$\overline{X}$	43,19	43,55	42,96	42,78	42,91	43,49	42,61	42,62	42,54	42,80
UCL- $\overline{X}$ =44,52	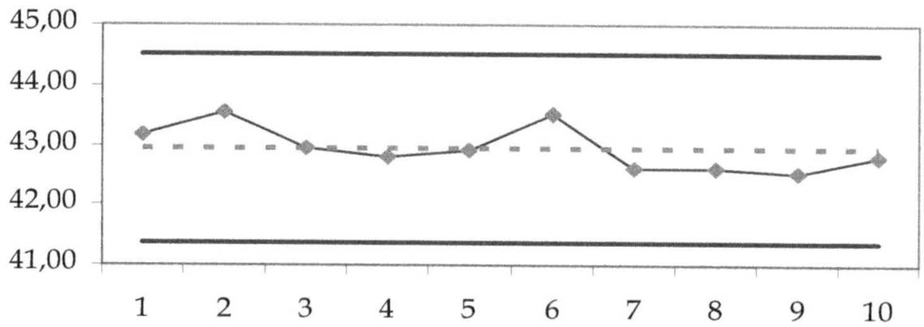									
LCL- $\overline{X}$ =41,37										
$\overline{\overline{X}}$ =42,94										
R	1,33	1,67	1,6	3	4,36	1,09	2,74	3,41	3,34	4,77
UCL- $\overline{R}$ =5,77	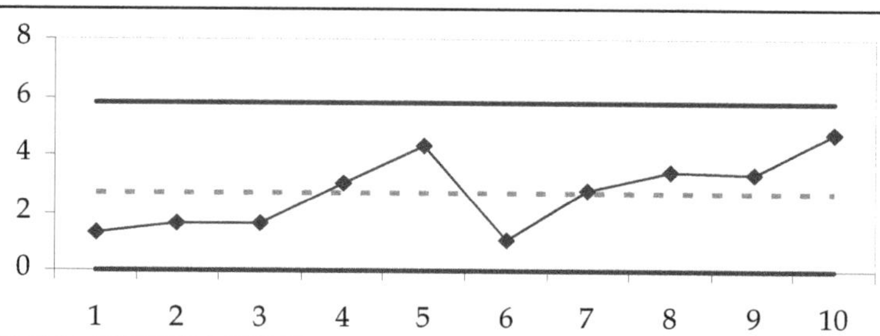									
LCL- $\overline{R}$ =0										
$\overline{R}$ =2,73										

Table 7. A control chart showing the amount of moisture in a sucuk production line

4.4 Application of scatter diagrams in traditional sucuk processing

The formation of lactic acid bacteria in fermented meat products prevents the formation of undesirable bacteria. The lactic acid produced during ripening decreases pH to 5.3. If the value of pH is below 5.3 the water holding capacity of meat proteins decreases and the product dries quickly. Table 8 shows changes in pH during the ripening process. The parameters given in Table 8 are obtained with these experimental data modeled with the logistic equation.

In this application, Logistic model was applied to determine the best fit for the experimental data of ripening of sucuk. Modeling was carried out using the least square method and the Microsoft Excel spreadsheet (Microsoft Office 2003, USA) was used to perform this task using the SOLVER tool based on the Generalized Reduced Gradient (GRG) method of iteration. This is a search method to minimize the sum of squares of the differences between the predicted and experimental data (Hii et al., 2009).

Logistic parameters			
y_0	x_0	a	b
5,43	2,38	0,93	3,44

Time (day)	pH_{exp}	pH_{pre}	$(pH_{exp}-pH_{pre})^2$
0	6,35	6,36	0,0001321
1	6,33	6,32	0,0001823
3	5,71	5,72	6,714E-05
6	5,50	5,47	0,0012100
9	5,43	5,44	5,581E-05
12	5,39	5,43	0,0017230
15	5,45	5,43	0,0004161
Sum			0,0037865

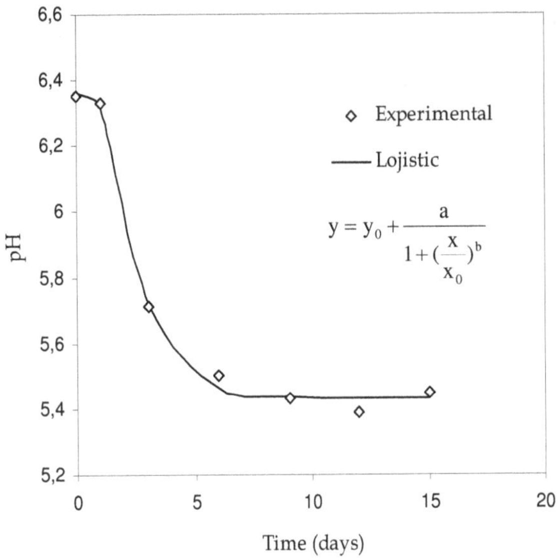

Table 8. Scatter diagram of pH during ripening

4.5 Failure mode and effect analysis of sucuk processing

Hazard analysis begins with identification of food safety hazards associated with the raw material. First, a complete list of hazards that could potentially be of concern is prepared. Cause analysis is based on determine potential hazard sources and classifying the causes (Arvanitoyannis & Traikou, 2005). This classification is done by fish bone diagram (Figure 5) and results are shown in Table 9.

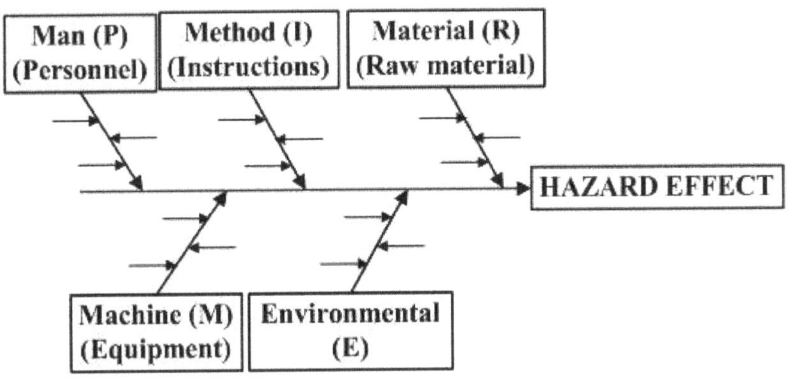

Fig. 5. Cause and effect analysis (Fish bone diagram)

A number of questions given in Figure 6 have to be answered for each hazard to identify significant hazards that could be of concern at each sucuk production step (ILSI, 2004). Hazard analysis starts questioning of the presence of a potential hazard whether it is significant or not in raw materials or in the processing steps. Questions and their results are shown in Table 9.

Sucuk processing basically consists of dough formation (mincing and kneading) and fermentation/ripening steps. One of the main hazards comes from properties of raw materials such as microorganisms, antibiotics, hormones and biogenic amines. Additives and spices may contain foreign matters, insects, mycotoxins etc. In fermentation and ripining process, residual nitrate and nitrite may have a potential chemical hazard. Metal contamination is a major hazard during mincing since these processes are mechanic. These hazards, as shown in Table 9., have to be tested and controlled in every batch. Results obtained from hazard analysis give a sign for the magnitude of hazard in a next step, moreover, whether it is a CCP or not.

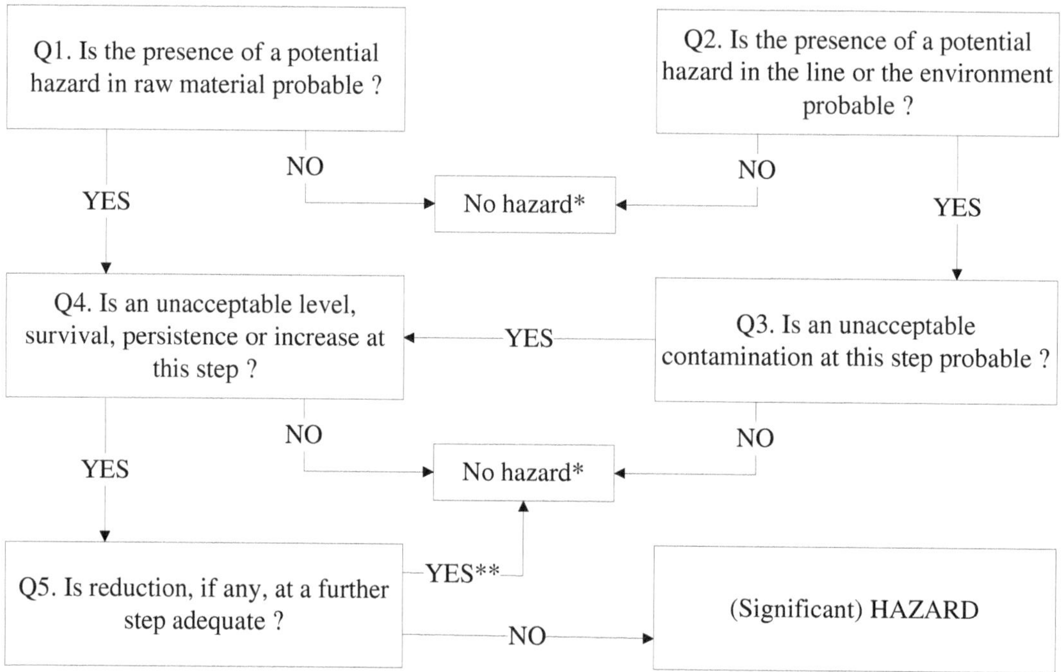

Fig. 6. Hazard analysis (decision tree)

It is generally agreed that risk assessment should be an independent scientific process, distinct from measures taken to control and manage the risk. The overall risk analysis process includes risk assessment, risk management and risk communication, and also involves political, social economic and technical considerations (ILSI, 2001; Serra et al, 1999; Sperber, 2001) reported that hazard analysis was qualitative and risk assessment was quantitative process. Therefore risk assessment after hazard analysis done has to be quantified. It was stated that risk assessment was a compound of probability and severity (Barendsz, 1998). In this study, probability and severity of the hazards are considered as a five class hazard score matrix. This is shown in Table 10. Significant hazards found in hazard analysis (Table 9) are used for determination of risk assessment by five class hazard score matrix which was given in Table 11. Microorganisms in both meat and additives are found to be 4th risk class (Table 11) by risk analysis after determining hazard analysis. Interestingly almost all processes are classified as 4th risk class.

ISO 22000-Food safety management system standard requires definition of all hazards starting from raw materials to finished products in the plant (clause 7.4.2. of ISO 22000-FSMS). In the mean time, the possible severity of unfavorable health effects and the likelihood of their occurrence have to be evaluated (clause 7.4.3. of ISO 22000-FSMS). After assessment of hazards, control measures have to be considered for preventing, eliminating, or reducing these food safety hazards to be defined acceptable level (clause 7.4.4. of ISO 22000-FSMS) (ISO, 2005).

Process name/step	Process descriptions	Potential Hazards	Cause analysis*		Hazard Analysis (Y/N)**					
			Causes (Sources and reasons)	Cause class	Q1	Q2	Q3	Q4	Q5	SH
Raw Material Reception (meat)	Meat is receptioned and analyzed (Microbiological, antibiotic)	B: microorganisms	Farm environment, slaughtering	R	Y	-	-	Y	N	Y
		C: antibiotics, hormones, biogenic amines (BA)	BA are generated in course of microbial and animal metabolism.	R	Y	-	-	Y	N	Y
		P: bone pieces	Slaughtering	R	Y	-	-	Y	N	Y
Raw Material Reception (Additives, Spices)	Additives and spices are receptioned and analyzed (Microbiological, foreign matter, insects)	B: microorganisms	Handling, processing	R	Y	-	-	Y	N	Y
		C: pesticide residues, mycotoxins	Mycotoxins produced by m.o. under undesirable storage and processing conditions.	R	Y	-	-	Y	N	Y
		P: metal	Agricultural harvesting	R	Y	-	-	Y	N	Y
Meat storage	Storage between 0-4 °C.	B: microorganisms	Temp. increase	P, M	-	Y	Y	Y	N	Y
Mincing	Spices and additives addition	B: microorganisms	Temp. increase during mincing	P, M	-	Y	Y	Y	N	Y
		C: insufficient nitrate and nitrite addition	Process formulation	P, M	-	Y	Y	Y	N	Y
		P: metal contamination	Equipment	M	-	Y	N	-	-	N
Conditioning	12 hr between 0-4 °C.	B: microorganisms	Temp. inc. during conditioning	M	-	Y	Y	Y	N	Y
Mincing and kneading	Addition of tail fat and mincing of meat dough	B: microorganisms	Temp. increase during mincing	M	-	Y	Y	Y	N	Y
		P: metal contamination	Equipment	M	-	Y	N	-	-	N
Filling	Filling into casings	B: microorganisms	Natural casings	R	-	Y	Y	Y	N	Y
		P: tearing, air pockets	Processing	R, M	-	Y	Y	Y	N	Y
Fermentation /ripining	Decrease in pH	B: microorganisms	Processing	M	-	Y	Y	Y	N	Y
		C: residual of nitrate and nitrite	Processing	M	-	Y	Y	Y	N	Y
Metal detection	Metal detection	P: metal residue	Metal analysis	M	-	Y	Y	Y	N	Y
Product storage	50% RH and 30 °C	B: microorganisms	Storage	M	-	Y	Y	Y	N	Y

*Fish bone diagram (Figure 6), ** Hazard analysis (Figure 7), SH: Significant hazard

Table 9. Failure mode and effect analysis of sucuk manufacturing process

Severity			Risk Classes				
Catastrophic	Death or lasting damage	E	3	4	4	4	4
Critical	Many concerned people and lasting or continuous damages	D	3	3	4	4	4
Serious	Many concerned people, no lasting damages	C	2	3	3	4	4
Low	Single case, no lasting damages or minimal concentration	B	2	2	3	3	4
Ignorable	Hazard to be discovered prior to consumption or minimal indisposition	A	1	2	2	3	3
			I	II	III	IV	V
Probability			Unlikely (< per 1 years)	Rare (per year)	Occasional (per semester)	Frequent (per month)	Very frequent (per week)

Risk classes	Control measures
	1. No measure necessary.
	2. Periodic measures are measures which often cover a one-time activity.
	3. General control measures and prerequisite programs
	4. Specific control measures are specifically developed and used to control the risk.

Table 10. Five-class hazard scoring matrix

4.5.1 Critical control points in the sucuk processing

Critical control points are location, operation, procedure, or process where control can be carried out to remove the hazards for food safety or to reduce them to an acceptable level. Critical control points of Bulgur processing were determined. A decision tree was used for determining steps which could be designated as critical control points (ILSI, 2004; Bolat, 2002; Lee & Hathaway, 1998; Sandrou &Arvanitoyannis, 2000a, 2000b; Arvanitoyannis & Mauropoulos, 2000) (Figure 7). Critical control points of sucuk processing are listed on Table 11.

After questioning, all processing steps of traditional sucuk manufacturing are found to be in CCP structure. Significant hazards at those processes have to be followed by special monitoring systems.

Critical limits are minimum and/or maximum values to which a biological, chemical, or physical parameter must be controlled at a CCP to prevent, eliminate, or reduce to an acceptable level to the occurrence of a food safety hazard. These limits show if the identified hazards can be put under control or not. Critical limits may be determined for factors like temperature, time, physical dimensions, etc. Critical limits for each critical control points for sucuk processing were evaluated on Table 12. These were taken from literature, legal provisions, or from comparable standard procedures. Identified CCPs have to be and to be controlled in HACCP plan as defined in clause 7.6.2. of ISO 22000-FSMS.

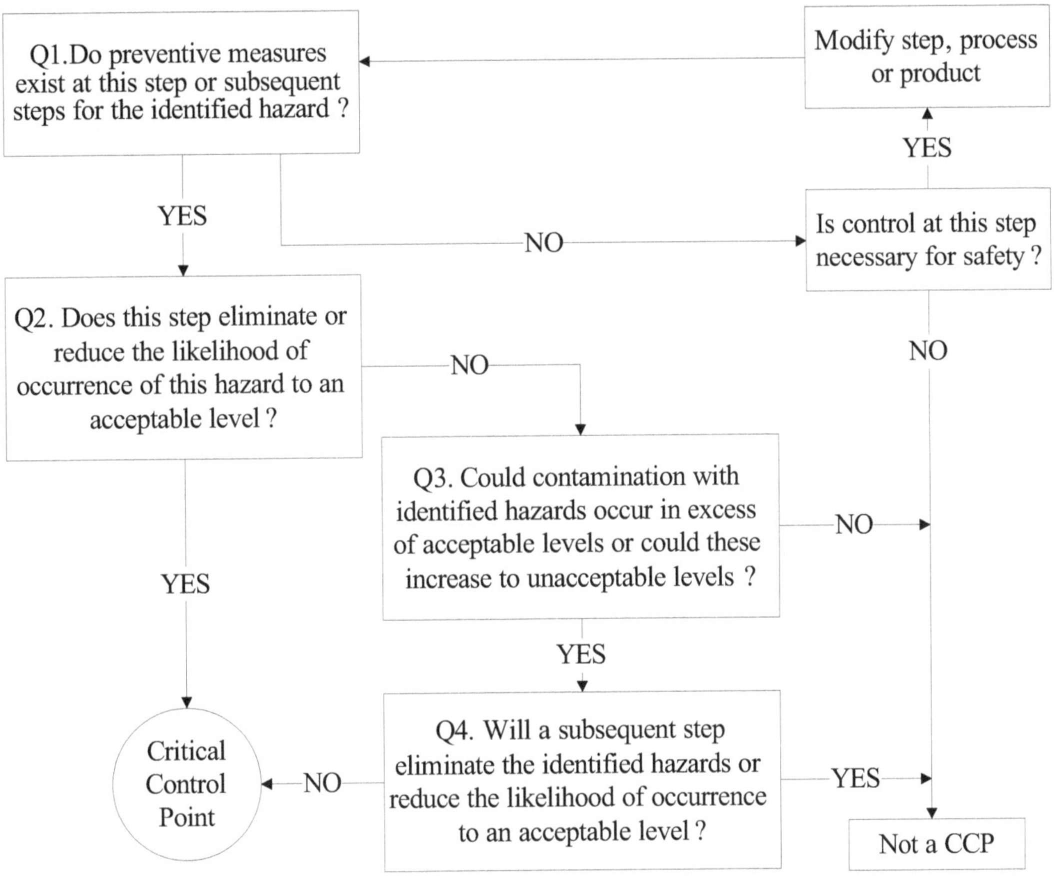

Fig. 7. CCP analysis (Decision tree)

4.5.2 Implementation of HACCP system-HACCP plan

Ideally, a HACCP study should be carried out as part of product and process development, so that potential hazards can be "designed out" at the earliest stage. In any case, a HACCP study results in a HACCP plan that should be correctly implemented to ensure that the appropriate control measures are put in place before products are put on the market.

The HACCP plan is a controlled document which consists of significant hazards, critical control points, critical limits for each hazard at each CCP, monitoring procedures for each hazard at each CCP, and corrective actions if critical limits are exceeded. Some hazards are considered to be control points (CPs) because the hazards can be controlled by prerequisite programs (Derosier et al., 2002).

Monitoring is systematic and planned observation to make sure that CCPs are under control. When monitoring results show that criteria are not met, appropriate and immediate precautions should be taken to correct the deviations. For example, corrective actions may be re-heating or re-operating, increasing the operation temperature, extending operation time, decreasing pH, changing equipment of measurement, changing equipment of process and maintaining, extra training for employees, revising HACCP documents, change in process flow, etc. Procedures should be improved for corrective actions (Arvanitoyannis & Traikou, 2005; Efstratiadis & Arvanitoyannis, 2000).

Process name /step	Significant hazards	Risk assessment*			Preventive actions/control measures	CCP analysis (Y/N)**				
		S	P	RC		Q1.	Q2.	Q3.	Q4.	no:
Raw Material Reception (meat)	B: microorganisms	E	IV	4	Certified suppliers with HACCP program, Microbiological analysis	Y	N	Y	N	1b
	C: antibiotics, hormones, biogenic amines (BA)	E	III	4	Chemical analysis	Y	N	Y	N	1c
	P: bone pieces	B	III	3	Physical observations	Y	Y	-	-	1p
Raw Material Reception (Additives, spices)	B: microorganisms	D	IV	4	Certified suppliers with HACCP program, Microbiological analysis	Y	N	Y	N	2b
	C: pesticide residues, mycotoxins	B	III	3	Chemical analysis	Y	N	Y	N	2c
	P: metal	B	II	2	Metal detector	Y	N	Y	Y	2p
Meat storage	B: microorganisms	E	III	4	Temp. control	Y	N	Y	N	3
Mincing	B: microorganisms	E	III	4	Temp. control	Y	N	Y	N	4b
	C: insufficient nitrate and nitrite addition	E	III	4	Chemical analysis	Y	N	Y	N	4c
Conditioning	B: microorganisms	E	III	4	Temp. control	Y	N	Y	N	5
Mincing and kneading	B: microorganisms	E	III	4	Temp. control	Y	N	Y	N	6
Filling	B: microorganisms	E	III	4	Temp. control	Y	N	Y	N	7b
	P: tearing	C	IV	4	Physical observations	Y	N	Y	N	7c
Fermentation/ripining	B: microorganisms	E	III	4	Temp. control	Y	N	Y	N	8b
	C: residual of nitrate and nitrite	E	III	4	Chemical analysis	Y	N	Y	N	8c
Metal detection	P: metal residue	E	III	4	Calibration	Y	Y			9
Product storage	B: microorganisms	E	II	4	Temp. control	Y	N	Y	N	10

*Risk assessment (Table9), **CCP analysis (Figure 8), S: severity, P: probability, RC: risk class

Table 11. Risk assessment and CCPs in the processing of sucuk

Natural casings must be controlled for each batch. Temperatures of storage, mincing, conditioning and fermentation processes have to be monitored. Monitoring results should be continuously recorded.

Verification is the effort to determine whether the HACCP plan is valid and whether the system operates as planned or the HACCP plan is scientifically and technically evaluated. All stages in the process should be documented in order to enable retrospective observation, verification, and validation of the HACCP system. A recording procedure should be

Process name/step	CCP No:	Significant hazards	Critical limits	Monitoring** M.	F.	R.	Corrective action
Raw Material Reception (meat)	1b	B: microorganisms	*	MA	EB	LT	Reject
	1c	C: antibiotics, hormones	No	CA	EB	LT	Reject
	1p	P: Bone pieces	No	CA	EB	LT	Reject
Raw Material Reception (Additives, spices)	2b	B: microorganisms	Usually no, depends on types of spice and additives	MA	EB	LT	Reject
	2c	C: pesticide residues, mycotoxins	No	CA	EB	LT	Reject
	2p	P: metal	No	CA	EB	LT	Reject
Meat storage	3	B: microorganisms	*	MA	EB	LT	Discard
Mincing	4b	B: microorganisms	*	MA	EB	LT	Discard
	4c	C: insufficient nitrate and nitrite addition	150 ppm nitrite, 300 ppm nitrate	CA	EB	LT	Discard
Conditioning	5	B: microorganisms	*	MA	EB	LT	Discard
Mincing and kneading	6	B: microorganisms	*	MA	EB	LT	Discard
Filling	7p	P: tearing, air pockets	No	PE	EB	LT	Discard
	7b	B: microorganisms	*	MA	EB	LT	Discard
Fermentation/ ripening	8b	B: microorganisms	*	MA	EB	LT	Discard
	8c	C: Biogenic amine	Depends on types of amines	CA	EB	LT	Discard
Metal detection	9	P: Metal residue	No	Metal detector	EB	LT	Discard
Product storage	10	B: microorganisms	*	MA	EB	LT	Discard

* Microorganisms limits: No E.coli, $5*10^2$ S. aureus, No Salmonella (Anon 2000)

** MA: Microbiological analysis, CA: Chemical analysis, PE: Physical examination, EB: Every batch, LT: Lab. technician M: Method, F: Frequency, R: responsible

Table 12. HACCP plan for the processing of sucuk

prepared documenting the methods applied and the procedures followed. Verification should be implemented through internal audits with involves reviewing the pre-requisites, the hazards and risk assessment, critical control points, and critical limits.

The followings should be included in the HACCP plan according to the clause 7.6.2. of ISO 22000-FSMS; food safety hazards to be controlled at the CCP, control measures, critical limits, monitoring procedures, corrective actions to be taken if critical limits are exceeded, responsibilities, authorities and records of monitoring.

4.5.3 Quality system for the sucuk processing

ISO 9000:2000-QMS consisted of quality systems that focused on documenting all quality assurance and improvement processes in a company (ISO, 1999). Although the ISO 9000:2000-QMS was originally developed for the manufacturing sector, it had been applied to many service organizations and was gaining some acceptance in the food industry.

As seen in Figure 1., ISO 9000-QMS standard is consisted of five main parts. Namely; these are Quality management system, Management responsibility, Resource management, Product realization, Measurement, analysis and improvement. Standard articles are in Deming's cycle (PDCA) are continuously improved. The standard is worked out by essential processes. The processes are classified as strategic, operational and supportive processes are shown in Table 2. As seen in Figure 1, those processes cover all articles of the standard and also some procedures along with these processes are mandatory.

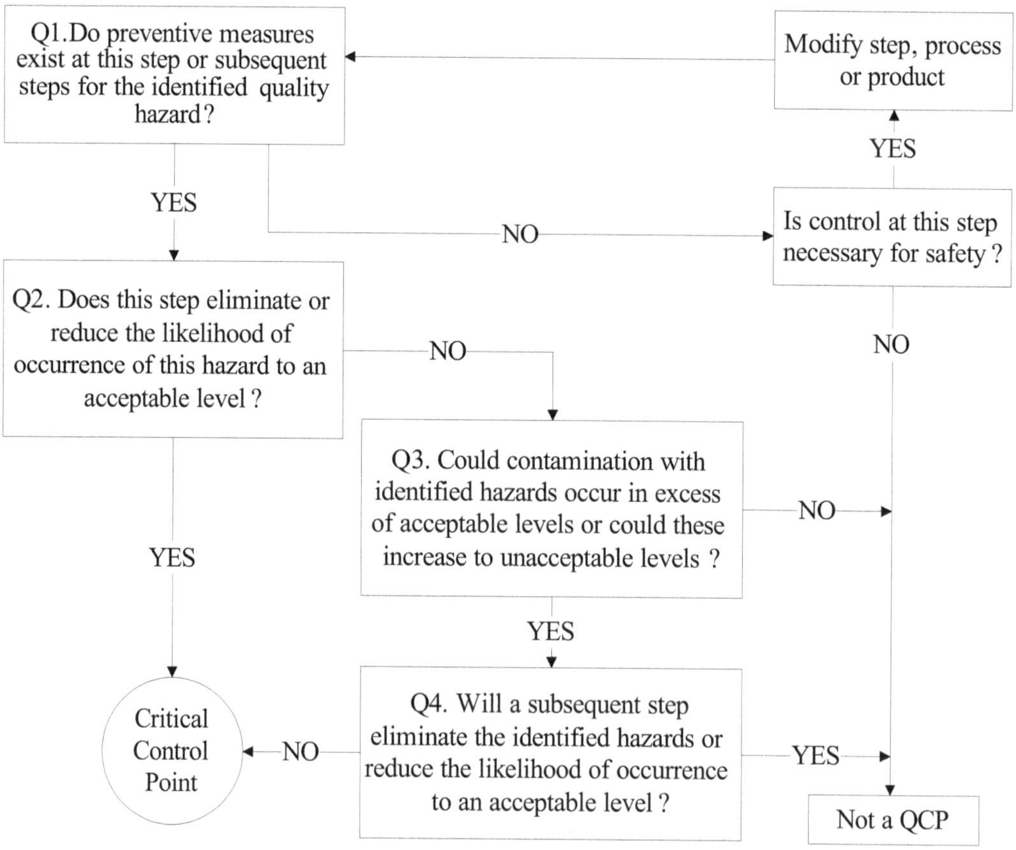

Fig. 8. Quality control points analysis (Decision tree)

Traditional sucuk processing is not a long-chain process. However, biological processes are usually involved in sucuk processing. Quality parameters of sucuk processing in small scale plants are affected by technological and administrative applications. Quality parameters of sucuk processing and quality hazards in the process are given in Table 13.

Quality control point (QCP) means a procedure where a control can be applied and a quality hazard (for example, taste, appearance, nutrition, color and so on) can be prevented, eliminated or reduced to acceptable levels (Figure 8).

Raw materials reception, mincing, conditioning, fermentation and ripening processes are analyzed as quality control points (Table 14). Defects on meat and additives directly affect quality, are however not able to be eliminated through the process. Color is an important quality parameter during many processes. Color of the sucuk is desired to be bright red color. This is usually controlled by temperature and other processing parameters as well as by addition of nitrite/nitrate. Critical limits, monitoring and corrective actions of quality parameters determined through the QCPs are given in Table 13.

Process name/step	Quality Hazard	Preventive actions/control measures	QCP analysis (Y/N)*				
			Q1.	Q2.	Q3.	Q4.	no:
Raw Material Reception (meat)	Rigor meat, dark or light red color, acidity	Effective supplier assurance	Y	N	Y	N	1
Raw Material Reception (Additives, spices)	Not having their specific color and flavor etc.	Effective supplier assurance	Y	N	Y	N	2
Meat storage	Color	Time and temp. control	Y	N	Y	N	3
Mincing	Color	Temp. control	Y	N	Y	N	4
Conditioning	Color, juiciness, drip loss	Temp. control	Y	N	Y	N	5
Mincing and kneading	Heterogeneous ingredients distribution	Cutter operation parameters control	Y	N	Y	N	6
Filling	Heterogeneous fat appearance on natural casings, bursting of casings	Casing control	Y	N	Y	N	7
Fermentation/ ripening	Dark red color, Water lost, Soft or hard texture formation, case hardening, pH	Time, temp. and relative humidity control	Y	N	Y	N	8
Metal detection							
Product storage	Water lost or gain	Temp. and relative humidity control	Y	N	Y	N	9

Table 13. QCPs in the processing of Sucuk

QCP No:	Process name /step	Quality parameter /hazard	Limits	Monitoring			Corrective action
				M.	F.	R.	
1	Raw Material Reception (meat)	Rigor meat, dark or light red color, acidity	Bright red color	VE	EB	LT	Reject
2	Raw Material Reception (Additives, Spices)	Not having their own specific color and flavor etc.	Their own specific color and flavor etc.	VE	EB	LT	Reject
3	Meat storage	Color	Bright red color	VE	EB	LT	Adjustment of nitrate level
4	Mincing	Color	Bright red color	VE	EB	LT	Adjustment of nitrate level
5	Conditioning	Color, juiciness, drip loss	Bright red color	VE	EB	LT	Adjustment of nitrate level
6	Mincing and kneading	Heterogeneous ingredients distribution	Mosaic appearance	VE	EB	LT	Reprocess
7	Filling	Heterogeneous fat appearance on natural casings, Bursting of casings	no	VE	EB	LT	Reprocess
8	Fermentation/ripining	Dark red color, Water lost, Soft or hard texture formation, Case hardening, pH	40 % water content, pH:5.4	VE & CA	EB	LT	Reprocess
9	Product storage	Water lost or gain	40 % water content	VE & CA	EB	LT	Reclassify

** VE: Visual examination, CA: Chemical analysis, EB: Every batch, LT: Lab. technician M: Method, F: Frequency, R: responsible

Table 14. Quality plan for the processing of Sucuk

5. Conclusion

The SPC techniques in food processing operations can play an important role of quality control and safety. The use of SPC techniques enables plant operators to take corrective actions quickly when needed before the variation affects significantly the CCPs of the plant. Traditional sucuk processing was used as a demonstrated process and some simple SPC techniques were used as the tools. Pareto analysis indicates that the priority problems of customer complaints. First five problems, namely off flavor, rancid, off color, poor texture and too oily cover approximately 90 % of total complaints. Control charts show that the process is in statistical control for moisture content in traditional sucuk production line. The control charts did not show out-of-control conditions in this study. Of course, we may expect out-of-limits. The pH change during ripening was modeled to Logistic equation. Scatter diagram of this change indicated a decrease and a leveling in pH after 5 days.

In this work, an effort was made for safety and quality parameter analyses (e.g. Failure mode and effect) of traditional sucuk production by describing and outlining the incoming hazards in every process stage, starting from raw materials to the final product. Hazard, cause and risk analyses for traditional sucuk production lead to have CCPs in every production steps. All production steps were also determined to be quality control points. A more efficient correction of the process is possible by use of these SPC tools.

6. References

Anon. (2000). Turkish Food Codex, Meat and meat products regulations. *National press*, no:24167

Arvanitoyannis, I. S. & Mauropoulos, A. A. (2000). Implementation of the hazard analysis critical control point (HACCP) system to Kasseri/Kefalotiri and Anevato cheese production lines. *Food Control*, 11: 31

Arvanitoyannis, I. S. & Traikou, A. (2005). A Comprehensive review of the implementation of hazard analysis critical control point (HACCP) to the production of flour and flour-based products. *Crit. Rev. Food Sci. and Nut.*, 45: 327

Arvanitoyannis, I.S. & Varzakas, T.H. (2008). Application of ISO 22000 and Failure Mode and Effect Analysis (FMEA) for Industrial Processing of Salmon: A Case Study. *Critical Reviews in Food Science and Nutrition*, 48:411–429

Arvanitoyannis, I.S. & Varzakas, T.H., (2007). Application of failure mode and effect analysis (FMEA), cause and effect analysis and Pareto diagram in conjunction with HACCP to a potato chips manufacturing plant. *International Journal of Food Science and Technology*, 42, 1424–1442

Ayranci, E & Dalgic, A.C. (1992). Moisture sorption isotherms of Pistacia terebinthus L. and its Protein Isolate. *Lebensmittel-Wissenschaft und –Technologie-Food science and technology*, 25, 482-483.

Banani, R. C.; Runu, C. & Utpal R. C. (2007). Validity of modified Gompertz and Logistic models in predicting cell growth of Pediococcus acidilactici H during the production of bacteriocin pediocin AcH. *Journal of Food Engineering*, Vol. 80, 1171-1175

Barendsz, A.W. (1998). Food safety and total quality management. *Food Control*, 9:2-3: 163

Bolat, T. (2002). Implementation of the hazard analysis critical control point (HACCP) system in a fast food business. *Food Rev. Int.*, 18: 337.

Bozkurt H. & Erkmen O. (2007). Effects of some commercial additives on the quality of sucuk (Turkish dry-fermented sausage). *Food Chemistry*, 101, 1465–1473

Bruce, H. L.; Scott, J. R. & Thompson, J. M. (2009). Application of an exponential model to early postmortem bovine muscle pH decline. *Meat Science*, Vol. 58, 39-44

Chase, R.B. & Aquilano, N.J. (1995). Production and Operations Management. *The McGraw Hill Companies*, Seventh Edition.

Codex Alimentarius Commission. (2003). Hazard Analysis and Critical Control Point (HACCP) system and guidelines for its application. In Food Hygiene Basic Texts. Rome: Food and Agriculture Organization of the United Nations, World Health Organization.

Daniela, S.R.; Aurora, M.C.; María, C.P.P.; Rodrigo, D. & Antonio M.L. (2009). Modeling survival of high hydrostatic pressure treated stationary- and exponential-phase Listeria innocua cells, *Innovative Food Science and Emerging Technologies*, 10, 135–141

Derosier, J.; Stalhandske, E.; Bagian, J.P.; & Nudell, T. (2002). Using Health Care Failure Mode and Effect Analysis™: The VA National Center for Patient Safety's Prospective Risk Analysis System. The Joint commission. *J. Qual. Imp.* 27(5): 248

Efstratiadis, M. M. & Arvanitoyannis, I. S. (2000). Implementation of HACCP to large scale production line of Greek ouzo and brandy: a case study. *Food Control,* 11: 19.

FAO. (1998). Food and Agriculture Organization/World Health Organization (FAO/WHO). (2001). Manuel on the application of the HACCP system in mycotoxin prevention and control. Food and Agriculture Organization of the United Nations, Rome.

Gao, Y.L.; Ju, X.R. & Ding, W. (2007). A predictive model for the influence of food components on survival of Listeria monocytogenes LM 54004 under high hydrostatic pressure and mild heat conditions. *International Journal of Food Microbiology*, 287-294

Grigg, N.P.; Daly, J. & Stewart, M. (1998). Case study: the use of statistical process control in fish product packaging. *Food Control*,Vol. 9, 289-297

Hii, C.L.; Law, C.L. & Cloke, M. (2009). Modeling using a new thin layer drying model and product quality of cocoa. *Journal of Food Engineering,* 90, 191–198

ILSI Europe. (2001). Principles of risk assessment of food and drinking water related to human health. Concise monograph series. Washington, DC: ILSI Press.

ILSI Europe. (2004). A simple guide to understanding and applying the hazard analysis critical control point concept. Concise monograph series. Washington, DC: ILSI Press.

ISO. (2005). ISO 22000: Food Safety Management Systems: Requirements. International Organization for Standardization, Geneva, Switzerland.

ISO. (1999). ISO 9000: Quality Management Systems: Requirements. International Organization for Standardization. Geneva, Switzerland.

Juran, J.M. & Gryna, F.M. (1998). Juran's Quality Handbook. 5th edition, (New York, McGraw-Hill)

Lee, J. A. & Hathaway, S. C. (1998). The challenge of designing valid HACCP plans for raw food commodities. *Food Control* 9: 111.

Mortimore, S. E. & Wallace, C. A . (1998). HACCP: A Practical Approach, 2nd edition, Aspen Publishers Inc, Gaithersburg, MD, USA.

Peng, Y. & Lu, R. (2007). Prediction of apple fruit firmness and soluble solids content using characteristics of multi spectral scattering images. *Journal of Food Engineering,* Vol.82, 142-152

Sandrou, D. K. & Arvanitoyannis, I. S. (2000b). Implementation of hazard analysis critical control point (HACCP) to the dairy industry: current status and perspectives. *Food Rev. Int.* 16:(1): 77.

Sandrou, D. K., & Arvanitoyannis, I. S. (2000a). Application of hazard analysis Critical control point (HACCP) System to the cheese-making Industry: a review. *Food Rev. Int.* 16:(3): 327.

Serra, J. A.; Domenech, E.; Escriche, I. & Martorell, S. (1999). Risk assessment and critical control points from the production perspective. *Int. J. Food Microb.*, 46: 9

Sperber, W.H. (1998). Auditing and verification of food safety and HACCP. *Food Control,* Vol.9, 157-162

Sperber, W.H. (2001). Hazard Identification: from a quantitative to a qualitative approach. *Food Control* 12: 223.

Srikaeo, K., & Hourigan, J.A. (2002). The use of statistical process control (SPC) to enhance the validation of critical control points (CCPs) in shell egg washing. *Food Control,* 263-273.

Wu,L.; Orikasa, T.; Ogawa, Y. & Tagawa, A. (2007).Vacuum drying characteristics of eggplants, *Journal of Food Engineering*, Vol. 83, 422-429

11

Processing and Quality Control of Herbal Drugs and their Derivatives

José Otávio Carréra Silva Júnior, Roseane Maria Ribeiro Costa,
Francisco Martins Teixeira and Wagner Luiz Ramos Barbosa
Universidade Federal do Pará, Instituto de Ciências da Saúde,
Faculdade de Farmácia Rua Augusto Corrêa n. 1,
Cidade Universitária Professor José da Silveira Neto, CEP: 66.075-110, Belém-Pa,
Brazil

1. Introduction

For thousands of years mankind has used the resources of flora in the treatment of various diseases. There are reports, for example, of the use of plants for therapeutic purposes dating back to 3000 BC in the Chinese work *Pen Ts'ao* by Shen Nung (Tyler, 1996; Ko, 1999). In 78 AD, the Greek botanist Pedanios Dioscorides described about 600 medicinal plants and this treaty remained as a reference source for more than fourteen centuries (Robbers et al., 1996; Tyler, 1996). The therapeutic properties of certain plants were discovered and propagated from generation to generation as a part of the popular culture through observation and experimentation by primitive people (Turolla & Nascimento, 2006).

In the sixteenth century, the Swiss physician Philippus Aureolus Theophrastus Bombastus von Hohenheim, known as Paracelsus (1493 - 1541), formulated the "Theory of Signatures" based on the latin proverb *similia similibus curantur,* which means "alike cures alike". According to this theory it was believed that the shape, color, flavor and odor of the plants were related to their therapeutical properties, giving clues to their clinical use. Some of these plants have become part of the allopathic and homeopathic pharmacopoeias since the nineteenth century, when their therapeutic basis started to be investigated (Elvin-Lewis, 2001). The isolation of morphine from *Papaver somniferum* in 1803 by the pharmacist Friedrich Wilhelm Adam Sertürmer marked the beginning of the extraction process of active ingredients from plants. Since then, other substances have been isolated, such as quinine and quinidine obtained from *Cinchona* sp in 1819, and atropine from *Atropa belladonna,* in 1831, which started to be used instead of plant extracts (Tyler 1996; Schulz, 2001).

The production of drugs by chemical synthesis, the growing of the economic power of pharmaceutical industries and the lack of scientific evidence on the efficacy of substances from plant origin combined with the difficulty of chemical, physico-chemical, pharmacological and toxicological control of plant extracts used so far, boosted their replacement by synthetic drugs (Rates, 2001). After the 1960s, there was a lack of interest from pharmaceutical companies and research institutes in the search for new substances from plant origin. This fact was due to the belief that the main active ingredients from known herbal drugs had already been isolated and all possible chemical modifications in these substances had already been performed (Schenkel et al., 2000). However, since the 1980s, technical advances and the development of new methods for isolation of active compounds from natural sources have enabled faster identification of substances in complex samples such as plant extracts. And so, there was a resurgence of interest in the research of these substances as prototypes for the development of new drugs from medicinal plants. According to Carvalho (2004), these medicinal plants are the ones which are selected and popularly used as medicine in treating diseases. They are defined by World Health Organization (WHO) 1978, as being any plant, which applied in a particular form and by any means to the human being, is capable of causing a pharmacological effect.

So, even after the development of large pharmaceutical laboratories and synthetic drugs, medicinal plants remained as an alternative form of treatment in various parts of the world. In the last decades, a revaluation of the use of herbal preparations was observed. These preparations are defined as any medication obtained and prepared, using only vegetable raw material with prophylactic, curative or diagnostic purposes, causing benefit to the user (Carvalho, 2004). Thus, some pharmaceutical companies began to make efforts toward the improvement of herbal medicines and their production on an industrial scale. This new development of herbal medicines, far from returning to the past, is characterized by the pursuit of industrial scale production, differently from the handmade forms which characterized its early stages (Turolla & Nascimento, 2006).

Currently, preparations derived from medicinal plants are widely used in many countries. In Africa, for example, 80% of the population depends on the use of these preparations, which represent alternatives to the high costs of synthetic drugs (Turolla & Nascimento, 2006).

The consumption of medicinal plants and herbal products has been somewhat surprising in recent years, constituting a promising pharmaceutical segment. This fact is primarily noted as a result of easy access, low cost and its popular or cultural compatibility (Tyler, 1996).

Medicinal plants are an important source of substances with biological activities. Many of them have become prototypes for the synthesis of a large number of bioactive compounds. Research indicates that Brazil is the world leader in plant diversity with about 55,000 described species and 350,000 to 550,000 estimated ones. From the cataloged ones, 10,000 species can be medicinal, aromatic or have other utilities (Borges et al., 2003).

Therefore there's a need to combine empirical knowledge about the popular use of medicinal plants with scientific research based on detailed studies of the plant species, as well as botanical, phytochemical, pharmacological, toxicological aspects, and the development of scientific and technological methodologies (Petrovick et al., 1997). The result of this scientific breakthrough is the development of a differential therapeutic herbal product, as unlike the traditional preparations obtained from plants in folk medicine, the scientific and technological grounding provide the development of herbal medicine (Wagner & Wiesenau, 2006; Leite, 2008).

So, the plant species that will be used in the development of phytotherapeutics deserves cares in its acquisition, like a previous unequivocal botanical identification, as popular names of the plants are very often regional, varying according to the region where they grow, so, it is very common that the same plant species has different vernacular denominations. On the other hand, different botanical species may have the same vernacular denomination, Furthermore, for a few different species, with some morphological similarity, the unequivocal distinction between them becomes very difficult; being not rare the cases of poisoning due to incorrect identification of the plant species (Farias,1985; Mengue, 2001).

Therefore it is indispensable the standardization of the starting material and intermediates in order to assure the quality of the product derived from them.

Standardization of material derived from plants represents a major challenge, especially for reproduction of biological effects. Botanical derivatives, when used for therapeutic purpose, are more complicated concerning the requirements of composition, constancy, stability, microbiological counts, etc. (Yunes et al., 2001).

The chemical standardization of derivatives of medicinal plants, like extracts and fractions, demands the application of methods and techniques that aim at detecting and characterizing substances that guarantee the quality of the plant material used, either by the aspect of the metabolic composition, chemical marker; or by the pharmacological activity, substances related to the activity of the plant, able to be quantified. However, studies prove that the plant secondary metabolism can vary considerably according to air temperature, water availability, ultraviolet radiation, nutrients, soil altitude and air quality in the place where the vegetable grows. Even mechanical stimulations or pathogens' attack can induce such variability, leading to the seasonal production of those potential markers (Gobbo-Neto, 2007).

The method used in the standardization of the starting material and derivatives must be validated considering the following parameters: specificity/selectivity, linearity, interval, precision, limit of detention, limit of quantification, accuracy and robustness, which must be determined and verified (Brazil, 2003).

The concern of regulatory agents about the standardization of herbal medicines provides the evaluation of important aspects such as efficacy and safety of these medications. The traditional use of various medicinal herbs based on folk knowledge and the belief that, being natural does not provoke adverse reactions, caused just a few of them to be evaluated through preclinical and clinical studies to prove their efficacy and safety (Turolla et al., 2006).

Vegetable raw material such as plants, pharmacogens or derivatives (extracts, tinctures, essential oils or dried products) has been widely used in drugstores and pharmaceutical industries. What worries most the scientific community is the use of new plant species as medicines without proven data about their biological action, non-toxicity (assessed in humans), side effects, safety, efficacy and others. Although these herbal medicines have natural active constituents, they should be assessed as drugs and therefore subjected to strict controls at every stage of their idealization, evaluation and development.

2. Definitions

2.1 Phytotherapy (Gaedcke & Steinhoff, 2003)

The term "phytotherapy" means the "prevention and treatment of human diseases using plants, parts of plants or preparations of plants".

The phytotherapy is a form of medicine that has grown noticeably over the years to the point that currently the world market for herbal medicines is around 44 billion dollars.

For Weiss and Fintelmann, it is a decisive aspect that the plant or parts of a plant which are used for pharmaceutical purposes are regarded as an active substance as a whole. Herbal medicinal products, in this regard, are always mixtures of a number of substances.

Phytotherapy has to be distinguished from other acknowledged therapeutic disciplines which also utilize plants such as homeopathy, invented by Samuel Hahnemann, and anthroposophy, whose background is on the Rudolf Steiner philosophy. The main difference

is that homeopathy is based on the principle "similia similibus curentur" - similar symptoms are healed by similar medicines. Besides that, homeopathy mostly uses very low doses. Efficacy is increased with the degree of dilution (potentiation).
Similar to homeopathy, anthroposophic medicine is based on a global approach to diseases. It focuses on the strong connection between human being and nature. Besides that, anthroposophy takes into account cosmological aspects when selecting the right medicine for individual cases of illness. In the same way as homeopathic medicines, anthroposophic medicines are mostly obtained from natural origin. They are partly manufactured according to the principles of homeopathy, sometimes also using heat (e. g. roasting, carbonization).
In contrast to homeopathy and anthroposophy, phytotherapy should definitely be understood as an allopathic discipline because the effects which are expected from herbal medicinal products are directed against the causes and the symptoms of a disease. Because of these important differences, phytoteraphy, in contrast to actual interpretation, in Germany for example, should not belong to the so-called "special therapeutic disciplines" or to "alternative medicine". It should, moreover, be classified as a regular discipline of natural orthodox science-oriented medicine, because the respective medicinal products have to comply with the same scientific requirements as those of the chemically defined substances in terms of quality, safety and efficacy.

2.2 Herbal drugs

For the term "herbal drug", the following definitions can be found in literature:
Drugs are herbal or animal organisms or organs transformed into a storable condition by drying. Furthermore, the definition comprises other matter extracted from plants or animals without organic structure such as resins, gums, fats, essential oils (Gaedcke & Steinhoff, 2003).
Drugs are complex active substances which are either used by patients as original herbal drugs or which serve as industrial starting materials for the manufacture of finished medicinal products or for the isolation of purified active substances or mixtures of substances. Drugs are either organized on a cellular basis, i. e. microorganisms, plants, animals or parts of these which have been dried or submitted to otherwise preservation or they are mixtures of substances which have been extracted from microorganisms, plants, animals or parts of these which do no longer have cellular structures, such as essential oils, resins, starch, fats, waxes, isolated mucous substances or animal toxins (Teuscher, 1997).
Herbal drugs are plants or parts of plants which have been transformed into storable conditions by drying, such as herba-, folium-, flos-, semen-, and radix drug (Hãnsel, 1991).
According to pharmaceutical linguistic rules, **herbal drugs** are dried or processed plants or parts of plants used for the manufacture of pharmaceutical preparations (Saller et al., 1995).
According to pharmaceutical linguistic rules, **herbal drugs** are dried herbal or animal starting materials (Bauer et al., 2002).
Herbal drugs are herbal matter used for pharmaceutical purposes. A "herbal drug" or a produced preparation therefore, is regarded as one active substance irrespective of the question of whether the active constituents of the herbal drug are known or not (Gaedcke & Steinhoff, 2003).
The definition for **herbal drug** in the European Pharmacopoeia is mainly whole, fragmented or cut, plants, parts of plants, algae, fungi, lichen in an unprocessed state, usually in a dried form, but sometimes fresh. Certain exudates that have not been subjected to a specific treatment are also considered to be herbal drugs. Herbal drugs are precisely defined by a

botanical scientific name according to the binomial system (genus, species, variety and author).
According to the definition of the European Pharmacopoeia, the expression "herbal drug" shall apply to herbal materials in dried as well as in fresh conditions, which from a specific point of view makes no sense. As a consequence, two kinds of herbal drugs would have to be distinguished, frist, the so-called "fresh herbal drug", which is a contradiction in itself (oxymoron) because the term "drug" implies that a material has been submitted to some kind of drying process, and second the so-called "dried herbal drugs" which due to the same reason, is linguistic nonsense.
Therefore, the starting materials used for the manufacture of herbal medicinal products should preferably be named "herbal drug" or "fresh part of plant".

2.3 Herbal medicinal products

Herbal medicinal products (Phytopharmaka) are regarding the active substance(s), more or less enriched preparations of plants or herbal drugs which, besides that, contain other concomitant substances exerting or not exerting therapeutic activity (Vogel, 1982).
Herbal medicinal products (Phytopharmaka) are those medicinal products which, as active substances, solely contain herbal drug preparations, such as comminuted parts of plants, extracts, pressed juices or distillates of plants. Isolated plant constituents such as digitoxin or menthol, as well as homeopathic medicinal products, are not regarded as herbal medicinal products.
Herbal medicinal products (Phytopharmaka) are complex preparations of herbal origin, i.e. galenic preparations of plants used within the sense of allopathic therapy. Isolated biogenic pure substances and complex preparations obtained from plants intended for use within alternative therapies such as homeopathy or anthroposophy do not fall within this definition (Teuscher, 1997).

2.4 Herbal drug preparations

According to the definition given in the European Pharmacopoeia Supplement 2000, herbal drug preparations are obtained by subjecting herbal drug to treatments such as extraction, distillation, expression, fractionation, purification, concentration and fermentation. These include comminuted or powdered herbal drug, tinctures, extracts, essential oils, fatty oils, expressed juice and processed exudates.
Extracts obtained from herbal drugs comply with the monograph on Extracts. Tinctures obtained from herbal drugs comply with the monograph on Tinctures.
Herbal teas comply with the monograph on Herbal teas.
Instant herbal teas consist of powder or granules of one or more herbal drug preparation(s) intended for the preparation of an oral solution immediately before use.
Extracts are preparations of liquid (liquid extracts and tinctures), semi-solid (soft extracts) or solid (dry extracts) consistency, obtained from herbal drugs or animal matter usually in a dry state.
Different types of extracts may be distinguished. Standardized extracts are adjusted within an acceptable tolerance to a given content of constituents with known therapeutic activity; Standardization is achieved by adjustment of the extract with inert material or by blending batches of extracts. Quantified extracts are adjusted to a defined range of constituents; adjustments are made by blending batches of extracts. Other extracts are essentially defined

by the production process (state of the herbal drug or animal matter to be extracted, solvent, extraction conditions) and their specifications.

Soft extracts are semi-solid preparations obtained by evaporation or partial evaporation of the solvent used for preparation.

Dry extracts are solid preparations obtained by evaporation of the solvent used for their production. Dry extracts usually have a loss on drying or water content not greater than 5 per cent m/m.

Liquid extracts are liquid preparations of which, in general, 1 part by mass or volume is equivalent to 1 part by mass of the herbal drug or animal matter. These preparations are adjusted, if necessary, so that they satisfy the requirements for the content of the solvent and, where applicable, for the constituents.

Tinctures are liquid preparations which are usually obtained using either 1 part of herbal drug or animal matter and 10 parts of extraction solvent or 1 part of herbal drug or animal matter and 5 parts of extraction solvent.

Different types of extracts may be distinguished. Standardized extracts are adjusted within an acceptable tolerance to a given content of constituents with known therapeutic activity; Standardization is achieved by adjustment of the extract with inert material or by blending batches of extracts. Quantified extracts are adjusted to a defined range of constituents; adjustments ar made by blending batches of extracts. Other extracts are essentially defined by the production process (state of the herbal drug or animal matter to be extracted, solvent, extraction conditions) and their specifications (Gaedcke & Steinhoff, 2003).

2.5 Classification of extracts in terms of their physical state

Depending on the physical state of an extract the following types can be distinguished:

- Liquid preparation: liquid extracts (fluid extract, tincture), oily macerates,
- Semi-solid preparations: soft extracts,
- Dry extracts: dry extracts.

The difference between fluid extract and tincture is that tinctures are not concentrated but diluted preparations.

The comminuted, mostly dried parts of the plant and the extraction solvent are combined in the extractor. This mixture is allowed to stand for several hours depending on the extraction process. Generally, extraction with additional extraction solvent is repeated until no more constituents are transferred to the extraction solution. In the next step, the extraction solution (miscella, eluate) is separated from the herbal drug residue. Since it contains the extractable herbal matter, the eluate represents an important intermediate product during the total manufacturing process.

If the extraction solvent is ethanol or water or a mixture of both, the preparations resulting after filtration are liquid extracts (fluid or tincture, depending on the grade of concentration). If the extraction is carried out with vegetable oils (e. g. rape oil or olive oil) oily macerates are obtained which are usually filled in soft gelatin capsules.

If the resulting preparation is a dry extract, processing of the eluate continues with cautious evaporation of the majority of the extraction solvent in the vacuum-evaporator. The resulting aqueous soft extract is evaporated to dryness using suitable drying aggregates, e. g. spray dryer, belt dryer or spray belt dryer. In most cases, suitable technical excipients such as maltodextrin, lactose or silicium dioxide have to be added. After grinding and sieving, flowable powder is obtained which can be further processed to tablets or coated tablets or filled in soft or hard gelatin capsules (Gaedcke & Steinhoff, 2003).

2.6 Ratio of the herbal drug to the extraction solvent

Maceration (extraction under steady-state conditions)

In this procedure, the ratio of the herbal drug to the extraction solvent is a decisive factor for the effectiveness (= extent) of the extraction. The quantity of extractable matter is increased with the quantity (mass, volume) of extraction solvent, as using higher amounts of extraction solvent, steady-state conditions are reached later.
The ratio of the herbal drug to the extraction solvent is, therefore, a relevant parameter for the quality of the extract and has to be exactly defined to ensure batch-to-batch conformity. It has to be specified as a fixed ratio, e.g. of 1:5 or 1:10.

Percolation (= exhaustive extraction)

In this extraction procedure, a fixed quantity of herbal drug (mass) is treated with a variable quantity (mass/volume) of extraction solvent until the extractable matter is completely transferred from the herbal drug matrix to the eluate (percolate). The ratio of the herbal drug to the extraction solvent may therefore vary from batch to batch within a certain range. It depends on the characteristics of the herbal drug (content of extractable matter, loss on drying, etc.). Herbal drug preparations manufactured by percolation procedures are described by the average quantity (mass/volume) of extraction solvent with a defined range, e.g. 1:12 (1:10 to 1:14).
This means that in case of tinctures the relevant factor for the quality of the preparation is the ratio of the herbal drug to the extraction solvent, and not the ratio of the herbal drug to the final tincture which is determined after the expression of the extraction solvent. Depending on the effectiveness of the expression process, the resulting ratio can be as follows:

- For tinctures 1:10 – a ratio of the herbal drug to the tincture of 1:7 to 1:9,
- For tinctures 1:5 - a ratio of the herbal drug to the tincture of 1:4 to 1:4, 5.

Subsequent filling-up to the initial ratio of the herbal drug to the extraction solvent of 1:10 or 1:5 is not in compliance with pharmacopoeial standards unless it is necessary for the adjustment of the preparation to a defined content of constituents or a group of constituents with known therapeutic activity (Gaedcke & Steinhoff, 2003).

3. Harvest and postharvest processing

Botanic is an essential area in the study of medicinal plants, which constitutes a very heterogeneous set of plants distributed in different taxonomic groups, with very different morpho-anatomic characteristics and whose unifying factor is their richness of pharmacologically active compounds. As a considerable proportion of medicinal plants are wild, the correct identification of plant material must be made by literature and consultation with experts and herbarium. The lack of scientific identification, or misidentification, will compromise the rest of the scientific work on the plant. So, for medicinal plant research, we should perform a harvesting for botanical identification and another one for phytochemical and pharmacological studies, each one with specific recommendations. From an anatomical standpoint, medicinal plants have aroused interest due to their abundance of secretory structures such as idioblasts, cavities, channels, laticifers and glandular trichomes, among others (Fahn, 1979; Evert, 2006), and the chemical diversity of their secretions which are rich in terpenes, alkaloids and phenolic compounds (Harbone, 1997). These secretions can be identified by conventional chemical analysis or by histochemical methods, which identify the compounds *in situ*, such as tests for lipids and terpenic substances, tests for phenolic compounds,tests for proteins, tests for alkaloids , tests for carbohydrates and tests for crystals.

3.1 Harvest

For each medicinal plant there is an appropriate time for harvesting the crop. The phytochemical monitoring of the active compounds allows the establishment of the right time to harvest. However, for plants whose active principles are not known yet, there are some general rules which can be applied. The bark should be harvested in spring, early summer and autumn. The humid environment facilitates the detachment of the bark. The bark should be carefully removed by cutting vertical segments. Care must be taken not to "roulette" the trunk, that is, to remove peels in horizontal cotes surrounding the trunk. This procedure prevents the circulation of the sap, resulting in the plant's death.

The underground organs: roots, rhizomes, tubers, bulbs of perennial plants should be harvested during winter, the dormant period, when the concentration of active principles reaches its maximum in these organs. The herbaceous plants and leaves are harvested when they start flowering. Some plants allow more than one cut. Sometimes, when there are well defined rainy and dry periods, the harvesting of the leaves is done during the dry season, allowing the plant to regenerate them during the rainy season. The shoot tips are harvested in full bloom and before seed formation. The flowers are cut before opening up completely, but sometimes the open inflorescences are harvested. The fruits are harvest "at once", i.e. before reaching the mature state. The seeds are harvested when ripe. If they are from fleshy fruits, the leftover pulp which surrounds them should be removed and the seeds dried. Periods of drought and rainfall influence the content of active principles. Thus, the alkaloid content decreases after the rain whereas the content of essential oils increases. The content of essential oils decreases after the drought. The concentration of active principles varies according to the time of the day. In general, glycosides reach their highest concentration in the afternoon, while essential oils reach their maximum level around noon. The exception is chamomile (*Matricaria recutita*), which reaches higher levels and better quality of essential oil during the night (Sharapin, 2000).

3.2 Post-harvest processing

The post-harvest processing aims at the conservation of the physical, chemical, organoleptic and pharmacological characteristics of the plant drug. The inadequate post-harvest processing results in low quality raw material, with loss of active ingredients, increased microbial load and bad commercial presentation.

The loss of active ingredients involve: degradation by metabolic processes; active principles hydrolysis; decomposition by light; enzymatic decomposition; degradation of thermolabile substances by heat ; volatilization of essential oils and contamination by bacteria and fungi.

The first stage of post-harvest processing involves examination and manual separation of parts which are damaged, stained and with signs of attacks by insects and / or fungi. The next recommended step, is to wash the drug in running water.

The most important stage of post-harvest processing is undoubtedly drying. The industry uses dried plants, enabling their preservation for prolonged periods of time. The exceptions are plants used to obtain essential oils, homeopathic tinctures and some extracts like artichoke (*Cynara scolymus*), which are processed fresh.

The moisture content in fresh plants varies from 60% to 80%. The drying process reduces the moisture content to 5% - 12%. According to the plant organ, the weight losses during drying are:

- Leaves: 20% to 75%
- Bark: 40% to 65%
- Wood: 30% to 70%
- Roots: 25% to 80%
- Flowers: 15% to 80%

The drying process stops the degradation processes caused by yeasts or enzymes, prevents the development of microorganisms and oxidation and hydrolysis reactions. However, as it involves heat, there are losses of essential oils and volatile substances, as well as the risk of degradation of thermolabile substances during the process. Most medicinal plants can be dried at temperatures between 30°C and 60°C. Plants containing essential oils or volatile substances should be dried at temperatures below 40°C. In all cases good air circulation should be ensured, favoring the process.

The method of drying must be experimentally determined for each plant drug. The slow drying may cause harmful changes, by the action of enzymes, fungi and bacteria, before the process is completed. A very quick drying hardens the superficial layer of the cells and prevents the evaporation of water inside the organ, which also results in the action of enzymes (Sharapin, 2000).

3.2.1 Storage

However great care has been taken during harvesting and drying, the plants lose active ingredients by degradation during storage. Although the recommended time limit for storing leaves and shoot tips is from12 to 18 months, and for bark and roots from 12 to 36 months, some plants lose active ingredients soon. The conservation of vegetable raw material for a longer period of time depends on storage conditions. Appropriate conditions prevent the product from having contact with the sun, dust, rodents and insects and other degradation factors, thereby, impeding the loss of volatile principles. The material can be wrapped in burlap sacks or bales. The use of plastic bags should be avoided as it does not allow adequate ventilation. The bags should be labeled with the scientific name of the plant and the part used entry date, supplier name origin and approval of quality control.

3.2.2 Grinding

The grinding is intended to reduce the particle size of the plant drug, making it suitable for the next step of the process which is extraction. The extraction of a drug as a whole or divided into coarse fragments will be incomplete due to poor penetration of the solvent in the plant tissue. It will also be very slow, since the cell membranes act as real barriers hindering the extraction procedure. In the case of previously divided drugs, such membranes are partially destroyed, making the dissolution of the cellular components in the outer liquid easier and more efficient. However, the excessive division and the formation of very fine dust may cause problems during the extraction process. In the percolation process there is a powder compaction, which impedes the passage of the solvent, resulting in an incomplete extraction of the drug. In the maceration process the very fine particles might pass to the extract and bring it to a cloudy appearance. The milling process is preceded by screening to remove impurities. In this operation strange material, such as large pieces of wood, other types of metal are removed manually.

4. Microbiological quality control of drug plants and their derivatives

4.1 Raw material

The microbiological quality assurance of herbal medicines must necessarily involve a proper stance regarding the Good Agricultural Practice. Researchers have even recommended the cultivation indoors, with full control over the climate and the presence of pathogens, and the possibility of genetic enhancement combined with biotechnological studies, indicating a tendency to domestication instead of harvesting from the wild (Calixto, 2000, Blumenthal et al., 1998; Bauer & TitteI, 1996). Yet the benefits that the cultivation of medicinal plants may bring to the achievement of desirable objectives related to the eight Millennium Development Goals proposed by the United Nations (UN) and addressed by the World Health Organization (WHO, 2009) (See still missing basic needs - Table 1) indicate the strategic importance of these products to the various traditional communities. These communities include family farmers, indigenous communities, Maroons, and other groupings in a vulnerable socioeconomic position, which have a historical knowledge of the properties and use of various medicinal plants, as it has been noted by several academic papers focused on the etnopharmacy (Pieroni & Vandebroek, 2007; Yoney et al., 2010; Leonti, 2011).For the success of this strategy it is necessary to ensure these communities with the access to this information and know-how, since they supply raw materials. This connection apparently seems to be unattainable due to social, anthropological and cultural incompatibilities. But what we have observed in practice is the gradual development of market relations between the major urban centers and the more reserved communities, which generally seek to avoid contact with the outside elements. This fact demonstrates the tendency of many of these communities to open channels for knowledge and values exchange in order to facilitate the development and quality of life without their identity loss.

4.2 Regulatory aspects

Heterogeneity exists not only between countries but even within the same country in relation to the maximum microbial limits which are acceptable for herbal products. Moreover, the treatment or application of plant material also involves different microbial limits and surveillance strictness. In some countries, herbal drugs for oral, topical or episodic use, produced by infusions, decoctions and maceration, have different laws when compared to plant drugs presented as capsules, tinctures, tablets, extracts and syrups. However, in general, the tests used to verify the presence of microorganisms in plant drugs show no significant variation and follow the recommendations used for non-sterile pharmaceutical products (Table 1).

4.3 Tests

4.3.1 Sampling and sample preparation

Initially 10 ml or 10 g of sample are needed for the performance of the assays. In case of raw materials, an interesting strategy to homogenize the sample and facilitate the interaction with the culture medium used, is the previous hand-grinding with a properly sterilized mortar and pestle in a sterile environment such as a laminar flow biological safety cabinet. So, when our analysis objects are leaves, stems or other plant constituents in their raw state, the sample preparation becomes important. On the other hand, thinner powders interact well with the solutions used in the homogenization and in the adjustment to near-neutral pH (pH = 7.0), favoring the growth of microorganisms present in the sample. Therefore, the pharmaceutical form may provide different strategies for sample preparation. In some cases it may be necessary to use other previous procedures, such as the use of inactivating agents, if evidenced the presence of preservatives in cosmetics based on herbal medicines, for example. When there is doubt about the presence of substances with inhibitory microbial growth a preparatory test for assessing the inhibitory capacity can be used. Carry out a transfer of each of the viable strains of *Staphylococcus aureus, Pseudomonas aeruginosa, Salmonella, Escherichia coli* and *Candida albicans* to 5 ml of soyabean casein broth and incubate at 30°C-35°C for 24 hours for bacteria and at 20°C- 25°C for 24 hours in the case of *Candida albicans*, making decimal dilutions in buffered peptone solution to obtain a suspension containing 50 to 100 viable cells. Use 1 ml of the microorganisms' inoculum separately in the presence or absence of the sample and incubate again as described for bacteria and fungi. If there is massive growth of microorganisms, microbiological assays may be undertaken; in case of little or no growth of viable strains it is necessary to use inactivating agents, for example, 0.5% soy lecithin, 4% polysorbate 20, 0.1% polysorbate 80, among others.

	Japanese Pharmac.[a, b]		United States Pharmac.[c]			British Pharmac[b]		Latin Amer. Pharmac.	
	Category 1	Category 2	Source 1	Source 2	Source 3	Category 1	Category 2	Argentine[d]	Brazil[e]
Aerobic bacteria	10^7	10^5	10^5	10^4	10^2	10^7	10^5	$10^7/10^4$	$10^7/10^5/10^4$
Molds and yeasts	10^4	10^3	10^3	10^3	10	10^5	10^4	$10^4/10^2$	$10^4/10^3/10^2$
Enterobacteria and other Gram negative bacteria	*	10^3	10^3	*	*	*	10^2	$10^4/10^2$	$10^4/10^3/10^2$
Escherichia coli	10^2	absence	absence	absence	*	10^2	absence	absence	10^2/10/absence
Salmonella	absence	absence	absence	absence	*	*	absence	absence	absence
Staphylococcus	*	*	*	*	*	*	*	absence	*/*/absence
Pseudomonas	*	*	*	*	*	*	*	absence	*

[a] Certain species of *Bacillus cereus*, *clostridia*, *Burkholderia*, *Aspergillus* and *Enterobacter* are also necessary to be tested depending on the origin of the herbal drug raw materials.
[b] Category 1: Herbal drugs to which boiling water is added before use and Category 2: Other herbal drugs and their preparations.
[c] Source 1: Dried or powdered Botanicals and Botanicals to be treated with boiling water before use.
Source 2: Tinctures, Powdered Botanicals Extracts, Fluidextracts and Nutritional Supplements with Botanicals.
Source 3: Infusions/Decoctions.
[d] The first value represents raw materials and final products for infusion preparations and the second value represents final products for topical and oral use.
[e] The first value represents Herbal drugs to which boiling water is added before use, the second value represents Herbal drugs to which the extractive process made in cold temperature and the third value represents final products for oral use.
*The limits are not specified.

Table 1. Recommended microbial limits for herbal drugs and their products or botanical ingredients and products

4.3.2 Viable microorganisms count

After preliminary tests, pour 10 ml or 10 g sample into a container containing 90 ml of soyabean casein broth, nutrient broth, buffered peptone broth or other appropriate diluents. It is important to attempt to the fact that the pH should be near-neutral and the characteristics of the sample, such as raw materials from forest origin, may contain higher amounts of fungi and therefore prone to high levels of aflatoxins. So, an appropriate medium would be one that favors the growth of fungi capable of producing these substances. From this first dilution, transfer 1 ml to tubes containing 9 ml of the used diluent, for example, soyabean casein broth, so as to obtain serial dilutions of 10^{-1}, 10^{-2} and 10^{-3}. In some cases the number of dilutions can be increased to improve the counting (Figure 1). From each dilution, transfer volumes of 0.1 to 0.5 ml to Petri dishes in duplicate containing Soyabean Casein Agar or Sabouraud-Dextrose Agar for counting bacteria and fungi, respectively. The spreading is accomplished with the aid of Drigalski spatula or a sterile glass rod. In case of bacteria, the incubation should be at 30°C-35 °C for 48 to 72 hours; for fungi, temperatures from 20°C to 25 °C for 5-7 days at least. Antibiotics are commonly used in the culture medium in order to inhibit the growth of undesirable microorganisms. Therefore, amphotericin B is added to the culture medium for bacterial growth (Soyabean Casein Agar or Nutrient Agar) and chloramphenicol to the culture medium for fungi growth (Sabouraud-Dextrose Agar or Potato Agar).

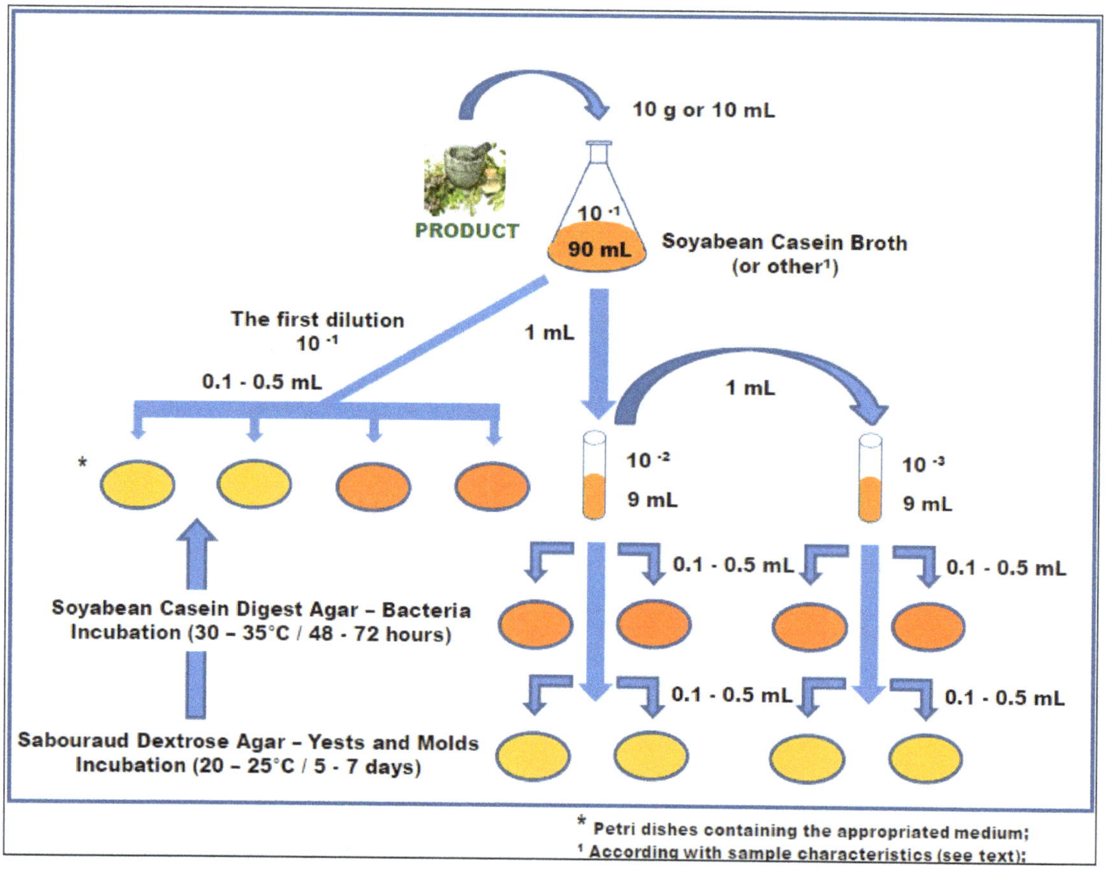

Fig. 1. Viable microorganism count

4.3.3 Search for undesirable microorganisms

Using appropriate enrichment medium, the same amount of sample used for the enumeration of microorganisms (10ml or 10 g of sample in a container containing 90 ml of medium) is used for the detection of pathogens. For detection of *Escherichia coli* and *Salmonella* sp., lactose broth is used and for the latter, after enrichment in lactose broth, the procedure is incubation in tetrathionate broth or selenite cystine broth for 24 hours at 30°C - 35 °C. In the case of *Staphylococcus aureus* and *Pseudomonas aeruginosa*, soybean casein broth is used for enrichment, which should also occur for 24 hours at 30°C - 35 ° C. Then, aliquots are transferred to culture medium for isolation and differentiation and subsequent use for conventional biochemical assessments (Figure 2 and 3).

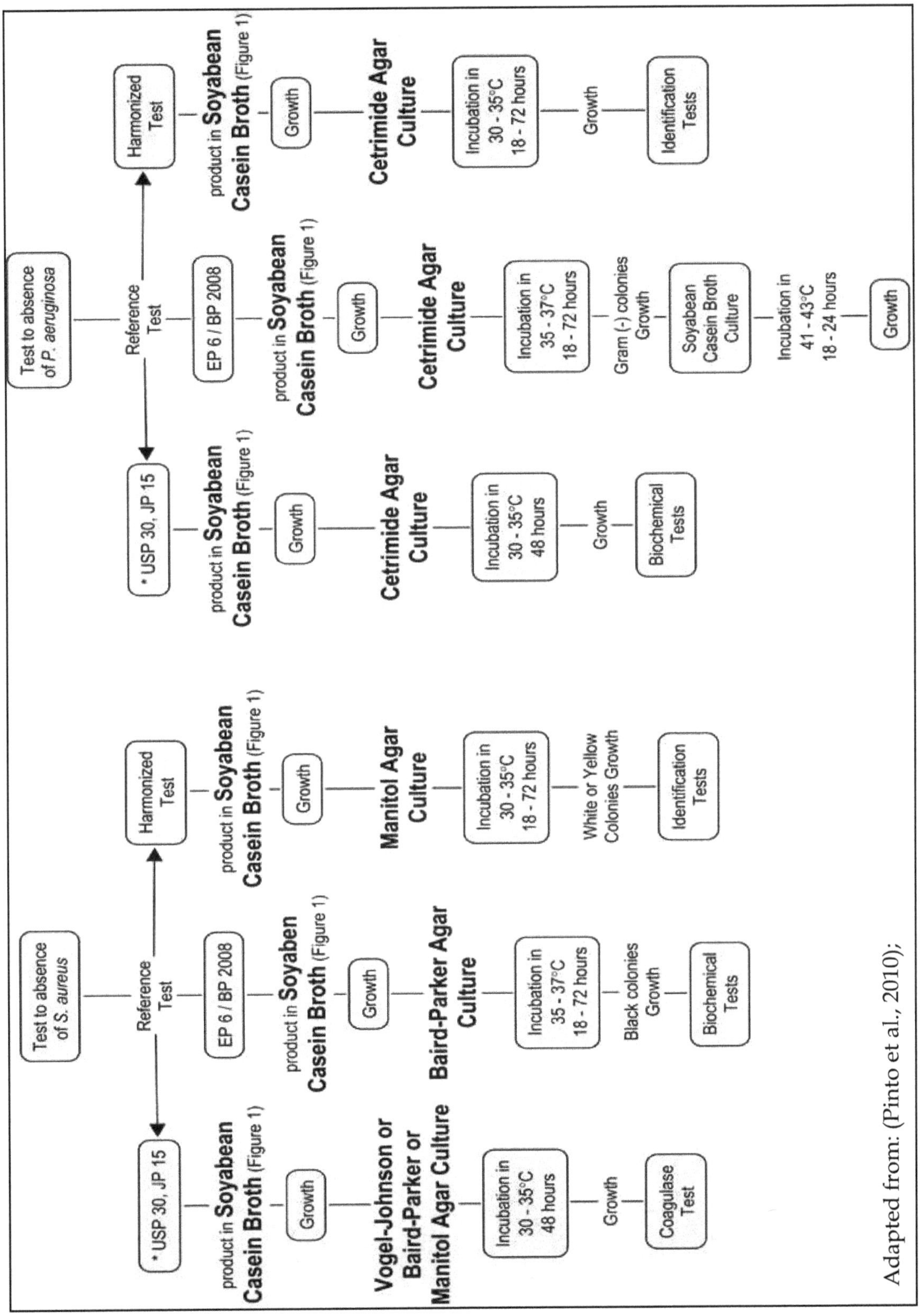

Adapted from: (Pinto et al., 2010);

Fig. 2. Enrichment and selective medium to *S. aureus* and *P. aeruginosa*

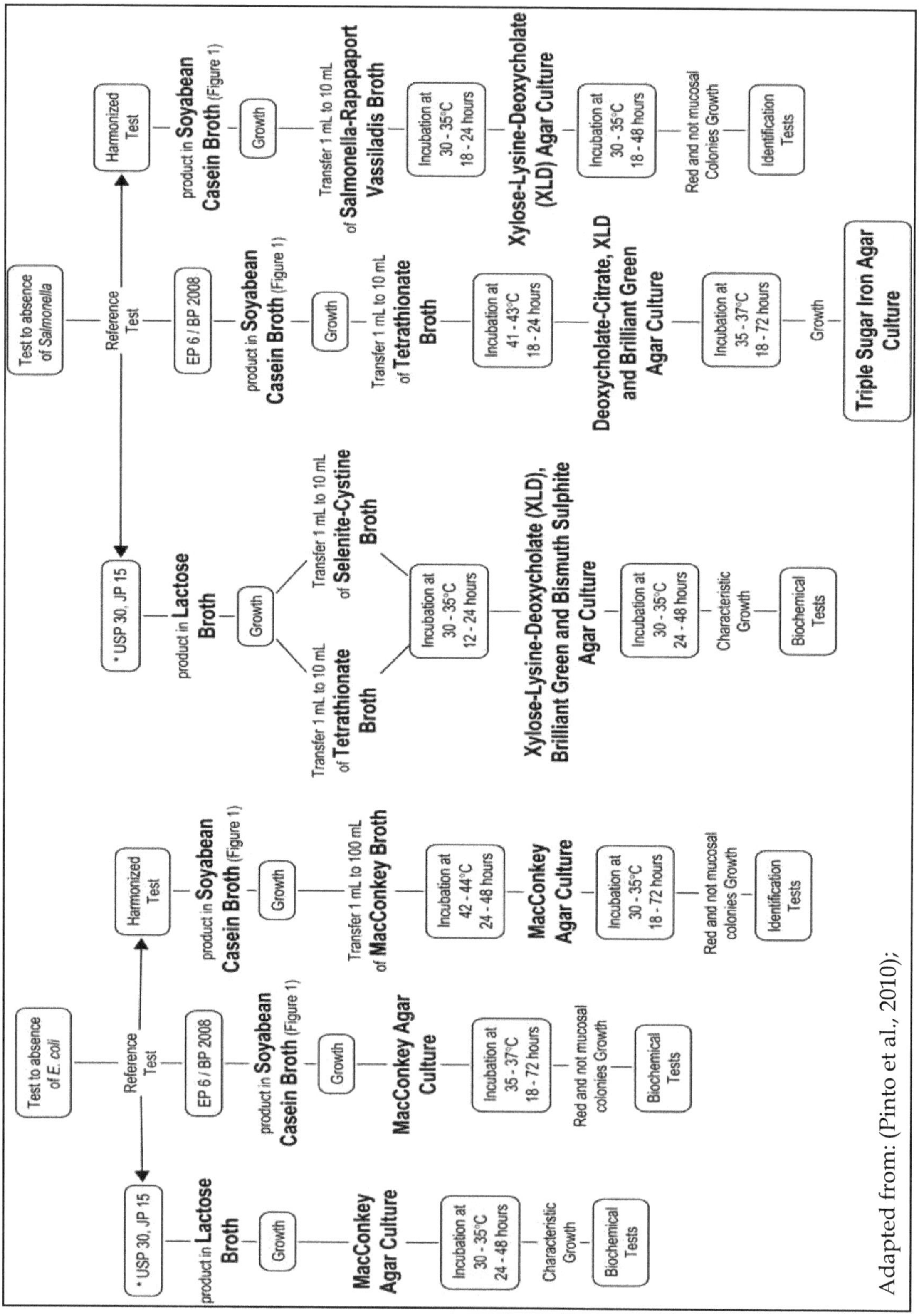

Fig. 3. Enrichment and selective medium to *E. coli* and *Salmonella*

5. Physical, chemical and physico-chemical controls of quality of herbal drugs and/or their derivatives: Tinctures and extracts

To ensure quality for vegetable raw material, the WHO, 1992 recommends that the pharmacopoeia specifications for the plant material must include:

- Botanical name, with reference to the authors;
- Specification of the part used;
- Morphological description, macro and microscopic examination;
- Determination of particle size distribution;
- Determination of total ash or sulfated ash (residue on ignition) and acid insoluble ash;
- Determination of extractable matter;
- Determination of water and loss on drying;
- Determination of essential oils;
- Identification by thin layer chromatography;
- Quantitative determination of active constituents;
- Limit tests for heavy metals;
- Determination of pesticide residues.

5.1 Botanical name

The botanical identification is essential to characterize the plant species. This identification cannot be made through popular names since the same species may have different common names and different species may be designated by the same common name. The identification of the plant is given by its "scientific name". The scientific name is always a Latin binomial, a term identifying the gender and both of them together identifying the species. The Latin binomial is followed by the name of the author of the botanical description, usually abbreviated. Finally, the identification is completed with the name of the botanical family to which the plant belongs.

5.2 Specification of the used part

The drug, i.e., used part of the plant, must be specified, for example, inflorescence, leaves, roots, wood or seeds. The specification is described in the language of the country and in Latin. The European Pharmacopoeia adopts as the title of the drug monograph, its name in Latin and as the subtitle, its name in English (or French, depending on the edition). The Brazilian Pharmacopoeia adopts as a title the popular name of the plant and as the subtitle, the specification of the used part, in Latin. Both pharmacopoeias complete the identification with the botanical name of the plant and specifications related to the content of active principles. The European Pharmacopoeia includes the scientific name of the plant when describing the drug, while the Brazilian Pharmacopoeia emphasizes it before the description.

5.3 Morphological description, macro and microscopic examination

A monograph of a plant drug describes the macroscopic, microscopic and organoleptic characteristics. The characteristics described should be compared to the drug sample, as a first step to establish its identity and purity. Whenever possible, authentic samples of the drug should be used as reference samples. The organoleptic characteristics (odor and flavor) often represent a practical guidance regarding the identity and purity of the drug. If the odor and taste vary considerably from the drug prescribed, the drug may be considered out of specification.

The macroscopic characteristics include the shape, size, color, texture, fracture aspects and characteristics of the cut surface. These features are useful for determining the identity and purity of the drug in question. However, since the judgment of these characteristics is very subjective, comparisons to authentic samples should be taken to avoid doubts.

The microscopic characteristics are viewed under a microscope, with or without the addition of chemical reagents. Microscopic analysis is indispensable for powdered drugs. This analysis helps to identify the drug and may be crucial in the identification of adulterants. However to ensure the identification of the drug, the microscopic analysis should be supplemented with data from chemical and physico-chemical analysis, Figures 4 and 5 (Alves, 2008; Alves et al. 2010).

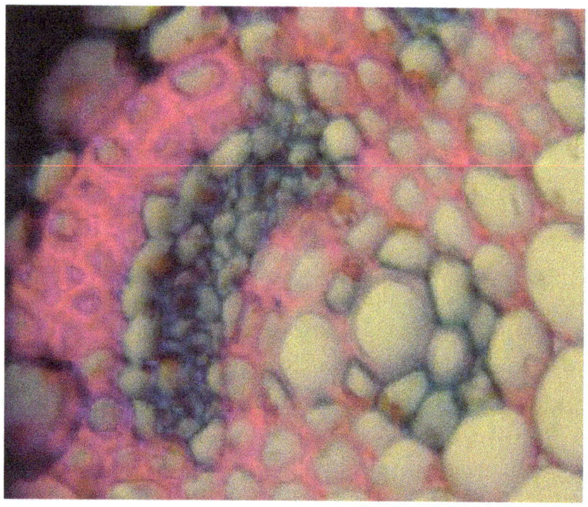

Fig. 4. *Arrabidaea chica* (Humb. & Bonpl.) B. Verlt. (Bignoniaceae). Cross section of the petiole. Detail of the vascular system and sclerenchyma; external phloem; xylem; internal phloem; sclerenchyma; parenchyma cells

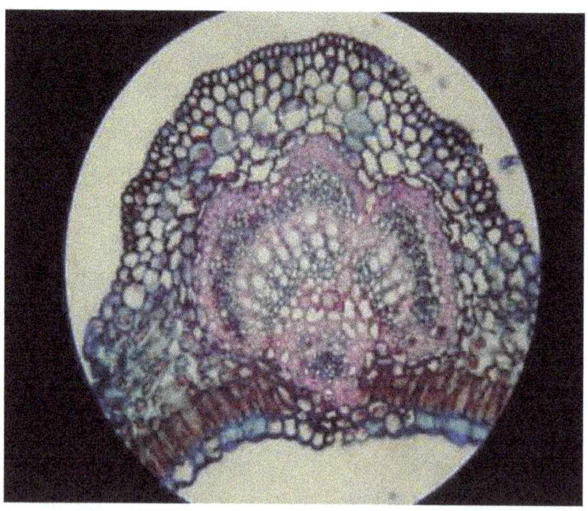

Fig. 5. *Arrabidaea chica* (Humb. & Bonpl.) B. Verlt. (Bignoniaceae). Cross section of the basal lamina. Upper epidermis; lower epidermis; angular collenchyma; fundamental parenchyma; sclerenchyma; phloem; xylem; palisade parenchyma e cuticule

5.4 Determination of particle size distribution

The particle size distribution of herbal drugs determines the contact surface available for interaction with the solvent used to obtain the plant derivative. It is a preliminary and important parameter for choosing the appropriate extraction process, as it has a direct influence on its efficiency (Santos et al., 2000).

Procedure for determination of particle size distribution: an electromagnetic sieve shaker is used. About 10 g of powdered plant material are subjected to a series of sieves with mesh size opening ranging from 2.00 mm to 125 µm, and agitated for 30 minutes. The particle size is analyzed in triplicate and evaluated by quantifying the percentage of powder retention in each sieve (Brazilian Pharmacopoeia V, 2010)

5.5 Determination of ash

The determination of ash includes the determination of total ash, sulfated ash, also called residue on ignition and determination of acid-insoluble ash. The total ash involves determining both the physiological and the non-physiological ash and consists of measuring the amount of non volatilized residue after the drug calcination. Sulfated ash is represented by non volatilized residue after calcination with concentrated sulfuric acid. The metals contained in the drug are converted to sulfates, as these are more stable to heat, and allow more accurate results than those obtained by simple calcination. The acid-insoluble ash is the residue obtained after boiling the residue obtained in the determination of total ash and sulfated ash with dilute hydrochloric acid, filtrating to remove the soluble and igniting the remaining insoluble matter. This procedure determines the level of silica, especially sand and siliceous earth present in the drug.

Procedure for determination of total ash: Accurately 3 grams of the powder is transferred to porcelain crucibles which were previously calcined, cooled and weighed. The samples are charred in a muffle furnace at 450 °C for 2 hours. After cooling in a desiccator, they are weighed on an analytical balance. This procedure is repeated until obtaining constant weight. The ash percentage obtained in triplicate, is calculated in relation to the dried drug (Brazilian Pharmacopoeia V, 2010).

5.6 Determination of extractable matter

The determination of extractable matter is carried out when there are no suitable methods to determine the active constituents of the drug by chemical or physico -chemical processes. Substances extracted with water, with ethanol in various dilutions and, more rarely, with ether are usually determined. The method is based on the solubility of active substances in a given solvent, and when these are not known, on the pharmacological activity of the extract obtained as a solvent.

5.7 Determination of water and loss on drying

The presence of excessive amounts of water in plant drugs is responsible for the growth of bacteria and fungi as well as the hydrolysis of constituents. The pharmacopoeial monographs limit the water content, especially in drugs that have the facility to absorb it, or in which the excessive amounts of water cause deterioration. With few exceptions, the water content in vegetable drugs should vary between 8% and 14%.

The water content can be determined by the gravimetric method, where the drug is desiccated to constant weight in an oven. The heating also causes the loss of volatile substances. For this reason it cannot be applied to drugs that contain such substances. In this case the azeotropic method may be applied, which consists of distilling the drug sample with toluene or xylene. This method requires special equipment and it is more difficult to carry on than the gravimetric method.

Procedure for determination of water loss on drying and gravimetric method: Exactly 3 grams of powdered plant are transferred to a weighing bottle. The sample is subjected to a temperature of 105° C for two hours followed by cooling in desiccators and weighted (Costa, 1982; Brazilian Pharmacopoeia V, 2010). The operation is repeated until obtaining constant weight. The results of three determinations are evaluated in terms of weight percentage on the sample amount using the equation (Brazilian Pharmacopoeia V, 2010):

$$\%\ \text{loss} = \frac{\text{Wb-Wa}}{\text{Ws}} \times 100 \qquad (1)$$

Where:
Ws = sample weight (g)
Wb = weight of the weighing bottle containing the sample before drying (g)
Wa = weight of the weighing bottle containing the sample after drying (g)

Another method that can be applied is the Karl Fischer Method, which is based on the quantitative reaction between water and anhydrous solution of iodine and sulfur dioxide dissolved in pyridine and methanol (Karl Fischer reagents). Usually the excess of reagent is incorporated to the sample, and after waiting for the time required to the quantitative reaction, the reagent excess is titrated with a standard solution of water in methanol. This technique (of unrestricted use) is especially recommended for samples which slowly release their content in water.

5.8 Determination of essential oils

Essential oils are volatile constituents found in many plants and characterized the mixture of terpenes, sesquiterpenes and their oxygenated derivatives and, sometimes, aromatic compounds, which volatilize at room temperature and are oily. Essential oils usually contain pharmacologically active substances. The determination of essential oils is carried out by hydrodistillation collecting the distillate in a graduated tube, in which the aqueous phase is automatically separated from the oily phase and returns to the distillation flask. When the essential oil has a density near to that of water or when the phase separation is difficult, a previously measured quantity of a solvent with low mass density and a suitable boiling point (e.g. xylene) is added in the graduated tube to dissolve the essential oil and facilitate the separation.

5.9 Identification by thin layer chromatography

The TLC is a simple, efficient method and requires no sophisticated devices for its implementation. The method is used for the characterization of plant drugs, their extracts and tinctures, and indicates the presence of the drug or its extracts in a pharmaceutical formulation. When the active principles of the drug are not known, the identification should be made using the substances which are characteristics of the plant, even without pharmacological activity.

These substances, called markers (or positive markers), should be selected among the substances that are characteristic of the plant. Its use, however, should be limited to the identification of plant material, extracts and tinctures. The markers may also serve to identify the presence of the drug in a pharmaceutical formulation. However, when the markers are not the substances responsible for the pharmacological action of the drug they cannot be used for quantitative measurements. The existence of stained spots or bands with the same Rf of the reference substances, in the chromatogram of the sample is not sufficient to identify the drug.

The existence of other stained spots or bands and their position in relation to the position of the reference substances used must also be described. The use of reference substances that are not the plant constituents is useful in determining the occurrence of counterfeits. These substances are called negative markers. So, *Arnica montana* extracts are analyzed by comparison with rutin solutions, a substance that does not occur in this plant. The appearance of a spot in the chromatogram of the extract with the same Rf and color of rutin indicates a possible forgery with *Calendula officinalis* flowers.

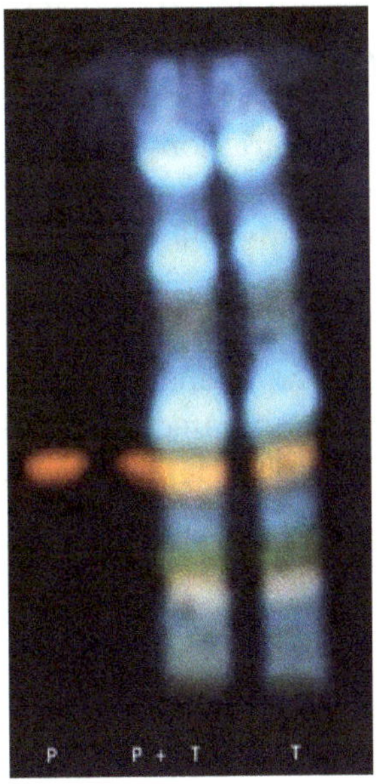

Fig. 6. TLC analysis of the tincture of *Calendula officinalis* L. Eluent I: ethyl acetate; formic acid; acetic acid; water (100:11:11:26); developer: NP/PEG 4000. Observation under light UV 365 nm; P- rutin standard ; T- Calendula tincture (Nunes, 2008; Nunes et al., 2009)

5.10 Quantitative determination of active principles

The selection of a method for quantitative determination of active principles in phytotherapeutics depends on the monograph of the drug in matter, which must to be considered as a whole designed to assure a satisfactory quality to the product. Many times the selection of a quantification method falls on a less specific technique, which despite the ease in performing, shows high precision, as for example, the acid-base volumetric determination of alkaloids, or titration in non aqueous solutions. If analytical equipments are available, among other more elaborated methods, the ultraviolet spectroscopy, a fast and simple technique with relative low cost, can be employed to quantify markers which present at least a chromophore, a functional group that absorbs light between 200nm 400nm. However, some molecules do not present such group and in this case it is worth, to introduce a chromophore in the molecule or to adopt another quantification technique.

Sometime it is not possible to isolate or get the marker in adequate conditions to be used in the method, and it is possible to characterize and quantify a group of substances of the same metabolic class to which the pharmacological activity of the plant can be associated. This is the case of the alkaloids of a species from Himatanthus genus, to which antispasmodic activity is alleged, and that were characterized and quantified as total alkaloid fraction in relation to the yoimbine (Barros, 2010). The method was developed in laboratory and validated according to both Brazilian and International regulation (ANVISA, 2003; IHC, 2005), taking into account the following parameters: selectivity, verified by analysis of the reference substance in comparison with the sample and their solvent (Methanol), in the same wavelength, where the absorption of the sample and the substance and the transparency of the solvent can be observed; the linearity, characterized by the determination (R2) and correlation (r) coefficients of the reference substance, and also, by the statistical analysis of the residue of the concentration values used to evaluate this parameter. Using five from the seven yoimbine concentration values employed to determine the linearity of the method, a calibration curve was built to, in fact, quantify the marker in the sample. The repeatability, the intermediate precision and the accuracy of the method must also be verified. In Brazil, ANVISA determines a 5% limit to the variation of the accuracy of a quantification method, which should not be lower than 95%. Other parameters that validate the developed method are detection and quantification limits. The following figures illustrate the selectivity (Figure 7), the linearity (Figure 8) e the analysis of residue (Figure 9) extracted from *Himatanthus* sp. (Barros, 2010).

Currently, in Brazil the regulation agency recommends for the registration of phytotherapeutical the use of more elaborated methods, which demand techniques like High Performance Liquid Chromatogrphy (HPLC) or Gas Chromatography (GC), for the quantification of markers.

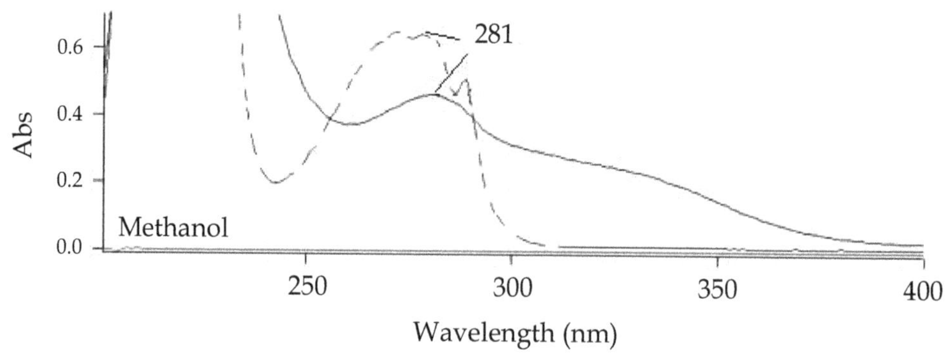

Fig. 7. Selectivity of the method developed with 22μg/mL Yoimbine as reference, (- - -), in relation to the alkaloid fraction of the aqueous extract of Himatanthus sp at 30 μg/mL (-) and to solvent methanol, observed from 200nm to 400nm (absorbance vs wavelength)

5.11 Limit tests for heavy metals

The limit test for heavy metals consists in verifying if the content of metallic impurities that react colorimetrically with sulfide ion does not exceed the limit specified in the monographs in terms of micrograms of lead per gram of test sample. Similarly, the reaction with thioacetamide may be employed for determining the limit of heavy metals in terms of lead.

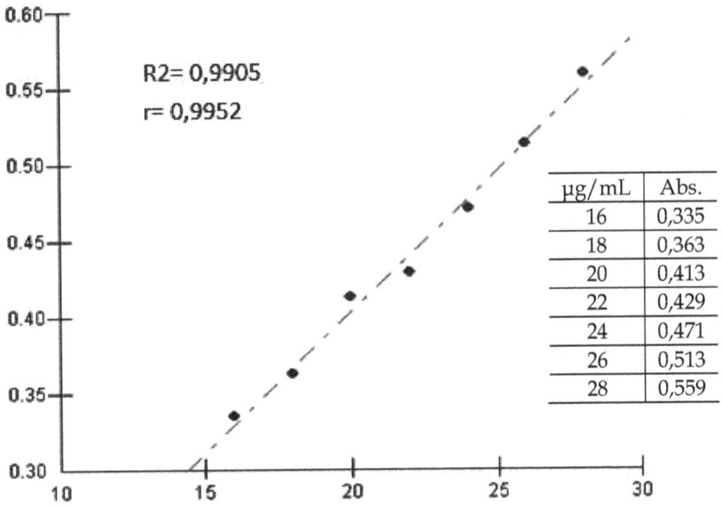

µg/mL	Abs.
16	0,335
18	0,363
20	0,413
22	0,429
24	0,471
26	0,513
28	0,559

Fig. 8. Graphical representation of the linearity of the method using Yoimbine in methanol at 281nm, the detail concentrations and its respective absorbance (absorbance vs concentration)

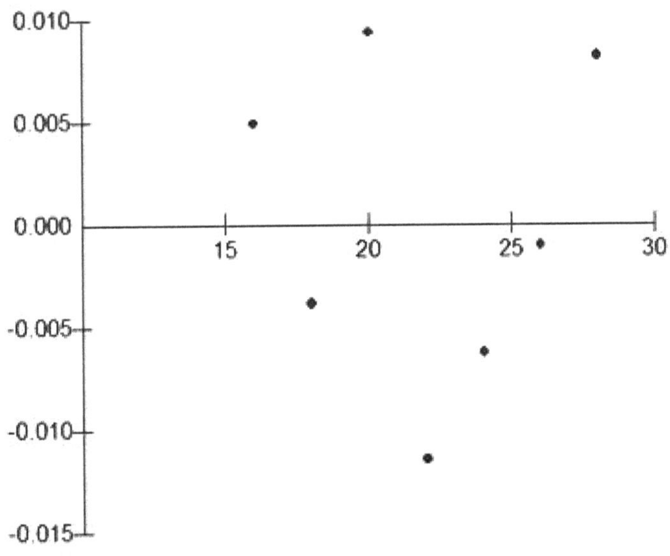

Fig. 9. Graphical representation of the residues analysis of the concentration values of Yoimbine solutions at 16, 18, 20, 22, 24, 26 and 28 µg/mL used in the calibration curve and determination of linearity

Procedure: The tests are conducted in transparent flat-bottomed glass tubes, with a capacity of approximately 70 mL and the external mark corresponding to a volume of 45-50 mL with an internal diameter of 23 mm. The tubes used should be equal in both the inner diameter and in other aspects, since the comparison is direct. The tubes should be observed from above, against a white background. The standard volume used varies according to the specified in the monograph under analysis.

5.12 Determination of pesticide residues

The use of pesticides to protect growing plants used as food from destruction by insects has grown enormously. The perception of the serious danger that the indiscriminate use of pesticides represented has led the WHO to establish limits to their residues. Since then, numerous methods for pesticide residue analysis have been published in the literature. Medicinal plants as well as food plants are subjected to attack by insects and fungi. Weeds are responsible for the reduced yields. Plant drugs accumulate pesticide just as food plants from agricultural practices such as spray application, the capture of the treated soils or administration of fumigants during storage.

6. Other methods that can be used for quality control of herbal drugs and/or their derivatives, tinctures and extracts

6.1 The infrared (IR) and ultaviolet (UV) spectroscopy

Infrared radiation corresponds approximately to the portion of the electromagnetic spectrum lying between the regions of the visible and microwave. The most useful portion to organic chemistry is situated between 4000 cm-1 and 400 cm-1. This band when absorbed by an organic molecule, converts into a molecular vibration energy. The process is quantized, like a series of bands, as each change of vibrational energy level corresponds to a series of changes in rotational energy levels (Silverstein et al., 2007). It is possible to obtain spectra of gases, liquids and solids in the infrared. Liquids can be examined in their pure state or in solution. The solvent should be fairly transparent in the region of interest so as not to interfere in the result. Volatile liquids are examined in closed cells with very thin spacers. Solid samples are examined in the form of airborne dust, pressed disk (KBr, ZnSe, etc.), or glassy film deposited on a transparent plate (Silverstein et al., 2007).

The infrared spectrum of a chemical compound is considered one of its most characteristic physic-chemical features and, because of this the infrared spectroscopy is extensively used to indentify compounds (Silverstein et al., 2007).

Another type of spectroscopy is performed in the ultraviolet (UV) region involving photons spectroscopy, and called spectrophotometry. Using a range between 200 to 400 nm the molecules undergo electronic transitions of molecular orbitals (Silverstein et al., 2007) The UV spectrophotometry is one of the most used methods in analytical determinations in various fields and may be applied to determinations of organic and inorganic compounds, for example, in the identification of the active principle of the drug. The molecular absorption spectroscopy is valuable for the identification of functional groups in the molecule. More important, however, are the applications of ultraviolet absorption spectroscopy for the quantitative determination of compounds containing chromophoric groups (Vinade & Vinade, 2005). Spectrophotometry in the UV region of the electromagnetic spectrum is one of the most used analytical techniques in terms of robustness, relatively low cost and large number of developed applications. It is based on the Beer-Lambert law, which is the mathematical basis for measuring radiation absorption by samples in solid, liquid or gaseous state in ultraviolet regions, visible and infrared electromagnetic spectrum (Perkampus, 1992). In determining the parameters of quality control of herbal medicines, which are composed of a complex mixture of components and due to the limitations on sensitivity in this method it is often necessary to use preliminary steps for separation and concentration of the desired elements, with a consequent increase of sensitivity. Among these techniques, we can mention the liquid-liquid extraction, precipitation and solid-liquid extraction (Cheng and Bray, 1955).

6.2 Thermal analysis

Thermal analysis is a term used to describe the analytical techniques that measure the physical and chemical properties of a sample as a function of temperature, while the substance is subjected to a controlled temperature program. The sample is subjected to a temperature schedule that consists of a series of preselected segments in which the sample is heated or cooled at a constant rate or kept at a constant temperature (Giolito & Ionashiro, 1988).

In recent decades, the thermo analytical techniques have gained increasing importance in all areas of knowledge in basic and applied chemistry. This development in the use of this methodology really endowed with great potential, was favored by the availability of instruments controlled by microprocessors, capable of providing accurate information about the thermal behavior of materials in a relatively short time. These methods are widely used in quality control of natural and synthetic drugs, because they can quickly provide data on the stability of the analyzed material, in the presence of its thermal behavior (Giolito & Ionashiro, 1988). Other methodologies which are importantly increasing in Brazil are: thermogravimetry (TG), differential thermal analysis (DTA) and differential scanning calorimetry (DSC) which are used to study pre-formulation or drug excipient compatibility. Among several papers published in this area, the most outstanding ones are: application of thermogravimetry (TG) in quality control of Milon (*Cissampelos sympodialis* Eichi.) Minispermaceae (Aragão et al., 2002), thermal analysis and compatibility study of zidovudine with excipients (Araujo et al., 2003); study of thermal stability of metronidazole tablets (Souza et al., 2002); Thermal analysis study of captopril coated tablets by thermogravimetry (TG) and differential scanning calorimetry (DSC) (Bazzo & SILVA, 2005); thermoanalytical study of glibenclamide and excipients (Oliveira et al., 2004); thermoanalitycal study (TG, DTG and DSC) of *in natura* and processed coffee (Schnitzler et al., 2005); study, characterization and determination of the purity of commercial samples of saccharin (Schnitzler et al., 2005); determination of moisture content and ash content of commercial samples of guarana using conventional methods and thermal analysis (ARAÚJO et al., 2006); physicochemical characterization of fluid and spray dried extracts of *Symphytum officinale* L. (Silva Júnior, 2006; Silva Júnior et al., 2006), assessing the compatibility between fluoxetine and excipients used in the manufacture of capsules (Stulz & Tagliari, 2006); thermoanalytical study and drug-excipient compatibility of rifampicin and some medications used in the treatment of Tuberculosis (Alves, 2007), thermal stability and compatibility of hydroquinone (Tagliari et al., 2008).

7. Conclusion

The development of herbal medicines, as a rule, involves planning and obtaining intermediate preparations as required steps for processing vegetable raw material into a finished product, which will provide the desired pharmaceutical presentation. Among the available intermediate preparations, Pharmacopoeias recommend the tincture or fluid extract. These liquid presentations can be utilized to obtain standardized dried extracts, which can be used in the production of various pharmaceutical forms. It is important that the starting material is stabilized in order to ensure the reproducibility of the process. It also has to be sufficiently pulverized so as to achieve optimum performance in the process of extracting the chemical constituents of pharmaceutical interest.

To obtain a derivative of any medicinal plant, being it herbal medicine in any form, quality control is required from the cultivation, management and harvesting of the plant species; passing through the production of intermediate product up to the final formulation. Following a set of criteria it is possible to characterize the raw plant, its derivative and the formulation, designating an adequate planning to be followed as to establish the parameters of quality control. When the approach is applied to the analysis of natural extracts, the study of pre-formulation becomes more difficult because often the available markers are altered as a function of pH, solvent polarity, temperature and interactions (excipient and vehicle). When formulating products containing natural ingredients it is essential to identify standardized markers or to develop methods for the quantification of purified chemical groups before, during and after the production process. Therefore, for the technological development of herbal medicines according to the requirements and specifications of the countries' laws, it is essential to establish protocols that ensure quality control of raw materials, vegetable products and ingredients used in their production, as well as validation of qualitative and quantitative techniques appropriate to the chemical markers chosen. Only then, we can get a finished product with assured quality.

8. Acknowledgment

The authors acknowledge the Federal University of Pará (UFPA), Foundation to Support Research and Development (FADESP), National Council for Scientific and Technological Development (CNPq), Brazilian Federal Agency for Support and Evaluation of Graduate Education (CAPES) and Pará Research Foundation (FAPESPA) by financial support to works realized.

9. References

Alves, M. S. M. , Mendes, P. C., Vieira, J. G. P., Ozela, E. F., Barbosa, W. L. R., Silva Júnior, J. O. C. Análise farmacognóstica das folhas de *Arrabidaea chica* (Humb. & Bonpl.) B. Verlt., Bignoniaceae. *Rev. bras. farmacogn.* [online]. 2010, vol.20, n.2, pp. 215-221.

Alves, M.S.M. Caracterização farmacognóstica, química, físico-química e estudos preliminares de pré-formulação da *Arrabidaea chica* (Humb. & Bonpl.) B. Verlt. 2008. Dissertação (Mestrado em Ciências Farmacêuticas), Faculdade de Farmácia, Universidade Federal do Pará, Belém.

Alves, R. Estufo termoanalítico e de compatibilidade fármaco-excipiente de refampicina e alguns medicamentos utilizados na terapêutica da tuberculose. Dissertação de mestrado - Universidade de São Paulo, São Paulo 2007.

Aragão, C.F.S.; Souza, F.S.; Barros, A.C.S.; Veras, J.W.E.; Barbosa Filho, J.M.; Macedo, R.O. aplicação da termogravimetria (TG) no controle de qualidade da milona (*Cissampelos sympodialis* Eichl.) Menispermaceae. Revista Brasileira de Farmacognosia, v. 12, supl., p.60 - 61, 2002.

Araújo, A. A.; S. Mercuri, L. P.; Seixas, S. R. S.; Storpitis, S.; Matos, J. R. Determinação dos teores de umidade e cinzas de amostras comerciais de guaraná utilizando métodos convencionais e análise térmica. Brazilian Journal of Pharmaceutical Sciences, v. 42, n.2, abr/jun., 2006.

Araújo, A.A.S. Análise térmica e determinação dos parâmetros cinéticos de preparações farmacêuticas e novas especialidades de zidovudina. 225f. Tese (Doutorado em Ciências Farmacêuticas) - Faculdade de Ciências Farmacêuticas - USP, São Paulo, 2003.

Bauer, K. H., Frömming, K. H., Füher, C.: Lehrbuch der Pharmazeutischen Technologie, 7th ed. Stuttgart, 2002.

Bauer, R., Tittel, G. Quality assessment of herbal preparations as a precondition of pharmacological and clinical studies. Phytomedicine 2: 193-198. 1996.

Bazzo, G.C.; Silva, M.A.S. Estudo termoanalítico de comprimidos contendo captopril através de termogravimetria e calorimetria exploratória diferencial. Revista Brasileira de Ciências Farmacêuticas, vol. 41, n.3, 2005.

Blumenthal, M., Brusse, W. R., Goldberg, A., Gruenwald, J., Hall, T., Riggins, C. W., Rister, R. S. *The Complete German Commission E Monographs. Therapeutic Guide to Herbal Medicines*. The American Botanical Council, Austin, TX, USA. 1998

Borges, L.; Sciliar, M.; Almeida, S. Biodiversidade brasileira e produtos industriais, Belo Horizonte: UFMG, 2003. Disponível em http://www.icb.ifmg.br/~ibem/aulas/grad/tge/biodiv/2002/prodindust/. Acesso em 12 nov.2006.

Brasil. RE nº899 de 29 de maio de 2003. Dispõe sobre o Guia para validação de métodos analíticos e bioanalíticos. Ministério da Saúde. Agência Nacional de Vigilância Sanitária. Disponível em: HTTP://e-legis.anvisa.gov.br.

Calixto, J. B. Efficacy, safety, quality control, marketing and regulatory guidelines for herbal medicines (phytotherapeutic agents). Braz. J. Med. Biol. Res. 33(2): 179-189. 2000.

Carvalho, J.C.T. Fitoterápicos anti-inflamatórios: aspectos químicos, farmacológicos e aplicações terapêuticas. Tecmed. São Paulo, 2004.

Cheng, K.L.; Bray, R.H. 1-(2-pyridylazo)-2- naphthol as a possible analytical reagent. Analytical Chemistry, v. 27, p. 782, 1955.

Costa, A.F. Farmacognosia. 3 Ed. v. 3. Fundação Calouste Gulbenkian: Lisboa, 2000.

Elvin-Lewis, Memory. Should we be concerned about herbal medicines? *J. Ethnopharmacol.*, Amsterdam, v.75, p.141-164, 2001.

Evert, R. F. Esau´s plant anatomy, Hoboken, New Jersey: J. Wiley, 2006.

Fahn A. Secretory tissues in plant. London: Academic Press, 1979.

Farias, M. R. et al, P.R. O problema da qualidade dos fitoterápicos. Caderno de farmácia, Vol. 1, nº 2, 73-82, 1985.

Farmacopéia Brasileira, V ed. São Paulo: Editora Atheneu, 2010.

Ferreira, L.A.; Leite, J.P.V. Desenvolvimento de formulações fitoterápicas. In: LEITE, J.P.V. Fitoterapia: bases científicas e tecnológicas. São Paulo: Editora Atheneu, p. 206-251, 2008.

Gaedcke, F. W. Steinholf, K. B. (2003). *Herbal Medicinal Products*. Stuttgart, Germany: CRC Press, ISBN: 0-8493-1023-7. p. 1-30.

Giolito, I.; Ionashiro, M. Nomenclatura em análise térmica: Parte II. Cerâmica, São Paulo, v. 34, p 163-164, 1988.

Gobbo-Neto, L. Lopes, N. Plantas medicinais: Fatores de influência no conteúdo de metabólitos secundários. Quimica Nova, Vol. 30, nº2, 374-381, 2007.

Hãnsel, R.: Phytopharmaka. Grundlagen und Praxis, 2nd ed. Berlin, 1991.

Harbone, J. B. Plant secondary metabolism. In: Crawley M. J. (ed.) Plant ecology. 2 ed. Berlin: Blackwell Publishing, 1997, p. 132-155.

International Conference on Harmonization (2005), in: Procedings of the Conference on Harmonization (ICH), Comission of the Euro Communities.

Leite, J.P.V. (2009). *Fitoterapia: Bases Científicas e Tecnológicas*.São Paulo: ATHENEU, ISBN: 978-85-7379-237-9, p. 3-119.

Leonti, M. The future is written: Impact of scripts on the cognition, selection, knowledge and transmission of medicinal plant use and its implications for ethnobotany and ethnopharmacology. J. Ethnopharmacol. 19 [Epub ahead of print]. 2011.

Nunes, K. M. Caracterização química e físico-química e estudos preliminares de planejamento da formulação fitoterápica semi-sólida contendo *Calendula officinalis* L. 2008. 141 f. Dissertação (Mestrado em Ciências Farmacêuticas) - Universidade Federal do Pará, Belém 2008.

Nunes, K.M. et al. Padronizacao da Tintura de *Calendula officinalis* L. para seu Emprego em Formulacoes Semi-solidas Fitoterapicas. Latin American Journal of Pharmacy, n. 28, v. 3, p. 344-350, 2009.

Oliveira, G.G.G.; Ferraz, H.G.; Matos, J.D.R. Estudo termoanalítico de glibenclamida e alguns excipientes utilizados em formas farmacêuticas sólidas. In: 2° Congresso Panamericano de Análise térmica e Calorimetria. Poços de Caldas, 2004.

Perkampus, H. H.; UV-VIS Spectroscopy and its Applications, Springer-Verlag: Berlin, 1992.

Petrovick, P.R.; Gonzalez Ortega, G.; Bassani, V.L. From a medicinal plant to a pharmaceutical dosage form. A (still) long way for the Brazilian medicinal plants. Ciência e Cultura. v. 49, n.5/6, p. 364-369, 1997.

Pieroni, A. & Vandebroek, I. Traveling cultures and plants: the ethnobiology and ethnopharmacy of migrations. New York, Berghahn Books. 2007.

Pinto, M. T. J.; Kaneko, T. M.; Pinto, A. F. Controle Biológico de Qualidade de Produtos Farmacêuticos, correlatos e Cosméticos. Terceira Edição. 2010. Editora Atheneu.

Rates, S.M.K. Plants as source of drugs. Toxicon, Amsterdam, v.39, p.603- 613, 2001.

Robbers, J.E.; Speedie, M.K.; Tyler, V.E. *Pharmacognosy and pharmacobiotechnology*. Baltimore: Willians & Wilkins, 1996. p.1-14.

Santos, E.V.M. Extração de matérias-primas vegetais. In: SHARAPIN, N. Fundamentos de tecnologia de Produtos Fitoterápicos. Cyted, Santafé de Bogotá, 2000. p. 27-60.

Schenkel, E.P.; Osmann, G.M.; Mello, J.C.P.; Mentz, L.A.; Petrovick, P.R., orgs. *Farmacognosia*: da planta ao medicamento. 2.ed. Florianópolis. UFSC; Porto Alegre: UFRGS, 2000. cap.15, p.291-320.

Schnitzler, E.; Beninca, C.; Kobelnik, M.; Sotelo, G.F.C.; Carneiro, P.I.B. Estudo, caracterização e determinação do grau de pureza de amostra comerciais de sacarina. Publicatio UEPG. Ciências exatas e da terra, ciências agrárias e engenharias. Ponta Grossa, 2005.

Schnitzler, E.; Pereira, C.A.; Carvalho Filho, M.A.S. Estudo termoanalitico (TG, DTG e DSC) dos cafés *in natura* e processados. Publicatio UEPG. Ciências exatas e da terra, ciências agrárias e engenharias. Ponta Grossa, v. 11, n. 1, p. 61-66, 2005.

Schulz, V.; Hansel, R.; Tyler, V.E. Medicinal plants, phytomedicines, and phytotherapy. In: *Rational phytotherapy*: a physician's guide to herbal medicine.4.ed. New York, Berlin: Springer, 2001. cap.1, p.1-39.

Sharapin, N. Fundamentos de tecnologia de Produtos Fitoterápicos. Cyted, Santafé de Bogotá, 2000. p. 145-157.

Silva Júnior, J.O.C.; Vieira, J.L.F.; Barbosa, W.L.R.; Pereira, N.L. Caracterização físico-química do extrato fluido e seco por nebulização de *Symphytum fofficinale* L. Revista Brasileira de Farmacognosia, v.16 (supl.): Dez. 2006.

Silva Júnior, José Otávio Carréra. Obtenção e avaliação de forma farmacêutica semi-sólida fitoterápica contendo extrato seco por nebulização de *Shymphytum officinale* L. (confrei). Tese de doutorado / FCFRP- USP. 2006.

Silverstein, R.M.; Webster, F.X.; Kiemle, D.J. Identificação espectrométrica de compostos orgânicos. 7. Ed. Tradução: Ricardo bicca de Alencastro – Rio de Janeiro: LTC, 2007. p. 70-122.

Souza, F.S.; Macedo, R.O.; Veraz, J.W.E. Estudies of cimetidine préformulated and tablets for TG and DSC coupled to the photovisual system. Thermochim. Acta, v. 392-393, p. 99-106, 2002.

Stulzer, H.K.; Tagliari, M.P. Avaliação da compatibilidade entre a fluoxetina e excipientes usados na fabricação de cápsulas pela farmácia magistral. Visão Acadêmica. Curitiba, v.7, p. 15-23, 2006.

Tagliari, M.P.; Stulzer, H.K.; Kelmann, R.G.; Kuminek, G.; Silva, M.A.S. Estabilidade térmica e compatibilidade da hidroquinona. Revista Cosmetics & Toiletries. Vol.20, n°2, 2008.

Tuescher, E. : Biogene Arzneimittel, 5th Ed. Stuttgart: Wissenschaftliche Verlagsgesell-schafth mbH; 1997.

Turolla, M.S.R.; Nascimento, E. Inforomações toxicológicas de alguns fitoterápicos utilizados no Brasil. Brazilian Journal of Pharmaceutical Sciences, v. 42, n.2, abr/jun.,2006.

Tyler, V.E. Natural products and medicine: an overview.In: Balick, M.J.; Elisabetsky, E.; Laird, S.A., eds. *Medicinal resources of the tropical forest, biodiversity and its importance to human health.* New York: Columbia University Press, 1996. p.3-10. (Biology and resource management series).

United States Pharmacopoeia. 30 ed. Rockville: The United States Pharmacopeia Convention, 2006.

Vinadé, M.E.doC.; Vinadé, E.R.doC., Métodos espectroscópicos de analise quantitativa, editora UFSM, 2005.

Vogel, G.: Pflanzliche Arzneimittel aus medizinischer und pharmakologischer Sicht. In: Qualität pflanzlicher Arzneimittel, Stuttgart: Wissenschaftliche Verlagsgesell-schafth mbH; 1982. p. 19-30.

Wagner, H.; Wiesenauer, M. Fitoterapia: fitofármacos, farmacologia e aplicações clínicas. 2ª edição. São Paulo: Pharmabooks, 2006.

WHO World Health Organization. Quality Control Methods for Medicinal Plant Materials. Geneva: Organização Mundial de Saúde, 1992.

WHO. Health in the millennium development goals. (World Health Organization) (http://www.who.int/mdg/goals/en/, acessado em 25 de Julho de 2009).

Yoney, A., Prieto, J. M., Lardos, A., Heinrich, M. Ethnopharmacy of Turkish-speaking Cypriots in Greater London. Phytother. Res. 24(5): 731-740. 2010.

Yunes, A. R.; Pedrosa, C.R.; Filho, C. V. Fármacos e fitoterápicos: a necessidade do desenvolvimento da indústria de fitoterápicos e fitofármacos no Brasil. Química Nova. v. 24, n.1, p. 147 -152, 2001.

12

Allergen Extract Analysis and Quality Control

Samuele E. Burastero
*San Raffaele Scientific Institute, via Olgettina, 58, Milan
Italy*

1. Introduction

The increase in allergic diseases in Westernized Countries is an established phenomenon, which has been extensively documented by several large epidemiologic studies (Sicherer and Leung, 2010). Allergies affect nowadays a proportion of the general population as large as one out of five individuals. The most prevalent clinical expression of allergies include respiratory allergies, such as allergic rhinitis and asthma (Chu et al., 2010), skin allergies, such as atopic dermatitis (Spergel, 2010a), and food allergies (Chafen et al., 2010). The pathogenesis of allergic diseases, and the reasons for their increased incidence is partially known and include environmental and genetic factors (Kuriakose and Miller, 2010). In all cases, the hallmark of all these *bone fide* allergic diseases is the presence of specific antibodies of the immunoglobulin E (IgE) isotype against protein antigens, which are indicated as allergens on the basis of their capability to elicit allergic reactions. The presence in the biological fluid of IgE to a given allergen is indicated as "sensitization" to that allergen. In most cases, IgE are measured in serum, where they are more easily detected and also on the ground that allergy is a systemic condition, with clinically relevant expression in different individuals at different target organs (*e.g.*, lower respiratory tract in the case of allergic asthma, nasal mucosa in the case of allergic rhinitis, *etc.)* (Pucci and Incorvaia, 2008) depending on organ-specific characteristics, which have been only partially identified.

The correct identification of sensitizing allergens is required to put in action the most efficient strategies to counteract the clinically relevant effect of allergies as well as their remarkable effects on the quality of life (Cummings et al., 2010). Useful measures include allergen avoidance, when applicable, proper symptomatic therapy and, most importantly, allergen specific immunotherapy, which is the only intervention capable to actually modify the pathogenic mechanisms of allergic diseases and their natural history, known as the allergy march (Spergel 2010b).

IgE can be measured *in vivo* with prick testing and *in vitro* with immunochemistry testing. Notably, as compared to immunochemistry testing of other immunoglobulin classes, specific enhanced procedures have to be used for allergen specific IgE determination, due their concentrations in biological fluids, which is in the range of ten to hundred thousand times lower as compared to the most represented immunoglobulins, *e.g.*, those belonging to the IgG isotype. A major issue to be considered in allergen-specific IgE determination is the quality of the antigen to be used for testing. Indeed allergens, which are encountered by patients in natural context are complex mixtures of relatively heterogeneous proteins. This fact poses several problems to Manufacturers of allergen extracts, including the standardisation of procedures used to obtain them from raw allergen sources and the possibility that they are not fully representative of the actual contents in terms of allergen components, as compared to environmental allergen sources. In the last twenty years the advent of molecular allergology has introduced revolutionary changes in the possibility to properly diagnose and treat allergic individuals by using single allergen components rather than allergen extracts. Molecular allergology has also made it possible to standardize allergen extracts themselves, which can now be used with a much higher knowledge about their appropriateness as diagnostic or therapeutic tools in patients with sensitization profiles defined at the level of single allergen components.

Allergen products require registration by government institutions (Becker et al., 2006), such as the FDA in the United States and the Paul Ehrlich Institute in Germany. Basic researchers, physicians, regulatory authorities and manufacturers have long tried to define a common methodology to standardize allergen vaccines (Terho and Frew, 1995; van Ree et al., 2008)

The quality of mite and pollen allergen extracts is better defined today than it was in the past, and the quality of food and epithelial allergen extracts has also improved (Fernandez-Caldas et al., 2006; Ferrer et al., 2005). However, further improvement is needed, particularly for food allergen extracts, since preliminary studies have shown efficacy also in this hi-impact clinical application, using sublingual food allergen extracts (Enrique et al., 2005).

Thus, the heterogeneity of allergen extracts used for diagnosis and immunotherapy makes it necessary to develop methodologies to assess their potency and ensure their consistency, stability and safety. In general terms it is essential to apply standardization in order to control all aspects of the production process, including the variability intrinsic to the source materials and the consistency and reproducibility which have to be granted for the sake of safety and efficacy in the clinical use (diagnosis, immunotherapy, quantification of environmental allergens).

Nowadays, different types of standardizations are still largely used by different laboratories and manufacturers, which variably addresses crucial issues underlying these preparations, such as the qualifications applied to collectors of raw materials, the establishment of manufacturing procedures in compliance with good manufacturing practice (GMP) regulations, and the choice of formulations of allergen extracts intended for clinical use (Larsen and Dreborg, 2008).

Although a limited number of major allergens (King et al., 1994) stimulate IgE production in a greater part of patients, any antigen in a given source material has the potential to elicit an IgE response. Thus, on one side it is essential to ensure that all protein allergens in the allergenic source material, to which humans are exposed in real life, are actually contained in the raw material used for diagnosis or immunotherapy. On the other side, since the IgE binding capacity of an allergen extract is related to the content of one or a few major allergens, it is also important that the standardization procedure ensures consistency, not only in the overall IgE binding potency, but also in the relative and absolute content of single major allergens. Due to this complexity in the composition of allergen extracts, the use of standards is a key element in standardization (Lowenstein, 1987). In Europe, each laboratory and manufacturer establishes In-House Reference (IHR) preparations for each source material. The IHR must be thoroughly characterized by *in vitro* methods as a basis for equilibration of subsequent batches. These methods have traditionally been based on whole extracts, whereas only in the last decade reference to single allergen components has been progressively introduced. Although it is still widely supported the notion that the biological activity of allergen extracts (also known as "allergenicity" or "reactogenicity") has to be determined in humans by *in vivo* methods, *i.e.* prick testing, it is time for all stake-holders to be put in the position to compare each new batch by using *in vitro* methods exclusively. In order for this advancement to be achieved, international standard (IS) preparations should be made available and *in vitro* methods should be validated by international health authorities for each allergen source. All laboratories in the world should be put in the condition to compare the allergen contents of extracts, which are used in everyday clinical practice to diagnose and treat such a large proportion of the population. This chapter describes the principles and problems related to standardization of allergen extracts for research and clinical use.

2. Mechanisms of allergy

The immune system of allergic individuals is erroneously reacting against innocuous molecular markers of environmental elements, as if they were markers of invaders, *i.e.*, virus, bacteria or parasites, which could potentially impair the integrity of vital functions. Allergen specific IgE are the immunological heralds of such a reactivity, which was evolutionarily developed in mammals to react against parasites (Chinen and Shearer, 2007). Circulating basophils (and tissue resident mast cells) are the short-term reacting effector cells, which are activated when allergen-specific IgE, bound to their membranes via Fc epsilon receptor type I (indicated as "cytophilic IgE"), are triggered by allergen binding to release inflammatory mediators stored within secretory granules (Abramson and Pecht, 2007; Holowka et al., 2007; Macglashan, 2005). Remarkably, the action of these mediators takes place within a few minutes since allergen recognition, and includes as dramatic changes of the local tissue as increased permeability of the microvasculature, egress of several types of inflammatory cells, mainly lymphocytes and eosinophils, secretion of large amounts of fluid secretion from mucosal glands and contraction of smooth muscle fibres (Barrett and Austen, 2009; Hamid and Tulic, 2009; Holgate, 2008). The latter may induce bronchial constriction, which is clinically expressed as asthma. Allergy therapies include not only symptomatic drugs, which provide release to the short-term effects associated to the release of these mediators (Al Suleimani and Walker, 2007; Bush and Saglani; Novak, 2009), but also allergen avoidance and specific immunotherapy. Only allergen avoidance and specific immunotherapy can radically modify the course of allergic diseases. However, avoidance, which *per se* is always dramatically effective, can in most cases rather help patients to live together with allergy than preventing its effects (Dykewicz and Hamilos, 2010; Hamilton, 2010; Simons, 2010), due to the fact that exposure to most sensitizing allergens in the population is virtually unavoidable. In contrast, immunotherapy is a disease modifying intervention, which can change the pathogenesis of the underlying allergic condition (Akdis and Akdis, 2010). For all allergy therapies the proper identification of the sensitizing allergens is a prerequisite for success (Hamilton) and only the careful standardization of hundreds of allergens identified until now allows put in action accurate and effective therapeutic interventions (Mothes et al., 2006; Pittner et al., 2004; Valenta et al., 2007). In particular, in the case of immunotherapy, the performance of the diagnostic procedures is mostly crucial, since it influences the appropriateness of years-long procedures patients have to undertake (Hankin and Lockey, 2010) in order for their immune system to modify reactivity to armless antigens (Abramson et al.; Calamita et al., 2006; Radulovic et al., 2010). In front of this widely accepted circumstances, the determination of allergen specific IgE is still performed with criteria which do not allow to distinguish rather common occurrences which make it difficult or impossible to properly define the sensitization profile of allergic patients. Indeed, approximately 75% of allergic individuals are poly-sensitized, *i.e.* they produce IgE reacting with multiple allergen sources (Scala et al., 2010). This polyreactivity can in some cases be attributed to IgE reacting to major allergen components in different allergen sources, *i.e.*, it is associated with *bona fide* multiple allergies in clinical terms. However, in as much as one third of cases IgE react to multiple allergen components to the presence of IgE to evolutionarily conserved, structurally homologous allergen components, which are collectively indicated as panallergens (Hauser et al., 2010). In particular, the most common panallergen, profilin, has been found targeted by IgE is as many as 50% of subjects sensitized to grass and birch pollens (Chapman et al., 2007). On a clinical stand point, as a food allergen profilin usually elicits mild reactions, such as oral allergy syndrome, is not modified by processing and is especially important in allergy to some fruits, such as melon, watermelon, banana, tomato, citrus fruit and persimmon (Santos and Van Ree, 2010). In front of this well-defined scenario, diagnosis with allergen extracts cannot distinguish subjects sensitized to major allergens of those extracts from subjects sensitized to one profilin cross-reacting in one extract with profilin of one or more extracts tested in parallel. There are several negative outcomes stemming from this situation, among them the most disturbing are the following: patients do not receive suitable information to evaluate their allergic disturbances and are not prescribed proper immunotherapy. In fact, although allergen specific immunotherapy with single allergen components is not yet commercially available, yet the limits of extract-based diagnosis are certainly capable to negatively affect the management of extract-based immunotherapy. Most allergists do not prescribe immunotherapy to patients with a polysensitization pattern, without investigating whether this pattern is ascribed to a real multiple allergies rather that to cross-reactivity via panallergens, despite the fact that clinical benefits have been reported in immunotherapy-treated polysensitized subjects (Ciprandi et al., 2010a; Ciprandi et al., 2010b). Thus, the present knowledge of the pathogenesis of allergic diseases has dramatically improved on the ground of increased cloning of allergen components but it is still waiting a thorough change in the clinical management of patients, due to the poor application of molecular allergology to the principles of allergen standardization. Along this line, the natural history itself of allergic diseases may be more efficaciously dissected by using allergen components than extract. For instance, a functionally relevant T-cell response to conserved regions of panallergens was demonstrated to underlie the possibility in single patients allergic to one given allergen to react against another allergen source expressing a homologous, conserved component, such as a profilin. These results suggested that a reciprocal modulation of the response to one sensitizing allergen can occur following natural exposure to or immunotherapy with another allergen and may certainly have relevance in the management of patients with multiple allergies (Burastero et al., 2004). Thus, extract-based diagnosis and immunotherapy need to be standardized also on the ground of the possibility to properly monitor the evolution of allergic disturbances. In the next future all stake holders, patients first, will have to fully exploit the remarkable advancements that molecular allergology allowed to achieve over in-house reference extracts based allergology of the previous century.

3. Standardisation of allergens for allergy diagnosis

The diagnosis of allergic disease requires, besides a detailed history and physical examination, the determination of allergen-specific IgE (Hamilton, 2010). In order for this diagnosis to be properly performed, preparations containing allergens have to be utilized, both for *in vivo* and for *in vitro* testing. *In vivo* the presence of IgE can be detected with a low-cost procedure, which provides results in a matter of minutes, known as prick testing. Prick testing is performed by creating a 1-mm deep wound with a skin pricker, which put in contact single solutions containing each allergen to be tested with skin mast cells. These mast cells mediators include histamine and leukotrienes, which promptly increase the permeability of local vessels and generate erythema and oedema, a local effect read locally as "wheal and flare reaction". By measuring the size of the wheal, the extent of the degranulation is semi-quantitatively assessed, and can be used as an approximate measure of IgE levels. A part from the efficacy of the allergen extract used for prick testing, several other individual factors affect the results of this procedure, such as individual reactivity to histamine, age and sex of the pricked person, the site of reaction, the presence of non specific irritants, such as environmental pollutants, the season of the year, etc. (Bordignon and Burastero, 2006). This biological background has long represented a major limit in the possibility to accurately assess the allergen content of preparations containing allergens for diagnostic purposes.

In fact, allergen extracts are complex mixtures of protein materials obtained by Manufacturers from relevant allergen sources and the possibility to easily assess skin reactivity by sensitized subjects has long represented the criterion for assessing the appropriateness of each preparation (Fernández-Caldas et al., 2009). Indeed, this biological approach has obvious advantages over more complex analytical approaches, since it warrants to any Manufacturer the possibility to validate the allergen extracts they commercialize. However, this method also brings about a peculiar and an extremely complex set of standardisation problems, which -incidentally- are not shared by the remaining pharmaceutical industry. Firstly, in the absence of any obvious general criterion to assess the allergen content with a simple analytical approach, as the one that could be applied to measure the active substance in any drug preparation, each Manufacturer is encouraged by trivial commercial reasons to maintain strictly confidential all the relevant details of preparation procedures. This confidentiality is often used to claim that one given specific preparation is better performing as compared to that of competitors on several grounds. The latter include the efficiency of allergen recognition by patients IgE, the representativeness of the allergen source found in the environment in real life by patients, the capability to trigger clinically relevant symptoms and, last but not least, batch-to-batch consistence. As a matter of fact, all these criteria are rather difficult to verify on a scientific ground, not only because they are related to totally or partially unveiled industrial procedures but also because they are applied to complex protein mixtures.

Indeed, several studies have reported differences among commercially available diagnostic products for skin prick testing, see for instance Pagani *et al.* (Pagani et al., 2009). Another study quantified and compared the allergen content of different grass pollen preparations for skin prick testing (SPT) used in Europe (Sander et al., 2009). Strikingly, protein concentrations ranged from 15 to 427 μg/ml, and the concentration of Phl p 5, a major grass allergen, ranged from 0.15 to 18.3 μg/ml (Sander et al., 2009). Major allergens are allergen components within a given allergen source, which are recognized by the majority of patients sensitized to that allergen source, as established by gold standard criteria (Grier et al., 2002). Gold standard criteria include the appearance of clinical symptoms upon environmental allergen exposure and thus represent the most incontrovertible parameter of efficacy. Yet, extracts are still preferred to allergen components on the ground that conformational epitopes may not be properly expressed in single *E. coli* cloned and expressed protein allergens (Pomes, 2009), that glycosilation, which contribute to allergenicity (Shakib et al., 2008), is not maintained in recombinant allergens, and that a panel of several, yet to be completely defined, allergen components has to used to replace the comprehensive repertoire of protein allergens within an extract. Along this line, the quantification of single allergen components is considered an unsatisfactory criterion to define the characteristics of allergen extracts. Extracts in the United States are more homogenous with respect to total allergenic potency than the extracts produced in Europe, mainly because the FDA provides the same standardized reagent for internal use by all manufacturing companies (Slater, 2004). However, great differences have also been shown among non-standardized mold allergen extracts in the USA (Esch, 2004).

4. Standardisation of allergens for immunotherapy of allergic diseases

Specific immunotherapy is the practice of administering gradually increasing doses of allergen vaccines to reduce allergic symptoms and the need for medications. Thus, immunotherapy is the only curative intervention in the treatment of allergies, since it can modify allergen-driven immunological responses and restoring, to a certain degree, the Th1/Th2 balance (Akdis and Blaser, 2001). B and T lymphocytes, blocking antibodies, IL-10 and other cytokines play an important role in the response to specific immunotherapy (Chinen and Shearer, 2004). Effective allergen immunotherapy depends on the accuracy of the diagnosis and on the usage of well-characterized allergen extracts. The latter should ideally be prepared according to a patient-tailored approach, whereby only allergen components one given patient is sensitized to are administered (Vrtala, 2008). Although available allergen preparations do not allow this approach, yet numerous double-blind placebo-controlled studies using unmodified aqueous allergens (Gurka and Rocklin, 1988) and allergoids (Ferreira et al., 2006) (modified allergens) have demonstrated efficacy. Sublingual immunotherapy, using drops of aqueous allergen extracts under the tongue and then swallowed (Radulovic et al., 2010), or tablets (Bufe et al., 2009; Dahl et al., 2008) with similar type of extracts, also appear to be clinically beneficial, particularly for grass-induced rhinoconjunctivitis.

The comparison of different products from different companies at national and international levels is complicated due to the lack of international standards, similarly to the above quoted problems related to diagnostic products. Larenas-Linnemann and Cox (Larenas-Linnemann and Cox, 2008) reviewed the information obtained on unit definition and dosage of allergens from European manufacturers of allergen extracts used for sublingual immunotherapy (SLIT). They concluded that the monthly maintenance dose the manufacturers recommended for SLIT was 5-45 times higher than the recommended dose for subcutaneous immunotherapy. However, since each manufacturer in Europe uses its own in house reference preparations and its own units to express potencies, the comparison of different products from different companies at national and international levels is almost impossible. The amount of major allergens has started to be used, which represent a major improvement at least in principle, to overcome a *bona fide* anarchism, which is strongly supported by Manufacturers, in my opinion, for mere commercial reasons. In fact, in the absence of simple international units, such as microgram o micromoles, every manufacturer is legitimated to predicate the better performances of each own product, on the basis on not-verifiable statements and procedures. As a matter of fact, details on the procedures for allergen standardization, which are listed and described in paragraphs below, are never made publicly available on the ground of industrial protection issues. Thus, an inviolable system tends to self-perpetuate, which is hard to be challenged by the physiological dialectic, which should drive scientific issues towards their solution. Along this line, far from promoting the usage of homogeneous testing to quantify major allergen contents (*e.g.*, same protocols, same monoclonal antibodies for capture and detection in sandwich ELISA, *etc.*) most commentators and opinion leaders support the notion that since the reference extracts and antibodies used can influence the outcome of such assays (Larsen and Dreborg, 2008) basically there is no strong scientific basis to move from good old in-house reference units to micrograms of major allergens. This position certainly makes it less embarrassing to comment on the fact that the maintenance doses of the commercially available vaccines have been found to range from 0.2 to 21.6 μg in terms of Phl p 5 content (Larenas-Linnemann and Cox, 2008) which should per se indicate that in house reference should be limited to internal quality control procedures. Moreover, doctors and patients should be made really aware of what they are actually continuously administering or assuming, respectively, for the average two to four years treatment time, rather than counting on the reassuring, only partially verifiable statements of Manufactures.

5. Standardisation of allergens for measuring their environmental amount

The measurement of allergens in the environment is a well-established approach to assess the level of exposure of sensitized individuals in real life settings. This applies mainly to dust mite, animal allergens, cockroach, and molds. Epidemiologic studies, population surveys, and birth cohort studies have plainly defined levels of allergen exposure in Western populations and found strong associations between exposure and the development of asthma (Arbes et al., 2003; Heinrich et al., 2006; Illi et al., 2006; Sears et al., 2003; Sporik et al., 1999; Woodcock et al., 2004; Zock et al., 2006). Guidelines have been developed to indicate exposure levels that are risk factors for sensitization (Platts-Mills et al., 1997). Allergen assays are used for testing the efficacy of allergen avoidance procedures and devices and for monitoring clinical trials of avoidance and the efficacy of remediation (Morgan et al., 2004; Platts-Mills et al., 2000; Woodcock et al., 2004). These assays are used in the US indoor air quality industry for evaluation of allergen exposure in homes, the workplace, and public buildings. In this context, although allergen measurements have become routine, the same issues, which are commented above about the lack of international standard apply here. However those tests, which are routinely used to this aim necessarily include the usage of allergen components (mainly in recombinant form) in order to run the standard curves, since the latter are the core element of the assay itself, rather than prick testing. Thus, the quantification of allergen content in the environment, even in the absence of international standards, is expressed in conventional amounts of major allergen by all available assays (Hamilton, 2005), rather than according to the obscure and bizarre in-house reference units which still prevail in the diagnostic and immunotherapy fields.

6. International efforts to standardized allergens

The widespread use of allergen measurements in the fields of allergy, indoor air quality, and environmental exposure assessment has created an urgent need for internationally recognized purified allergen standards and for validated and certified immunoassays. Due to the common generalized mind-set by manufactures, immunotherapy products are still licensed based on their total potency as established by in-house, non-comparable reference units. Nevertheless, allergists increasingly use specific allergen measurements for dosing of immunotherapy. Maintenance doses of 5 to 20 mg of major allergen are associated with clinical improvement after immunotherapy, and natural allergenic products are being formulated, at least in part, based on specific allergen content (Nelson, 2007; van Ree, 2007). Allergen concentrations should be monitored not only to establish dose-response relationships between allergens and treatment efficacy but also to compare allergenic products from different manufacturers, and to formulate recombinant allergen diagnostics and vaccines (Becker et al., 2006; Chapman et al., 2000; Scheiner et al., 1994; van Ree, 2007). Although the progressive characterization of major allergen components and the development of techniques to quantify them, such as ELISA systems based on monoclonal antibodies, have led more manufacturers to provide information on the major allergen content of their extracts, identification of major allergen content is not currently mandatory, except for a limited number of extracts, such as cat and ragweed. The World Health Organization and some other regulatory government institutions now recommend that allergen manufacturers state the content of representative major allergens in mass units for their allergen products (Nelson, 2000). However, differences in assays and methodologies for measuring the major allergens still preclude direct comparisons among products of different manufacturers (Alvarez-Cuesta et al., 2006). In fact, although recombinant allergens are being used to develop new diagnostics and vaccines, yet the structural and immunologic properties of cloned allergen components had not been systematically compared with those of their natural counterparts in international collaborative studies. The World Health Organization (WHO)/International Union of Immunological Societies Allergen Standardization Sub-committee has been influential in coordinating international standardization. The committee established WHO-approved international standards for dust mite, dog hair, and birch, timothy, and short ragweed pollens and produced the WHO position paper that recommended the use of standardized allergen vaccines of defined allergen content for dosing in immunotherapy (Bousquet et al., 1998; Platts-Mills and Chapman, 1991). This approach was also endorsed by a position statement from the American Academy of Allergy, Asthma & Immunology (Cox et al., 2010). In 1999, the WHO/International Union of Immunological Societies Allergen Standardization Sub-committee initiated a specific program aimed to develop highly purified allergens that could be used for the standardization of *in vitro* assays which is the underlying issue in the implementation of this approach. This provided the genesis for a European Union–funded study entitled "Development of certified reference materials for allergenic products and validation of methods for their quantification" (acronym: CREATE) (van Ree et al., 2008).

The aim of the European Union CREATE project was to produce international standards of purified allergens with verifiable allergen content. Such standards would enable allergen manufacturers, academic organizations, and government and regulatory agencies to use a common international standard for specific allergen measurements. A second aim was to compare the specificity, sensitivity, and reproducibility of ELISAs for allergen analysis. Allergens were selected for the project based on the following criteria: (1) the allergen was a major allergen of well-documented clinical importance; (2) purified natural and recombinant forms of the allergen were available in greater than 20-mg amounts from academic or commercial laboratories; (3) there was strong evidence that the recombinant allergen had equivalent IgE binding to its natural counterpart and there was extensive structural data on the allergen; and (4) ELISA kits to measure the allergen were available from 1 or more laboratories.

To carry forward with this project, eight major allergens originating from four of the most important inhalant allergen sources were selected: Bet v 1 from birch pollen, Phl p 1 and Phl p 5 from grass pollen, Ole e 1 from olive pollen and Der p 1 and 2 and Der f 1 and Der f 2 from house dust mites. Three allergens were found to be suitable as biological reference materials; the rest, except rPhl p 1a, did indicate potential for optimization, but only if specific aspects of their protein expression processes will be modified. As a result of this study, recombinant Bet v 1 and Phl p 5 are being produced under Good Manufacturing Practice and presently being evaluated by the European Directorate for the Quality of Medicines as biologic reference preparations to be included in the European Pharmacopoeia as international standards. Consequently, at least for these allergens, standardization will become global and will hopefully permit comparisons among different manufacturing sources (Himly et al., 2009).

A detailed account of the aims, scope, and methods used in the CREATE project has been published elsewhere (van Ree et al., 2008)

7. Techniques for the standardization of allergen products

Allergen products, which are routinely used to diagnose and treat allergic diseases have been used for over 100 years. The quality of these allergen products is a key issue for both diagnosis, environmental monitoring of allergen levels and specific immunotherapy, and the standardization of allergen extracts is of primary importance to improve their quality and offer physicians worldwide a reliable method to diagnose and treat such widespread diseases as food allergies and allergic respiratory diseases. In particular, effective diagnosis and treatment, using skin test reagents and specific immunotherapy requires the optimal amount of allergens for testing and the maintenance dose of vaccine for treatment, respectively. Although a tremendous amount of information is available to implement this objective, internationally accepted rules are still lacking. The unavoidable empirical steps, which are preliminary to the production of allergen extracts form natural allergen sources are usually considered the only relevant aspect of the whole standardisation process, since this position is instrumental to support the concept that quantification of allergen component in weight (or molar) units are non-applicable and misleading. Obviously, any single step in the preparation of allergen extract has to treasure decades of previous consolidated experience in as trans-disciplinary expertises as zoology, palynology and biochemistry. Yet, the final products of such processes will have to be validated by international standards, in order to make it possible to evaluate their allergenic potency and compare the corresponding preparations of different Manufacturers, if quality is something different from a jealously kept secret of happy few.

8. Collection of raw source materials

Inhalant allergens are present in airborne particles derived from natural allergen sources. These particles constitute the material which humans are exposed to. The selection of raw material is finalized to provide extracts containing the same active allergens patients will encounter in real life in a manageable form. Although in most cases, the optimal source material is rather obvious, in some cases the allergen source is still debated (for instance, for cat allergy it is not yet established whether the best allergen source is saliva or dander and, in the case of mouse allergy, urine or dander). In principle, the source materials should be specific and include all relevant components in sufficient amounts to be recognized by serum IgE from the whole population displaying clinical symptoms when exposed to the corresponding allergen in a real life setting (Lowenstein, 1987). Collectors must be qualified to verify the identity and quality of the source materials, so that only specifically identified allergenic source materials that do not contain avoidable foreign substances should be used in the manufacture of allergenic extracts and methods should be applied to trace the materials from their origin. This includes complete identity labelling and certification from competent collectors. Avoiding non-allergenic, contaminant material is particularly crucial also on the basis of the fact that same doubts were raised about the possibility that immunotherapy extracts could raise sensitization to previously non-sensitizing protein components. Along this line, the processing and storage of source materials should be performed to ensure that no unintended substances, including microbial organisms, are introduced into the materials. Records should describe source materials in as much detail as possible, including the particulars of collection, pre-treatment, and storage.

8.1 Pollens

The natural sources of inhalant allergens from plants are the pollens. Pollen may be obtained either by collection in nature or from cultivated fields or greenhouses. The collection may be performed by several methods, such as vacuuming or drying flower heads followed by pulverizing. In brief, anthers, which are long, slender filaments in a flower that have two lobes at the top, are best collected from intact, partially opened buds. The pollen may be cleaned either by passing through sieves of different mesh sizes or by flotation. Finally, pollens are dried under controlled conditions and stored in sealed containers at -20°C. The maximum level of accepted contamination with pollen from other species is 1% by number. Pollen should be devoid of flower and plant fragments, with a limit of 5% by weight. Pollens may show large modifications in quantitative composition depending on season and location of growth. In order to achieve a relatively constant composition, harvests from different years and sites of collection should be pooled for the production of allergen extracts, after thorough *in vitro* characterization.

8.2 House dust mites

House dust mites are grown in cultures and the source materials for mite allergen extracts can be represented by either pure bodies or whole mite cultures. Extracts based on whole mite cultures include eggs, larvae, and faecal particles as well as mite decomposition material and contain all the material to which mite-sensitized individuals are exposed under natural conditions. The culture medium should ideally be antigen free or, alternatively, contaminants from the culture medium should be shown not to be allergenic. The pure mite body extracts avoid extensive contamination with debris from the culture medium. In one clinical study, vaccines based on whole mite cultures and pure mite body extracts have shown similar clinical efficacy (Wahn et al., 1988).

8.3 Mammals

Allergens of mammalian origin may be present in various sources (typically, dander, serum, saliva, or urine). The allergens to which humans are exposed depend on the normal behaviour of the animal and the optimal source of allergens from mammals should be systematically investigated using a large panel of sera from patients sensitized to each given

animal. Notably, no matter if they are derived from dander or deposited from body fluids, most mammal allergens are present in the fur. Only healthy animals must be used for collecting allergens, and *post-mortem* collection is allowed only in exceptional cases and if stringent precautions to minimize decomposition were taken.
The optimal source materials are often dander, because hair proteins are insoluble. Use of whole pelt would increase the proportion of serum proteins, which are generally of low allergenic activity. In the case of the popular dog allergen extracts, remarkable differences were reported when deriving the material from different dog breeds (Larsen and Dreborg, 2008; Lindgren et al., 1988), a mixture of material from different breeds should be selected representing a balanced content of the major allergens (Uhlin et al., 1984).

8.4 Insects

The most common insect allergen is hymenoptera venom, which is brought in contact with the human immune system by sting. In this case, the purified venom itself is the best allergen source. In more uncommon cases the route of exposure may be biting or even inhalation. In this cases whole insects (including insects debris) and saliva are the proper allergen source, respectively.

8.5 Fungi

Allergens should be extracted by moulds, provided that they are grown under strictly controlled conditions (Larsen and Dreborg, 2008). The harvested raw materials should consist of mycelia and spores. In order for fungal cultures to maintain constant composition, it is recommended that extracts are derived from several independent cultures of the same species obtained from established fungal culture banks, i.e., American Type Culture Collection. All batches should be derived from the same strain to secure a stable composition, since it is well established that they may vary even under apparently analogous growth conditions (Steringer et al., 1987; Wallenbeck et al., 1984). The cultivation medium should be devoid of allergenic ingredients (i.e., serum proteins) and any safety measures should be taken to avoid contamination by any microorganisms, including other fungi

8.6 Foods

The supply of standardized material for the preparation of food allergen extract is limited, due to the complexity of this area. In fact, foods are often derived from various subspecies, grown under a broad variety of conditions reflecting geographical variation. Moreover, foods are often cooked prior to ingestion, and the cooking procedures may differ geographically. Consequently, the source of allergen exposure is highly variable both in qualitative as well as in quantitative terms (Lemanske and Taylor, 1987). The possibility to prepare sets of food allergen extracts reflecting the local species, the habit of cultivation, harvesting, storing, and cooking is a conceptual academic attitude which is raising more problems than those it can solve. For this reason, unsatisfactory results have been observed from commercially available reagents, which have resulted in many clinicians using untreated foods from retail trade for diagnosis by the prick–prick method (Dreborg and Foucard, 1983). Examples are fresh fruit, cow's milk, and hen's egg. Undiluted cow's milk and hen's egg have the best-documented diagnostic properties (Verstege et al., 2005). In this scenario, the usage of purified food allergen components, in either natural of recombinant form appears as a by far more suitable approach to circumvent these limitations. Moreover, the characterization of the profile of sensitization to single allergen components allow to add up important clinical information, which cannot be extrapolated from diagnosis with whole extracts. For instance, the appearance of IgE to defined allergen components was documented in cohorts of milk allergic children (Hochwallner et al., 2010; Ott et al., 2008), which allows to follow up the clinical evolution of milk allergy. Another added value stems from the possibility to distinguish sensitizations associated with different profile risk. For instance, individuals with sensitization to nut allergen extract may have IgE to Cor a 1, cross-reacting birch allergens of the Bet v 1-like, PR-10 protein family or to Cor a 2, cross-reacting with profilins from several different allergen sources (fagales, grasses, pellitory, etc.). Alternatively, a positive skin prick test, or in vitro specific IgE determination assay, may be associated to the presence of IgE to the Lipid Transfer Protein Cor a 8. The former situation is associated with limited clinical symptoms (for instance, oral allergic syndrome) whereas the latter may be associated with severe systemic reactions. These two strikingly divergent scenarios, which can be referred to the acid and heat sensitivity of profilins and PR-10, *versus* the resistance to physical stimuli of lipid transfer proteins cannot be distinguished by extract-based diagnosis.

9. Preparation of allergen extracts

Allergens to be used for diagnostic purposes have to be as intact as possible in terms of molecular structures, which are recognized by allergic patients' IgE. Thus, any preventative measure has to be taken to prevent denaturation in the preparation and storage of allergen to be used for diagnosis or immunotherapy. On this basis, organic solvents, elevated temperatures, and extreme pH and ionic conditions should be carefully avoid whenever possible. The extraction should be performed under conditions resembling the physiological conditions (*i.e.*, physiological pH and ionic strength) and suppressing possible proteolytic degradation and microbial growth (Lowenstein et al., 1981; Lowenstein and Marsh, 1981, 1983). As a matter of fact, the optimal extraction time is usually a compromise between yield and denaturation of the allergens, and in general, the processing time is minimized and extraction performed at low temperatures. Low molecular weight, i.e., below 5000 Dalton, non-antigenic material is removed from the extract by conventional biochemical techniques, such as dialysis, ultra-filtration, or size exclusion chromatography. However, it should be kept in mind that any substance excluded from the final product must be directly shown to be non-allergenic, before being systematically discarded. The final extract should be stored either lyophilized or at low temperatures (i.e., -20°C to -80°C). Often 50% glycerol and non-allergenic proteins (*e.g.*, certified human serum albumin) are used as stabilizers.

9.1 IHR preparations

In Europe, the in-house reference preparations (IHR) are prepared by individual laboratories or Manufacturers, whereas in the United States, the US Food and Drug Administration (FDA) authorizes general standards of some common allergens for the purpose. IHR are specifically used by Manufacturers/laboratories for equilibration of the potency and composition of each batch of manufactured extract. By this procedure the batch-to-batch standardization is performed by comparison to the IHR using *in vitro* techniques exclusively.

Usually, three batches of the extract are produced in order to verify consistency and reproducibility of the production processes. The three batches are compared and, if

consistency is achieved, one is selected to represent the new IHR, which is subsequently dispended into freeze-dried aliquots of suitable size.
The IHR is defined by the determination of the dry weight, protein content and composition, with particular reference to major allergen content and total allergenic activity by *in vivo* and *in vitro* methods. The evaluation of total allergenic activity by skin prick testing is usually performed only occasionally, *i.e.*, not for all batches, and has been shown to correlate with major allergen content (Dreborg and Einarsson, 1992). In general, the use of major allergen determination with a validated assay is considered sufficient to validate results of IHR units, when combination with a specific IgE potency assay is available. However, if *in vitro* methods alone are used for the establishment of the potency of the IHR, comparison is best made with the international standards (IS), which is not available for all allergens (see below).

9.2 International standards

Besides IHR reparation, allergen extract standardization requires the use of an internationally defined standard for each source material, indicated with the acronym IS. IS of allergen extracts can be obtained from the National Institute of Biological Science and Control, NIBSC, London, United Kingdom (Health Protection Agency, 2010), and are produced under the auspices of the WHO according to guidelines established by the Allergen Standardization Sub-Committee under the International Union of Immunological Societies (IUIS). IS enable comparison of specific activities of products from different manufacturers and can be used as calibrators by new producers and laboratories.
IS are presently available for the following allergen extracts: *Ambrosia artemisiifolia* (short ragweed) (Helm et al., 1984), *Phleum pratense* (timothy grass) (Gjesing et al., 1985), the house dust mite *Dermatophagoides* pteronyssinus (Ford et al., 1985), *Betula verrucosa* (birch), and *Canis familiaris* (dog) (Larsen et al., 1988)

9.3 Units and measure

The strength or potency of an allergen extract (allergenicity or reactogenicity) corresponds the extent of the response it will elicit in human allergic subjects, to be considered as a representative population of all individual with clinically relevant symptoms when exposed to that given allergen. Allergic patients react to allergen extracts with different strength because they are differently sensitized, *i.e.*, they have different IgE levels to different allergen components within the extract. Thus, the degree of sensitivity differs from patient to patient as well as for each allergen in the extract. Since extracts from different producers differ in composition there is no straightforward relationship between potency and response when comparing products from different Manufacturers and their potency cannot be compared in a satisfactory manner. Prick skin testing of human allergic subjects is the prevalent *in vivo* method for the assessment of allergen extract potency (Platts-Mills and Chapman, 1991) and also constitutes the standard underlying the determination of biological units of allergen extract potency. In this context, criteria of patient selection are obviously crucial, since potency measures will be dependent on pattern of sensitization in the panel of selected patients, Moreover, besides the characteristics of the sensitization to single allergen components, several other *in vivo* factors have been reported to variably influence prick test readings, such as age, sex, site of pricking, environmental pollution, season of the year (Bordignon and Burastero, 2006). According to the Nordic Council on Medicines HEP were adopted as the Nordic Biological Unit for allergens, which imply to determine the concentration of allergen inducing a weal of the same size as that of histamine dihydrochloride, 10 mg/mL, as evaluated by a skin test run in parallel, in a panel of at least 20 patients attending an allergist who poses a diagnosis of allergy to the allergen of interest. The median concentration corresponds to 10,000 biological units (BU) (Dreborg et al., 1987). With proper patient selection this Unit has been shown to be relatively reproducible between different regions of Europe (Dreborg et al., 1987). European manufacturers use their own company-specific units, most of which are based on the same method. In the United States, the FDA uses a unit based on intra-dermal testing with the allergen extract and subsequent measurement of the flare rather than the weal size. This intradermal end point is expressed as the number of threefold dilution producing a summed erythema diameter of 50 mm. The mean value of 15 individuals defines the potency of the allergen extract, which is expressed in Allergy Units (AU). Later on, the Center for Biologics Evaluation and Research (CBER) in the United States proposed the Bioequivalent Allergy Unit (BAU). The method for assigning BAU is named ID50EAL. According to ID50EAL the intradermal dilution for 50 mm sum of erythema diameters determines the allergy unit (Turkeltaub, 1987).

In this context, labelling of the potency of allergen extracts based on the microgram amount of single allergen components, as progressively characterized by molecular cloning, to begin with the most representative major allergens, represented a revolutionary change in the field. Indeed, the major allergen content was found to correlate with the biological activity (Dreborg and Einarsson, 1992). If the same antibodies and methodology are used in the immunochemical determination of major allergen content determination of major allergen content can replace other methods for potency declaration.

Until a few years ago, each manufacturer used to express the allergenicity of each preparation using exclusively In-House Reference Units, without any reference to major allergen content. In my opinion, this scientifically unacceptable situation was strongly supported on a commercial ground, likely because allowed each manufacturer to prevent direct comparison between corresponding preparations of competitors. For more than a couple of decades this circumstance prevented allergists to know how far a given preparation was performing as compared to the corresponding preparations of the same allergen source from other manufacturers. Several surrogate markers were introduced, to compensate for this indefensible deficiency, including the bizarre ratio between the amounts of allergen used by each manufacturer in sublingual versus subcutaneous immunotherapy (Burastero, 2005; Gidaro et al., 2005). Even now that information of major allergen contents has become a unavoidable requisite on a cultural ground, although not yet a regulatory requirement (Moingeon, 2006), a sort of intellectually ambiguous position is maintained, by publicly supporting the notion, in congresses and meetings, that since different immunochemical methods are used to quantify such parameters, than it is still legitimate for each manufacturer to claim best performance of its own preparation regardless the amount of major allergens. As a matter of fact, extract potency can only be compared if at least uniform test methods and reference extracts are used (Larenas-Linnemann and Cox, 2008), which is by far a more acceptable, although in-development situation, than any alternative anarchism. Thus, even if in most cases the composition of test materials and the specificity of anti-allergen antibodies vary between laboratories, the content of a single major allergen does allow comparison of overall potency between marketed allergen extracts by far superior to any previously available methods.

Rather than persisting in old methods on the ground that the new ones has limits, new techniques will have to be developed and extensively applied in the next future to answer to the following questions: a) How far is one given extract qualitatively representative of the repertoire of allergen components which are actually encountered in real life by sensitized patients in different areas of the world? b) How much is each allergen component quantitatively represented?

10. Stability testing

Criteria, methods, and limits for stability are established in a not satisfactory fashion. In Europe, a total allergenic activity in the interval between 30 and 300% of the arbitrarily defined in house reference titre is accepted. In contrast, US authorities limit the variability to 50–200% of the labelled activity. The underlying problems in this context are obviously related to the lack of precision in methods used of allergenicity measurement. For stability assessment the extract should be stored at several different temperatures to assure safe storage at room temperature, in a refrigerator, and at 20°C. Accelerated degradation studies designed to measure the kinetics of breakdown of the allergen extract can be performed by incubation at multiple high temperatures.

The reference for stability testing is usually the In-House Reference Units itself, a strategic choice, which allows each Manufacturer to safely claim superior stability of its own product without the risk that controversy can be raised. The application of assays providing results in milligram or molar amounts of major allergens are highly needed also for the proper evaluation of stability of allergen extracts from different Manufacturers.

11. Batch-to-batch control

Having established an In-House Reference Preparation, batch-to-batch standardization is still performed by calibrating new freeze-dried batches in bulk with the IHR before dispensing into vials for distribution. Batch-to-batch standardization usullay include the steps indicated in Table 1

Although these sophisticated immunochemistry assays are helpful, they do not allow a straightforward comparison between different extracts, which could be performed with standardized assays based on the weight or molar amounts of major allergens.

12. Other techniques used for standardization

Beyond the use of monoclonal antibodies, other physico-chemical approaches have been explored for allergen standardization and offer new possibilities. Evaluation of mass spectrometry (MS) has been performed to determine its capacity to characterize the composition of allergen extracts (Heick et al., 2010; Houston et al., 2010). One advantage offered by the use of MS includes the measurement of several different allergenic components (allergens and isoforms) simultaneously rather than measuring individual allergens. This is advantageous while working with allergen preparations that contain a wide group of IgE binding proteins, such as mite extracts. Additionally, MS-based methods are available to discriminate between allergen isoforms, which is difficult to accomplish using immunologic based methods. This method could also be useful for the standardization of allergoids, since measuring major allergens is not possible in these preparations due to their chemical modification with aldehyde. The issues with MS-based protocols are that they are not quantitative and are not addressed in regulatory policies. Similarly, proteomic approaches are extremely informative about the composition in major and minor allergens within complex extracts, although they do not allow provide quantitative results (Corti et al., 2005).

Scope	*Full description*	*Acronym*	*Ref.*
Determination of dry weight			
Assessment of allergenic composition to ensure the presence in the final product of all allergens present in the source material	Cross-(radio)-immunoelectrophoresis	CIE/CRIE	(Lowenstein, 1978)
	Sodium dodecyl-sulfate polyacrylamide gel electrophoresis	SDS-PAGE	(Laemmli, 1970)
	Immunoblotting	IB	(Kyhse-Andersen, 1984)
	Isoelectric focusing	IEF	(Brighton, 1975)
Quantification of specific major allergens	Quantitative immunoelectrophoresis	QIE	(Lowenstein, 1978)
	Enzyme-linked immunosorbent assay	ELISA	(Engvall and Perlmann, 1972)
Quantification of the total allergenic activity	Radioallergosorbent test	RAST	(Ceska et al., 1972)
	RAST-inhibition		

Table 1. Steps in batch-to-batch control of allergen extracts

13. Recombinant allergens and allergen components

Allergen extracts are complex mixtures of substances, including mainly antigenic glycoproteins and variable amounts of non-antigenic, non-protein material, which may have some relevance in the trigger and in the establishment of the allergic reaction (Gutermuth et al., 2007; Traidl-Hoffmann et al., 2005). Since the beginning of the Nineties, allergen components has started to be characterized by molecular biology tools, namely by allergen cloning (Valenta et al., 1991), and the complex scenario of the composition of the clinically most important allergen sources has been gradually unveiled (Heiss et al., 1999; Kazemi-Shirazi et al., 2002; Valenta et al., 1999). For instance, presently as many as 50 allergen components from the *Phleum pratense* grass species have been identified (http://www.allergome.org/). *Phleum pratense* is a representative species in the group of grasses, which are known to trigger allergic symptoms. It has been extensively demonstrated that the homology among corresponding allergen components from different grasses is so high that, in the immune system perspective, the derived cross-reactivity of grass specific IgE make it possible to simplify grass allergy diagnosis to the point that one single species can be used as representative of the whole grass family (van Ree et al., 1998). A similar consideration has been extrapolated for *Fagales* (Van Ree et al., 1999). Thus, on one side it is acceptable to narrow down the number of species of a given family of allergenic plants to one representative species, on the other within each given species the complexity of the allergen components which are composing the extract has to be considered as comprehensively as possible. In fact, it is well established that individuals sensitized to one given allergen source are variably reacting with the different antigenic components of the raw allergen extract. For instance, grass allergic subjects mainly react against *Phl p 1* and *Phl p 5* allergen components, yet complex patterns of reactivity can be observed in single individuals (Rossi et al., 2001; Rossi et al., 2000). Remarkable advantages derived from the application of molecular allergology to the overall comprehension of allergic diseases pathogenesis, including the understanding the molecular characteristics of allergens, the study of allergen structures, the characterization of the humoral (or B-cell-mediated, or antibody-dependent) and cellular (or T cell- mediated) immune responses (Burastero et al., 2004). Moreover, sequence similarity searches have identified the biological functions of many allergens and allowed to characterize mechanisms involved in typical allergic phenomena such as airway hyper-responsiveness and airway inflammation correlated to allergen exposure. For instance, *Der p 1* is a glycoprotein with sequence homology and thiol protease function similar to the enzymes papain, actinidin bromelain and cathepsins B and H (Chua et al., 1988). Only a limited number of clinical trials have been performed until now to compare the efficacy of recombinant allergens as compared to raw allergen extracts, although clinical benefit when using the former either in native (Jutel et al., 2005; Pauli et al., 2008) or modified forms (Niederberger et al., 2007; Purohit et al., 2008) have been reported. Recombinant allergens will overcome some of the pitfalls of using natural allergen products for immunotherapy by enabling physicians to administer only the clinically relevant allergens, thus avoiding exposure to unnecessary antigens. In this context, although the recombinant allergen era has not started yet for immunotherapy, yet quality control criteria must include the quantification of major allergen content in allergen extracts, as an invaluable tool to compare extracts from different manufacturers used for diagnosis or immunotherapy (Larsen and Dreborg, 2008).

14. Conclusion

Methods to achieve the standardisation of allergens used for diagnostic or therapeutic purposes should be homogeneous throughout the world. The present situation, whereby different Manufacturers use different units generate confusion and unreliable information, which may imply either underestimation or overestimation of the potency of allergen extracts. These differences may depend on the variability of the raw material used, the production methods and the lack of batch-to-batch consistence of the preparation procedure. The determination of the content in major allergen is essential to overcome these difficulties. Results of the CREATE project highlight a few limitations of recombinant allergen-based methodologies, which could support the implementation of this approach. In principle, as different factors as incorrect folding, aggregation, poor solubility and insufficient stability may affect the possibility to use a given allergen component as reference standard (Chapman et al., 2008). Nevertheless, knowledge generated by molecular allergology cannot longer wait to be integrated in the know-how to be developed and applied in this scenario. Along this line, the European Medicines Agency (EMEA) recommends proving that each allergen extract contains the relevant allergens by antibody-based techniques or mass spectrometry. In this context, new promising techniques, such as nuclear magnetic resonance and small angle X ray scattering, can also be applied to characterize allergenic molecules in the laboratory.

Overall, this growing awareness is slowly affecting the methods by which allergen extracts are standardized. This is a necessary achievement in modern allergology, not only in the perspective of better patient care, but also under the prospect of definitely accompanying this discipline to the podium it deserves. Development of standardized methods to measure allergen content are also eagerly needed by the imminent improvement of specific immunotherapy, which will imply the usage of recombinant (or purified) allergen components, instead of allergen extracts. This step will definitely promote the development of internationally accepted, standardized methods to measure allergen content, and to quantify the homogeneity, folding, aggregation, solubility and stability of recombinant products.

There is no doubt about the fact that allergen standardization is a fast developing field, which will soon allow to complete the progress of allergology from the present transition status where much is still managed according to traditional approaches based on allergen extracts and old cuisine to the full implementation of molecular immunology. The dramatic social relevance of allergies will warrant the encouragement of the medical and scientific community to this transition.

15. References

Abramson, J., and Pecht, I. (2007). Regulation of the mast cell response to the type 1 Fc epsilon receptor. *Immunol Rev* Vol.*217*, pp.231-254.

Abramson, M.J., Puy, R.M., and Weiner, J.M. (2010). Injection allergen immunotherapy for asthma. *Cochrane Database Syst Rev*, No.8, pp.CD001186.

Health Protection Agency, (2010). Biological Reference Material.

Akdis, C.A., and Akdis, M. (2010). Mechanisms of allergen-specific immunotherapy. *J Allergy Clin Immunol* Vol.*127*, No.1, pp.18-27; quiz 28-19.

Akdis, C.A., and Blaser, K. (2001). Mechanisms of interleukin-10-mediated immune suppression. *Immunology* Vol.*103*, No.2, pp.131-136.

Al Suleimani, Y.M., and Walker, M.J. (2007). Allergic rhinitis and its pharmacology. *Pharmacol Ther* Vol.*114*, No.3, pp.233-260.

Alvarez-Cuesta, E., Bousquet, J., Canonica, G.W., Durham, S.R., Malling, H.J., and Valovirta, E. (2006). Standards for practical allergen-specific immunotherapy. *Allergy* Vol.*61 Suppl 82*, pp.1-20.

Arbes, S.J., Jr., Cohn, R.D., Yin, M., Muilenberg, M.L., Burge, H.A., Friedman, W., and Zeldin, D.C. (2003). House dust mite allergen in US beds: results from the First National Survey of Lead and Allergens in Housing. *J Allergy Clin Immunol* Vol.*111*, No.2, pp.408-414.

Barrett, N.A., and Austen, K.F. (2009). Innate cells and T helper 2 cell immunity in airway inflammation. *Immunity* Vol.*31*, No.3, pp.425-437.

Becker, W.M., Vogel, L., and Vieths, S. (2006). Standardization of allergen extracts for immunotherapy: where do we stand? *Curr Opin Allergy Clin Immunol* Vol.6, No.6, pp.470-475.

Bordignon, V., and Burastero, S.E. (2006). Age, gender and reactivity to allergens independently influence skin reactivity to histamine. *J Investig Allergol Clin Immunol* Vol.*16*, No.2, pp.129-135.

Bousquet, J., Lockey, R., Malling, H.J., Alvarez-Cuesta, E., Canonica, G.W., Chapman, M.D., Creticos, P.J., Dayer, J.M., Durham, S.R., Demoly, P., *et al.* (1998). Allergen immunotherapy: therapeutic vaccines for allergic diseases. World Health Organization. American academy of Allergy, Asthma and Immunology. *Ann Allergy Asthma Immunol* Vol.*81*, No.5 Pt 1, pp.401-405.

Brighton, W.D. (1975). Profiles of allergen extract components by isoelectric focussing and radioimmunoassay. *Dev Biol Stand* Vol.*29*, pp.362-369.

Bufe, A., Eberle, P., Franke-Beckmann, E., Funck, J., Kimmig, M., Klimek, L., Knecht, R., Stephan, V., Tholstrup, B., Weisshaar, C., *et al.* (2009). Safety and efficacy in children of an SQ-standardized grass allergen tablet for sublingual immunotherapy. *J Allergy Clin Immunol* Vol.*123*, No.1, pp.167-173 e167.

Burastero, S. (2005). Regarding Gidaro GB, Marcucci F, Sensi L, Incorvaia C, Frati F, Ciprandi G. The safety of sublingual-swallow immunotherapy: an analysis of published studies. Clin Exp Allergy 2005; 35:565-71. *Clin Exp Allergy* Vol.*35*, No.10, pp.1407-1408; author reply 1409.

Burastero, S.E., Paolucci, C., Breda, D., Longhi, R., Silvestri, M., Hammer, J., Protti, M.P., and Rossi, G.A. (2004). T-cell receptor-mediated cross-allergenicity. *Int Arch Allergy Immunol* Vol.*135*, No.4, pp.296-305.

Bush, A., and Saglani, S. (2010). Management of severe asthma in children. *Lancet* Vol.*376*, No.9743, pp.814-825.

Calamita, Z., Saconato, H., Pela, A.B., and Atallah, A.N. (2006). Efficacy of sublingual immunotherapy in asthma: systematic review of randomized-clinical trials using the Cochrane Collaboration method. *Allergy* Vol.*61*, No.10, pp.1162-1172.

Ceska, M., Eriksson, R., and Varga, J.M. (1972). Radioimmunosorbent assay of allergens. *J Allergy Clin Immunol* Vol.*49*, No.1, pp.1-9.

Chafen, J.J., Newberry, S.J., Riedl, M.A., Bravata, D.M., Maglione, M., Suttorp, M.J., Sundaram, V., Paige, N.M., Towfigh, A., Hulley, B.J., *et al.* (2010). Diagnosing and managing common food allergies: a systematic review. *JAMA* Vol.*303*, No.18, pp.1848-1856.

Chapman, M.D., Ferreira, F., Villalba, M., Cromwell, O., Bryan, D., Becker, W.M., Fernandez-Rivas, M., Durham, S., Vieths, S., and van Ree, R. (2008). The European Union CREATE project: a model for international standardization of allergy diagnostics and vaccines. *J Allergy Clin Immunol* Vol.*122*, No.5, pp.882-889 e882.

Chapman, M.D., Pomes, A., Breiteneder, H., and Ferreira, F. (2007). Nomenclature and structural biology of allergens. *J Allergy Clin Immunol* Vol.*119*, No.2, pp.414-420.

Chapman, M.D., Smith, A.M., Vailes, L.D., Arruda, L.K., Dhanaraj, V., and Pomes, A. (2000). Recombinant allergens for diagnosis and therapy of allergic disease. *J Allergy Clin Immunol* Vol.*106*, No.3, pp.409-418.

Chinen, J., and Shearer, W.T. (2004). Advances in asthma, allergy and immunology series 2004: basic and clinical immunology. *J Allergy Clin Immunol* Vol.*114*, No.2, pp.398-405.

Chinen, J., and Shearer, W.T. (2007). Advances in basic and clinical immunology in 2006. *J Allergy Clin Immunol* Vol.*120*, No.2, pp.263-270.

Chu, H.W., Lloyd, C.M., Karmaus, W., Maestrelli, P., Mason, P., Salcedo, G., Thaikoottathil, J., and Wardlaw, A.J. Developments in the field of allergy in 2009 through the eyes of Clinical and Experimental Allergy. *Clin Exp Allergy* Vol.*40*, No.11, pp.1611-1631.

Chua, K.Y., Stewart, G.A., Thomas, W.R., Simpson, R.J., Dilworth, R.J., Plozza, T.M., and Turner, K.J. (1988). Sequence analysis of cDNA coding for a major house dust mite allergen, Der p 1. Homology with cysteine proteases. *J Exp Med* Vol.*167*, No.1, pp.175-182.

Ciprandi, G., Cadario, G., Di Gioacchino, G.M., Gangemi, S., Gasparini, A., Isola, S., Marengo, F., Minelli, S., Ricciardi, L., Ridolo, E., *et al.* (2010a). Sublingual immunotherapy in children with allergic polysensitization. *Allergy Asthma Proc* Vol.*31*, No.3, pp.227-231.

Ciprandi, G., Incorvaia, C., Puccinelli, P., Scurati, S., Masieri, S., and Frati, F. (2010b). The POLISMAIL lesson: sublingual immunotherapy may be prescribed also in polysensitized patients. *Int J Immunopathol Pharmacol* Vol.*23*, No.2, pp.637-640.

Corti, V., Cattaneo, A., Bachi, A., Rossi, R.E., Monasterolo, G., Paolucci, C., Burastero, S.E., and Alessio, M. (2005). Identification of grass pollen allergens by two-dimensional gel electrophoresis and serological screening. *Proteomics* Vol.*5*, No.3, pp.729-736.

Cox, L., Nelson, H., Lockey, R., Calabria, C., Chacko, T., Finegold, I., Nelson, M., Weber, R., Bernstein, D.I., Blessing-Moore, J., *et al.* (2010). Allergen immunotherapy: a practice parameter third update. *J Allergy Clin Immunol* Vol.*127*, No.1 Suppl, pp.S1-55.

Cummings, A.J., Knibb, R.C., King, R.M., and Lucas, J.S. (2010). The psychosocial impact of food allergy and food hypersensitivity in children, adolescents and their families: a review. *Allergy* Vol.*65*, No.8, pp.933-945.

Dahl, R., Kapp, A., Colombo, G., de Monchy, J.G., Rak, S., Emminger, W., Riis, B., Gronager, P.M., and Durham, S.R. (2008). Sublingual grass allergen tablet immunotherapy provides sustained clinical benefit with progressive immunologic changes over 2 years. *J Allergy Clin Immunol* Vol.*121*, No.2, pp.512-518 e512.

Dreborg, S., Basomba, A., Belin, L., Durham, S., Einarsson, R., Eriksson, N.E., Frostad, A.B., Grimmer, O., Halvorsen, R., Holgersson, M., *et al.* (1987). Biological equilibration of allergen preparations: methodological aspects and reproducibility. *Clin Allergy* Vol.*17*, No.6, pp.537-550.

Dreborg, S., and Einarsson, R. (1992). The major allergen content of allergenic preparations reflect their biological activity. *Allergy* Vol.*47*, No.4 Pt 2, pp.418-423.

Dreborg, S., and Foucard, T. (1983). Allergy to apple, carrot and potato in children with birch pollen allergy. *Allergy* Vol.*38*, No.3, pp.167-172.

Dykewicz, M.S., and Hamilos, D.L. (2010). Rhinitis and sinusitis. *J Allergy Clin Immunol* Vol.*125*, No.2 Suppl 2, pp.S103-115.

Engvall, E., and Perlmann, P. (1972). Enzyme-linked immunosorbent assay, Elisa. 3. Quantitation of specific antibodies by enzyme-labeled anti-immunoglobulin in antigen-coated tubes. *J Immunol* Vol.*109*, No.1, pp.129-135.

Enrique, E., Pineda, F., Malek, T., Bartra, J., Basagana, M., Tella, R., Castello, J.V., Alonso, R., de Mateo, J.A., Cerda-Trias, T., *et al.* (2005). Sublingual immunotherapy for hazelnut food allergy: a randomized, double-blind, placebo-controlled study with a standardized hazelnut extract. *J Allergy Clin Immunol* Vol.*116*, No.5, pp.1073-1079.

Esch, R.E. (2004). Manufacturing and standardizing fungal allergen products. *J Allergy Clin Immunol* Vol.*113*, No.2, pp.210-215.

Fernandez-Caldas, E., Carnes, J., Gallego, M., Mari, A., and Pagan Aleman, J.A. (2006). Standardization of animal epithelia. *Arb Paul Ehrlich Inst Bundesamt Sera Impfstoffe Frankf A M*, No.95, pp.107-116; discussion 116, 155.

Fernández-Caldas, E., Zakzuk, J., and Lockey, R.F. (2009). Allergen Standardization and Characterization.

Ferreira, F., Briza, P., Infuhr, D., Schmidt, G., Wallner, M., Wopfner, N., Thalhamer, J., and Achatz, G. (2006). Modified recombinant allergens for safer immunotherapy. *Inflamm Allergy Drug Targets* Vol.5, No.1, pp.5-14.

Ferrer, A., Carnes, J., Gallego, M.T., Andreu, C., and Fernandez-Caldas, E. (2005). Characterization and improvement of apple extracts for the diagnosis of apple IgE-mediated allergy. *Ann Allergy Asthma Immunol* Vol.*95*, No.5, pp.462-467.

Ford, A., Seagroatt, V., Platts-Mills, T.A., and Lowenstein, H. (1985). A collaborative study on the first international standard of Dermatophagoides pteronyssinus (house dust mite) extract. *J Allergy Clin Immunol* Vol.*75*, No.6, pp.676-686.

Gidaro, G.B., Marcucci, F., Sensi, L., Incorvaia, C., Frati, F., and Ciprandi, G. (2005). The safety of sublingual-swallow immunotherapy: an analysis of published studies. *Clin Exp Allergy* Vol.*35*, No.5, pp.565-571.

Gjesing, B., Jager, L., Marsh, D.G., and Lowenstein, H. (1985). The international collaborative study establishing the first international standard for timothy (Phleum pratense) grass pollen allergenic extract. *J Allergy Clin Immunol* Vol.*75*, No.2, pp.258-267.

Grier, T.J., Hazelhurst, D.M., Duncan, E.A., West, T.K., and Esch, R.E. (2002). Major allergen measurements: sources of variability, validation, quality assurance, and utility for laboratories, manufacturers, and clinics. *Allergy Asthma Proc* Vol.*23*, No.2, pp.125-131.

Gurka, G., and Rocklin, R. (1988). Immunologic responses during allergen-specific immunotherapy for respiratory allergy. *Ann Allergy* Vol.*61*, No.4, pp.239-245.

Gutermuth, J., Bewersdorff, M., Traidl-Hoffmann, C., Ring, J., Mueller, M.J., Behrendt, H., and Jakob, T. (2007). Immunomodulatory effects of aqueous birch pollen extracts and phytoprostanes on primary immune responses in vivo. *J Allergy Clin Immunol* Vol.*120*, No.2, pp.293-299.

Hamid, Q., and Tulic, M. (2009). Immunobiology of asthma. *Annu Rev Physiol* Vol.*71*, pp.489-507.

Hamilton, R.G. (2010). Clinical laboratory assessment of immediate-type hypersensitivity. *J Allergy Clin Immunol* Vol.*125*, No.2 Suppl 2, pp.S284-296.

Hamilton, R.G. (2005). Assessment of indoor allergen exposure. *Curr Allergy Asthma Rep* Vol.*5*, No.5, pp.394-401.

Hankin, C.S., and Lockey, R.F. (2010). Patient characteristics associated with allergen immunotherapy initiation and adherence. *J Allergy Clin Immunol* Vol.*127*, No.1, pp.46-48, 48 e41-43.

Hauser, M., Roulias, A., Ferreira, F., and Egger, M. (2010). Panallergens and their impact on the allergic patient. *Allergy Asthma Clin Immunol* Vol.*6*, No.1, pp.1.

Heick, J., Fischer, M., and Popping, B. (2010). First screening method for the simultaneous detection of seven allergens by liquid chromatography mass spectrometry. *J Chromatogr A* Vol.*1218*, No.7, pp.938-943.

Heinrich, J., Bedada, G.B., Zock, J.P., Chinn, S., Norback, D., Olivieri, M., Svanes, C., Ponzio, M., Verlato, G., Villani, S., *et al.* (2006). Cat allergen level: its determinants and relationship to specific IgE to cat across European centers. *J Allergy Clin Immunol* Vol.*118*, No.3, pp.674-681.

Heiss, S., Mahler, V., Steiner, R., Spitzauer, S., Schweiger, C., Kraft, D., and Valenta, R. (1999). Component-resolved diagnosis (CRD) of type I allergy with recombinant grass and tree pollen allergens by skin testing. *J Invest Dermatol* Vol.*113*, No.5, pp.830-837.

Helm, R.M., Gauerke, M.B., Baer, H., Lowenstein, H., Ford, A., Levy, D.A., Norman, P.S., and Yunginger, J.W. (1984). Production and testing of an international reference standard of short ragweed pollen extract. *J Allergy Clin Immunol* Vol.*73*, No.6, pp.790-800.

Himly, M., Nony, E., Chabre, H., Van Overtvelt, L., Neubauer, A., van Ree, R., Buchheit, K.H., Vieths, S., Moingeon, P., and Ferreira, F. (2009). Standardization of allergen products: 1. Detailed characterization of GMP-produced recombinant Bet v 1.0101 as biological reference preparation. *Allergy* Vol.*64*, No.7, pp.1038-1045.

Hochwallner, H., Schulmeister, U., Swoboda, I., Balic, N., Geller, B., Nystrand, M., Harlin, A., Thalhamer, J., Scheiblhofer, S., Niggemann, B., *et al.* (2010). Microarray and allergenic activity assessment of milk allergens. *Clin Exp Allergy* Vol.*40*, No.12, pp.1809-1818.

Holgate, S.T. (2008). Pathogenesis of asthma. *Clin Exp Allergy* Vol.*38*, No.6, pp.872-897.

Holowka, D., Sil, D., Torigoe, C., and Baird, B. (2007). Insights into immunoglobulin E receptor signaling from structurally defined ligands. *Immunol Rev* Vol.*217*, pp.269-279.

Houston, N.L., Lee, D.G., Stevenson, S.E., Ladics, G.S., Bannon, G.A., McClain, S., Privalle, L., Stagg, N., Herouet-Guicheney, C., MacIntosh, S.C., *et al.* (2010). Quantitation of soybean allergens using tandem mass spectrometry. *J Proteome Res* Vol.*10*, No.2, pp.763-773.

Illi, S., von Mutius, E., Lau, S., Niggemann, B., Gruber, C., and Wahn, U. (2006). Perennial allergen sensitisation early in life and chronic asthma in children: a birth cohort study. *Lancet* Vol.*368*, No.9537, pp.763-770.

Jutel, M., Jaeger, L., Suck, R., Meyer, H., Fiebig, H., and Cromwell, O. (2005). Allergen-specific immunotherapy with recombinant grass pollen allergens. *J Allergy Clin Immunol* Vol.*116*, No.3, pp.608-613.

Kazemi-Shirazi, L., Niederberger, V., Linhart, B., Lidholm, J., Kraft, D., and Valenta, R. (2002). Recombinant marker allergens: diagnostic gatekeepers for the treatment of allergy. *Int Arch Allergy Immunol* Vol.*127*, No.4, pp.259-268.

King, T.P., Hoffman, D., Lowenstein, H., Marsh, D.G., Platts-Mills, T.A., and Thomas, W. (1994). Allergen nomenclature. WHO/IUIS Allergen Nomenclature Subcommittee. *Int Arch Allergy Immunol* Vol.*105*, No.3, pp.224-233.

Kuriakose, J.S., and Miller, R.L. (2010). Environmental epigenetics and allergic diseases: recent advances. *Clin Exp Allergy* Vol.*40*, No.11, pp.1602-1610.

Kyhse-Andersen, J. (1984). Electroblotting of multiple gels: a simple apparatus without buffer tank for rapid transfer of proteins from polyacrylamide to nitrocellulose. *J Biochem Biophys Methods* Vol.*10*, No.3-4, pp.203-209.

Laemmli, U.K. (1970). Cleavage of structural proteins during the assembly of the head of bacteriophage T4. *Nature* Vol.*227*, No.5259, pp.680-685.

Larenas-Linnemann, D., and Cox, L.S. (2008). European allergen extract units and potency: review of available information. *Ann Allergy Asthma Immunol* Vol.*100*, No.2, pp.137-145.

Larsen, J.N., and Dreborg, S. (2008). Standardization of allergen extracts. *Methods Mol Med* Vol.*138*, pp.133-145.

Larsen, J.N., Ford, A., Gjesing, B., Levy, D., Petrunov, B., Silvestri, L., and Lowenstein, H. (1988). The collaborative study of the international standard of dog, Canis domesticus, hair/dander extract. *J Allergy Clin Immunol* Vol.*82*, No.3 Pt 1, pp.318-330.

Lemanske, R.F., Jr., and Taylor, S.L. (1987). Standardized extracts, foods. *Clin Rev Allergy* Vol.*5*, No.1, pp.23-36.

Lindgren, S., Belin, L., Dreborg, S., Einarsson, R., and Pahlman, I. (1988). Breed-specific dog-dandruff allergens. *J Allergy Clin Immunol* Vol.*82*, No.2, pp.196-204.

Lowenstein, H. (1978). Quantitative immunoelectrophoretic methods as a tool for the analysis and isolation of allergens. *Prog Allergy* Vol.*25*, pp.1-62.

Lowenstein, H. (1987). Selection of reference preparation. IUIS reference preparation criteria. International Union of Immunological Societies. *Arb Paul Ehrlich Inst Georg Speyer Haus Ferdinand Blum Inst Frankf A M*, No.80, pp.75-78.

Lowenstein, H., King, T.P., Goodfriend, L., Hussain, R., Roebber, M., and Marsh, D.G. (1981). Antigens of Ambrosia elatior (short ragweed) pollen. II. Immunochemical identification of known antigens by quantitative immunoelectrophoresis. *J Immunol* Vol.*127*, No.2, pp.637-642.

Lowenstein, H., and Marsh, D.G. (1981). Antigens of Ambrosia elatior (short ragweed) pollen. I. Crossed immunoelectrophoretic analyses. *J Immunol* Vol.*126*, No.3, pp.943-948.

Lowenstein, H., and Marsh, D.G. (1983). Antigens of Ambrosia elatior (short ragweed) pollen. III. Crossed radioimmunoelectrophoresis of ragweed-allergic patients' sera with special attention to quantification of IgE responses. *J Immunol* Vol.*130*, No.2, pp.727-731.

Macglashan, D., Jr. (2005). IgE and Fc{epsilon}RI regulation. *Ann N Y Acad Sci* Vol.*1050*, pp.73-88.

Moingeon, P. (2006). Sublingual immunotherapy: from biological extracts to recombinant allergens. *Allergy* Vol.*61 Suppl 81*, pp.15-19.

Morgan, W.J., Crain, E.F., Gruchalla, R.S., O'Connor, G.T., Kattan, M., Evans, R., 3rd, Stout, J., Malindzak, G., Smartt, E., Plaut, M., *et al.* (2004). Results of a home-based environmental intervention among urban children with asthma. *N Engl J Med* Vol.*351*, No.11, pp.1068-1080.

Mothes, N., Valenta, R., and Spitzauer, S. (2006). Allergy testing: the role of recombinant allergens. *Clin Chem Lab Med* Vol.*44*, No.2, pp.125-132.

Nelson, H.S. (2000). The use of standardized extracts in allergen immunotherapy. *J Allergy Clin Immunol* Vol.*106*, No.1 Pt 1, pp.41-45.

Nelson, H.S. (2007). Allergen immunotherapy: where is it now? *J Allergy Clin Immunol* Vol.*119*, No.4, pp.769-779.

Niederberger, V., Reisinger, J., Valent, P., Krauth, M.T., Pauli, G., van Hage, M., Cromwell, O., Horak, F., and Valenta, R. (2007). Vaccination with genetically modified birch pollen allergens: immune and clinical effects on oral allergy syndrome. *J Allergy Clin Immunol* Vol.*119*, No.4, pp.1013-1016.

Novak, N. (2009). New insights into the mechanism and management of allergic diseases: atopic dermatitis. *Allergy* Vol.*64*, No.2, pp.265-275.

Ott, H., Baron, J.M., Heise, R., Ocklenburg, C., Stanzel, S., Merk, H.F., Niggemann, B., and Beyer, K. (2008). Clinical usefulness of microarray-based IgE detection in children with suspected food allergy. *Allergy* Vol.*63*, No.11, pp.1521-1528.

Pagani, M., Antico, A., Cilia, M., Calabro, D., Poto, S., Pecora, S., and Burastero, S.E. (2009). Comparison of different diagnostic products for skin prick testing. *Eur Ann Allergy Clin Immunol* Vol.*41*, No.1, pp.23-31.

Pauli, G., Larsen, T.H., Rak, S., Horak, F., Pastorello, E., Valenta, R., Purohit, A., Arvidsson, M., Kavina, A., Schroeder, J.W., *et al.* (2008). Efficacy of recombinant birch pollen vaccine for the treatment of birch-allergic rhinoconjunctivitis. *J Allergy Clin Immunol* Vol.*122*, No.5, pp.951-960.

Pittner, G., Vrtala, S., Thomas, W.R., Weghofer, M., Kundi, M., Horak, F., Kraft, D., and Valenta, R. (2004). Component-resolved diagnosis of house-dust mite allergy with purified natural and recombinant mite allergens. *Clin Exp Allergy* Vol.*34*, No.4, pp.597-603.

Platts-Mills, T.A., and Chapman, M.D. (1991). Allergen standardization. *J Allergy Clin Immunol* Vol.*87*, No.3, pp.621-625.

Platts-Mills, T.A., Vaughan, J.W., Carter, M.C., and Woodfolk, J.A. (2000). The role of intervention in established allergy: avoidance of indoor allergens in the treatment of chronic allergic disease. *J Allergy Clin Immunol* Vol.*106*, No.5, pp.787-804.

Platts-Mills, T.A., Vervloet, D., Thomas, W.R., Aalberse, R.C., and Chapman, M.D. (1997). Indoor allergens and asthma: report of the Third International Workshop. *J Allergy Clin Immunol* Vol.*100*, No.6 Pt 1, pp.S2-24.

Pomes, A. (2010). Relevant B cell epitopes in allergic disease. *Int Arch Allergy Immunol* Vol.*152*, No.1, pp.1-11.

Pucci, S., and Incorvaia, C. (2008). Allergy as an organ and a systemic disease. *Clin Exp Immunol* Vol.*153 Suppl 1*, pp.1-2.

Purohit, A., Niederberger, V., Kronqvist, M., Horak, F., Gronneberg, R., Suck, R., Weber, B., Fiebig, H., van Hage, M., Pauli, G., *et al.* (2008). Clinical effects of immunotherapy with genetically modified recombinant birch pollen Bet v 1 derivatives. *Clin Exp Allergy* Vol.*38*, No.9, pp.1514-1525.

Radulovic, S., Calderon, M.A., Wilson, D., and Durham, S. (2010). Sublingual immunotherapy for allergic rhinitis. *Cochrane Database Syst Rev*, No.12, pp.CD002893.

Rossi, R.E., Monasterolo, G., and Monasterolo, S. (2001). Measurement of IgE antibodies against purified grass-pollen allergens (Phl p 1, 2, 3, 4, 5, 6, 7, 11, and 12) in sera of patients allergic to grass pollen. *Allergy* Vol.*56*, No.12, pp.1180-1185.

Rossi, R.E., Monasterolo, G., Operti, D., Operti, R., and Berlen, R. (2000). Evaluation of IgE antibodies to recombinant pollen allergens (Phl p 1, Phl p 2, and Phl p 5) in a random sample of patients with specific IgE to Phleum pratense. *Allergy* Vol.*55*, No.2, pp.181-184.

Sander, I., Fleischer, C., Meurer, U., Bruning, T., and Raulf-Heimsoth, M. (2009). Allergen content of grass pollen preparations for skin prick testing and sublingual immunotherapy. *Allergy* Vol.*64*, No.10, pp.1486-1492.

Santos, A., and Van Ree, R. (2011). Profilins: Mimickers of Allergy or Relevant Allergens? *Int Arch Allergy Immunol* Vol.*155*, No.3, pp.191-204.

Scala, E., Alessandri, C., Bernardi, M.L., Ferrara, R., Palazzo, P., Pomponi, D., Quaratino, D., Rasi, C., Zaffiro, A., Zennaro, D., *et al.* (2010). Cross-sectional survey on immunoglobulin E reactivity in 23,077 subjects using an allergenic molecule-based microarray detection system. *Clin Exp Allergy* Vol.*40*, No.6, pp.911-921.

Scheiner, O., Breiteneder, H., Dolocek, C., Duchene, M., Ebner, C., Ferreira, F., Hoffmann, K., Schenk, S., Valenta, R., and Kraft, D. (1994). Molecular and functional characterization of allergens: basic and practical aspects. *Arb Paul Ehrlich Inst Bundesamt Sera Impfstoffe Frankf A M*, No.87, pp.221-232; discussion 233-224.

Sears, M.R., Greene, J.M., Willan, A.R., Wiecek, E.M., Taylor, D.R., Flannery, E.M., Cowan, J.O., Herbison, G.P., Silva, P.A., and Poulton, R. (2003). A longitudinal, population-based, cohort study of childhood asthma followed to adulthood. *N Engl J Med* Vol.*349*, No.15, pp.1414-1422.

Shakib, F., Ghaemmaghami, A.M., and Sewell, H.F. (2008). The molecular basis of allergenicity. *Trends Immunol* Vol.*29*, No.12, pp.633-642.

Sicherer, S.H., and Leung, D.Y. Advances in allergic skin disease, anaphylaxis, and hypersensitivity reactions to foods, drugs, and insects in 2009. *J Allergy Clin Immunol* Vol.*125*, No.1, pp.85-97.

Simons, F.E. Anaphylaxis. (2010). *J Allergy Clin Immunol* Vol.*125*, No.2 Suppl 2, pp.S161-181.

Slater, J.E. (2004). Standardized allergen extracts in the United States. *Clin Allergy Immunol* Vol.*18*, pp.421-432.

Spergel, J.M. (2010a). Epidemiology of atopic dermatitis and atopic march in children. *Immunol Allergy Clin North Am* Vol.*30*, No.3, pp.269-280.

Spergel, J.M. (2010b). From atopic dermatitis to asthma: the atopic march. *Ann Allergy Asthma Immunol* Vol.*105*, No.2, pp.99-106; quiz 107-109, 117.

Sporik, R., Squillace, S.P., Ingram, J.M., Rakes, G., Honsinger, R.W., and Platts-Mills, T.A. (1999). Mite, cat, and cockroach exposure, allergen sensitisation, and asthma in children: a case-control study of three schools. *Thorax* Vol.*54*, No.8, pp.675-680.

Steringer, I., Aukrust, L., and Einarsson, R. (1987). Variability of antigenicity/allergenicity in different strains of Alternaria alternata. *Int Arch Allergy Appl Immunol* Vol.*84*, No.2, pp.190-197.

Terho, E., and Frew, A.J. (1995). Type III allergy skin testing. Position statement for EAACI Subcommittee on Skin Tests and Allergen Standardization. *Allergy* Vol.*50*, No.5, pp.392-396.

Traidl-Hoffmann, C., Mariani, V., Hochrein, H., Karg, K., Wagner, H., Ring, J., Mueller, M.J., Jakob, T., and Behrendt, H. (2005). Pollen-associated phytoprostanes inhibit dendritic cell interleukin-12 production and augment T helper type 2 cell polarization. *J Exp Med* Vol.*201*, No.4, pp.627-636.

Turkeltaub, P.C. (1987). Biological standardization based on quantitative skin testing--the ID50 EAL method (intradermal dilution for 50 mm sum of erythema diameters determines the allergy unit). *Arb Paul Ehrlich Inst Georg Speyer Haus Ferdinand Blum Inst Frankf A M*, No.80, pp.169-173.

Uhlin, T., Reuterby, J., and Einarsson, R. (1984). Antigenic/allergenic composition of Poodle/Alsatian dandruff extract. *Allergy* Vol.*39*, No.2, pp.125-133.

Valenta, R., Duchene, M., Pettenburger, K., Sillaber, C., Valent, P., Bettelheim, P., Breitenbach, M., Rumpold, H., Kraft, D., and Scheiner, O. (1991). Identification of profilin as a novel pollen allergen; IgE autoreactivity in sensitized individuals. *Science* Vol.*253*, No.5019, pp.557-560.

Valenta, R., Lidholm, J., Niederberger, V., Hayek, B., Kraft, D., and Gronlund, H. (1999). The recombinant allergen-based concept of component-resolved diagnostics and immunotherapy (CRD and CRIT). *Clin Exp Allergy* Vol.*29*, No.7, pp.896-904.

Valenta, R., Twaroch, T., and Swoboda, I. (2007). Component-resolved diagnosis to optimize allergen-specific immunotherapy in the Mediterranean area. *J Investig Allergol Clin Immunol* Vol.*17 Suppl 1*, pp.36-40.

van Ree, R. (2007). Indoor allergens: relevance of major allergen measurements and standardization. *J Allergy Clin Immunol* Vol.*119*, No.2, pp.270-277; quiz 278-279.

van Ree, R., Chapman, M.D., Ferreira, F., Vieths, S., Bryan, D., Cromwell, O., Villalba, M., Durham, S.R., Becker, W.M., Aalbers, M., *et al.* (2008). The CREATE project: development of certified reference materials for allergenic products and validation of methods for their quantification. *Allergy* Vol.*63*, No.3, pp.310-326.

van Ree, R., van Leeuwen, W.A., and Aalberse, R.C. (1998). How far can we simplify in vitro diagnostics for grass pollen allergy?: A study with 17 whole pollen extracts and purified natural and recombinant major allergens. *J Allergy Clin Immunol* Vol.*102*, No.2, pp.184-190.

Van Ree, R., Van Leeuwen, W.A., Akkerdaas, J.H., and Aalberse, R.C. (1999). How far can we simplify in vitro diagnostics for Fagales tree pollen allergy? A study with three whole pollen extracts and purified natural and recombinant allergens. *Clin Exp Allergy* Vol.*29*, No.6, pp.848-855.

Verstege, A., Mehl, A., Rolinck-Werninghaus, C., Staden, U., Nocon, M., Beyer, K., and Niggemann, B. (2005). The predictive value of the skin prick test weal size for the outcome of oral food challenges. *Clin Exp Allergy* Vol.*35*, No.9, pp.1220-1226.

Vrtala, S. (2008). From allergen genes to new forms of allergy diagnosis and treatment. *Allergy* Vol.*63*, No.3, pp.299-309.

Wahn, U., Schweter, C., Lind, P., and Lowenstein, H. (1988). Prospective study on immunologic changes induced by two different Dermatophagoides pteronyssinus extracts prepared from whole mite culture and mite bodies. *J Allergy Clin Immunol* Vol.*82*, No.3 Pt 1, pp.360-370.

Wallenbeck, I., Aukrust, L., and Einarsson, R. (1984). Antigenic variability of different strains of Aspergillus fumigatus. *Int Arch Allergy Appl Immunol* Vol.*73*, No.2, pp.166-172.

Woodcock, A., Lowe, L.A., Murray, C.S., Simpson, B.M., Pipis, S.D., Kissen, P., Simpson, A., and Custovic, A. (2004). Early life environmental control: effect on symptoms, sensitization, and lung function at age 3 years. *Am J Respir Crit Care Med* Vol.*170*, No.4, pp.433-439.

Zock, J.P., Heinrich, J., Jarvis, D., Verlato, G., Norback, D., Plana, E., Sunyer, J., Chinn, S., Olivieri, M., Soon, A., *et al.* (2006). Distribution and determinants of house dust mite allergens in Europe: the European Community Respiratory Health Survey II. *J Allergy Clin Immunol* Vol.*118*, No.3, pp.682-690.

13

Quality Control of *Bupleurum* Species by Newly Established Eastern Blotting

Osamu Morinaga[1], Xiao-Wei Li[2] and Shunsuke Fujii[3]
[1]*Faculty of Pharmaceutical Sciences, Nagasaki International University*
[2]*School of Pharmaceutical Sciences, Peking University*
[3]*Graduate School of Health Management, Nagasaki International University*
[1,3]*Japan*
[2]*China*

1. Introduction

In the investigation of staining technique for several compounds, a polyvinyliden difluoride (PVDF) membrane was found as transfer membrane (Towbin et al., 1979), and applied to western blotting technique that utilizes antigen-antibody binding property for the specific and sensitive detection of peptides and proteins by immunostaining (Granger, 1988; Reig & Klein, 1988). In the case of low molecule compounds, thin-layer chromatography (TLC) immunoblotting of glycosphingolipids was reported using a nitrocellulose membrane (Towbin et al., 1984), but the transfer efficiency from TLC plate to the membrane was poor and not constant. Recently, the direct TLC immunostaining of glycolipids and glycosphingolipids was demonstrated without the blotting step from TLC plate to the membrane (Meisen, 2004; Suetake & Yu, 2003). Furthermore, TLC immunostaining of gangliosides (Miyamoto et al., 2006) and dot blot analysis of gangliosides on PVDF membrane (Chabraoui et al., 1993) were reported as the direct immunostaining. These immunostaining techniques were limitedly applied for glycolipids, glycosphingolipids and gangliosides because the other low molecule compounds were easily washed out into the buffer solution without fixing on the TLC plate or PVDF membrane.

Since small molecular compound such as saponin cannot fix on the PVDF membrane or TLC plate, no success of immunostaining for saponin has been reported. We reached to a new idea that a saponin was divided into two functional parts, sugar and aglycone moieties. Sugar parts in saponin could be oxidized to give aldehyde groups which were conjugated with carrier protein like bovine serum albumin (BSA) and then fixed onto the PVDF membrane as saponin-BSA conjugate because BSA was strongly binded on the membrane. In contrast, the aglycone part was recognized as epitope by monoclonal antibody (MAb) against saponin and then we succeeded to immunostaining of saponin on the PVDF membrane. The first success was reported on the immunostaining of solasodine glycosides by our group (Tanaka et al., 1997) followed ginsenosides (Fukuda, 1999, 2000, 2001). In 2001 we suggested a new name, [eastern blotting] for glycyrrhizin as a new immunostaining technique (Shan et al., 2001).

In eastern blotting the developed TLC plate was covered with PVDF membrane and all contents were blotted from TLC plate to the membrane by press and heating. After the blotting, the membrane was treated with sodium periodide and then immersed in BSA solution at alkaline condition for the preparation of hapten-BSA conjugate on the membrane. After blocking with skimmed-milk, the membrane was treated by MAb which recognize a hapten and then a second antibody labeled with peroxidase directed against first antibody. Finally a substrate is added resulting in staining (Fig. 1). Fig. 2 shows the mechanism of binding and immunostaining of saikosaponin a (SSa) onto the PVDF membrane as previously reported (Zhu et al., 2007). Eastern blotting could stain only hapten molecule on the PVDF membrane. However, since the transfer efficiency at blotting step was difficult to control, this method could not be applied for the quantitative analysis system. Therefore, we improved staining system into the direct staining without transfer to membrane from TLC plate. In this chapter we will discuss about a newly developed eastern blotting.

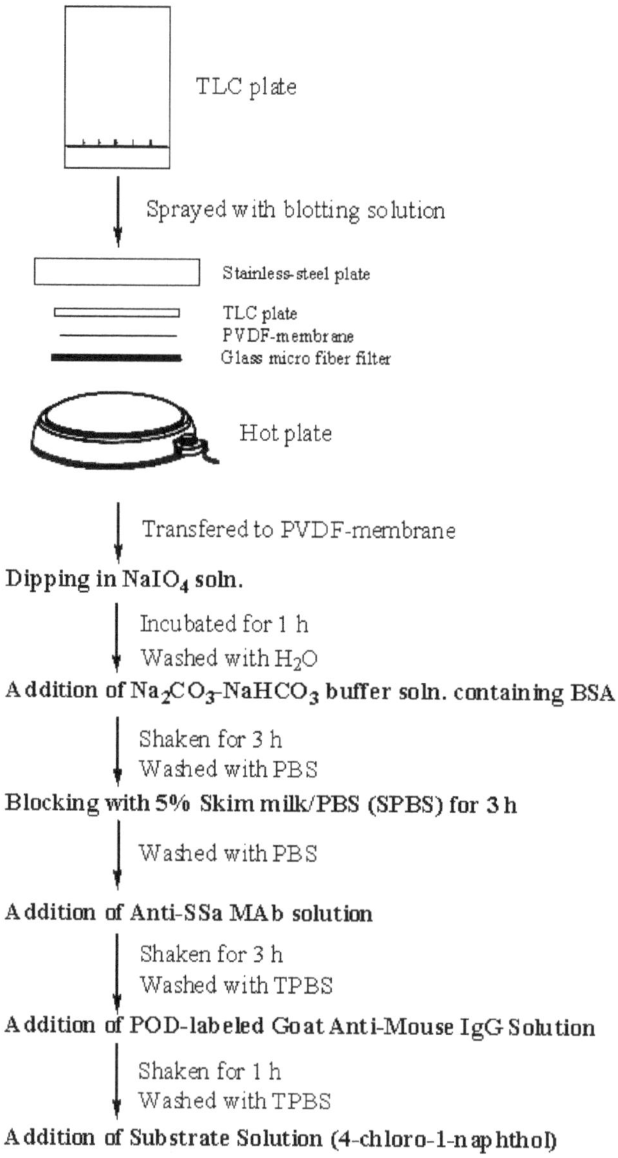

Fig. 1. Eastern blotting protocol

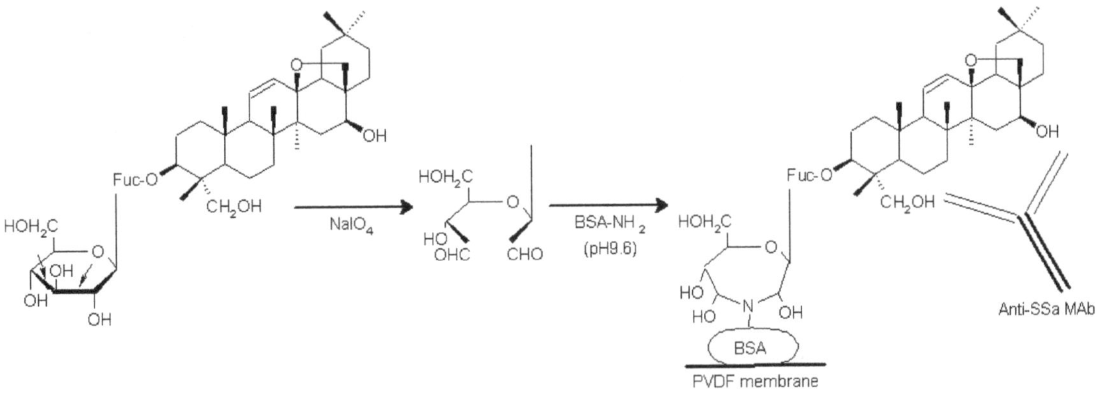

Fig. 2. Schematic diagram illustrating the immunodetection of SSa onto a PVDF membrane

Three major oleanane-saponins named saikosaponins such as SSa, SSc, and SSd (Fig. 3) and many minor saponins are isolated from the roots of *Bupleurum* species. SSa has anti-cancer, anti-inflammatory, corticosterone secreting and plasma-cholesterol decreasing activities. SSb_2 performs phagocytosis-increasing activity on macrophages. SSd shows liver protective effect, anti-inflammatory, immunoregulatory, virus inactivating and anti-cancer activities. Furthermore, in a prescription of Kampo medicine (Shosaikoto) containing Bupleuri radix, SSa, SSb_2, SSc, and SSd showed anti-tumor effects. Phytochemical and pharmacological analyses of Kampo medicine is extremely difficult due to combinatorial use of multiple herbs. In addition, because Kampo medicines are manufactured as highly standardized ethical drugs in Japan, a method of comprehensive analysis of the compounds for scientific quality control is urgently needed.

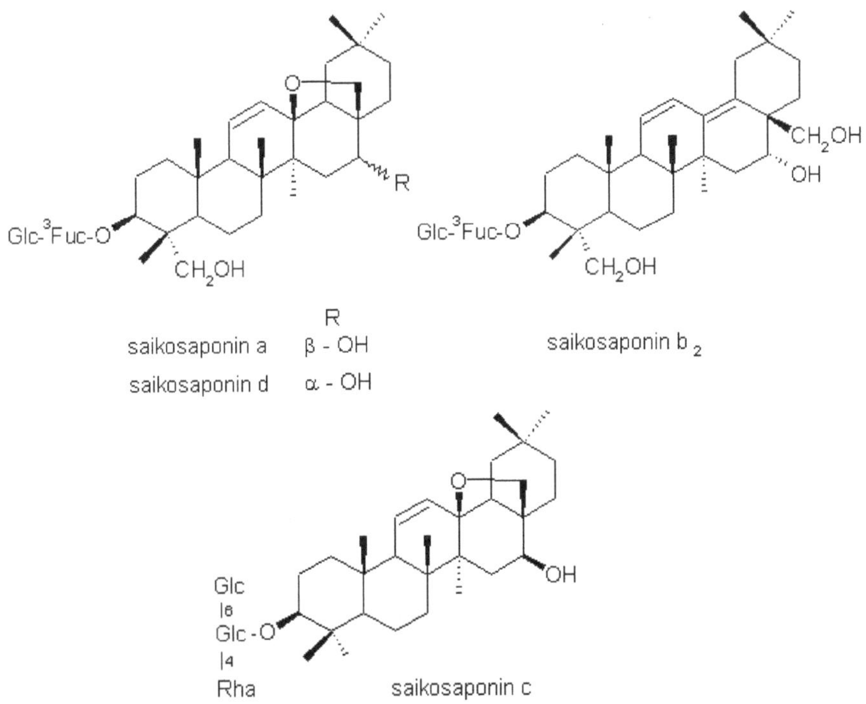

Fig. 3. Chemical structures of saikosaponins

Recently we prepared a specific MAb against SSa (Zhu et al., 2004) and a MAb having wide cross-reactivity to saikosaponins (Zhu et al., 2006), and developed an enzyme-linked immunosorbent assay (ELISA) system for quantitative measurement of SSa and/or total saikosaponins. However, it is difficult to gain the each content of SSa, SSb_2, SSc and SSd by these competitive ELISA methods. In pharmacological investigation of Kampo medicine, it is very important to grasp each bio-active compound concentration in each crude drugs prescribed individually, because individual saikosaponins have significant pharmacological effects as indicated above.

Therefore, we described here an unique approach, immunodetection of SSa, SSc, and SSd by new eastern blotting using anti-SSa MAb and its application to quantitative immunoassay using NIH Image for the estimation of saikosaponins in crude drugs and Kampo medicines containing Bupleuri radix for quality control as previously reported (Morinaga et al., 2006).

2. MAbs against SSa and saikosaponins and their developments for ELISA system

Immunizations, hybridizations and purifications of MAbs against SSa (1G6) and saikosaponins (3G10) and their developments of ELISA system for determination of SSa and total saikosaponins have been established (Zhu, 2004, 2006). Cross-reactivities are the most important factor in phytochemical investigations in which there are many structurally related compounds (see Table 1).

Compound	MAb-1G6	MAb-3G10
Saikosaponin a	100	100
Saikosaponin b_2	<0.25	63.77
Saikosaponin c	2.65	28.52
Saikosaponin d	3.76	15.62
Digitonin	<0.25	1.42
Solasonine	<0.25	<0.25
Solamargine	<0.25	<0.25
Glycyrrhizin	<0.25	<0.25
Ginsenoside Rb1	<0.25	<0.25
Ergosterol	<0.25	<0.25
Cholesterol	<0.25	<0.25
Sitosterol	<0.25	<0.25
Deoxycholic acid	0.45	<0.25

Table 1. Cross-reactivities (%) of anti-SSa MAbs (1G6) and (3G10)

Assay specificities were examined by competitive ELISA with various related compounds, then calculated following by Weiler and Zenk's method (Weiler & Zenk, 1976). The cross-reactivities (CR) of saikosaponins and related compounds were calculated by following equation.

$$CR\% = \frac{\mu g/ml \text{ of SSa yielding } A/A_0 = 50\%}{\mu g/ml \text{ of compound under investigation yielding } A/A_0 = 50\%} \times 100 \qquad (1)$$

A: absorbance in the presence of the test compound

A_0: absorbance in the absence of the test compound (10% MeOH)

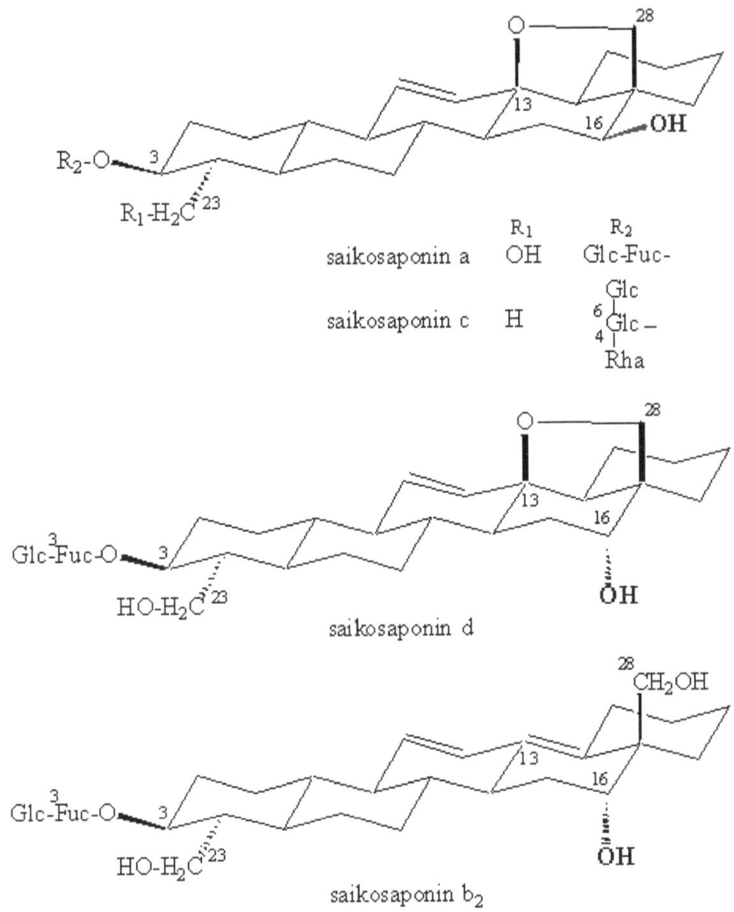

Fig. 4. Stereochemistry of saikosaponins

MAb-1G6 reacted only with structurally related SSc and SSd, weakly resulting in the high specificity of MAb. An undetectable cross-reaction with other steroidal compounds was shown. When compared the cross-reactivities between SSa having a β-hydroxyl group at the C-16 position and SSd (α-hydroxyl group), MAb-1G6 had cross-reactivities against SSd (see Fig. 4). From this, the hydroxyl group at the C-16 position is distinguished stereochemically by MAb-1G6.

MAb-3G10 cross-reacted with SSb_2, SSc and SSd at a rate of 63.8, 28.5 and 15.6%, respectively, easily suggesting that the ether ring between the C-13 and C-28 position in SSa might be opened in a mouse body during the immunization period, and then immunized. This wide cross-reaction is the major advantage of antibody reagent used in this ELISA, because when total saikosaponin concentrations in body fluid and/or in plant sample are needed, this MAb can be widely available, similarly to the results of anti-solamargine MAb (Ishiyama et al., 1996).

From these results, we decided that the concentration of the major saikosaponin, SSa, in the crude drug of Bupleuri radix can be analyzed by ELISA using MAb-1G6. On the other hand, when it is necessary to determine the concentration of total saikosaponins in the extracts of Kampo medicines, MAb-3G10 functions well for quantitative analysis because the ether ring at the C-13 and C-28 positions opens during the extraction process, as previously reported (Akahori, 1980).

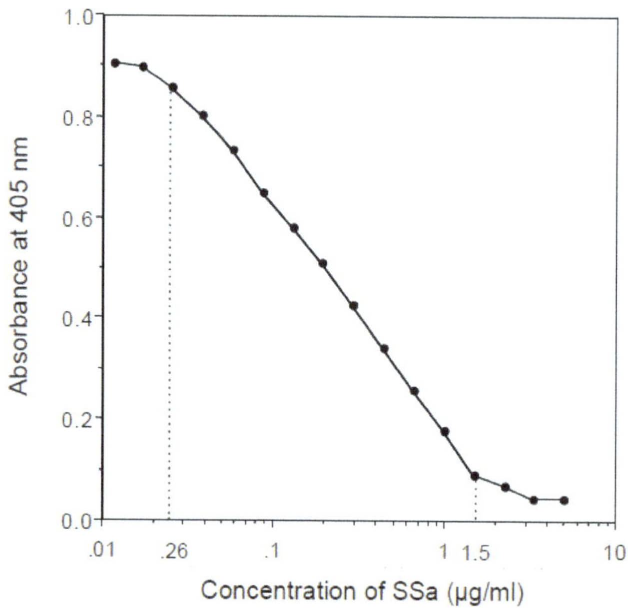

Fig. 5. Calibration curve of SSa by ELISA with MAb-1G6. Various concentrations of SSa were incubated with MAb-1G6 in the microtiter plate adsorbed with SSa-HSA (1 µg/ml). After washing with TPBS, the wells were again incubated with peroxidase-labeled anti-mouse IgG. Absorbance was measured at 405 nm

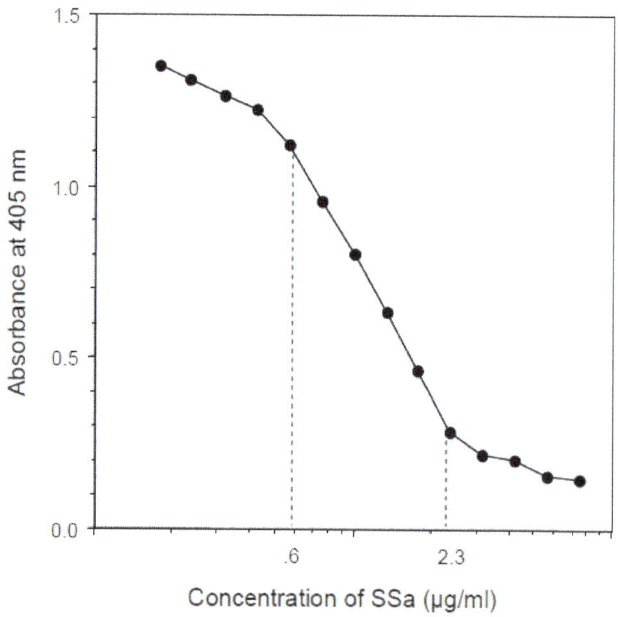

Fig. 6. Calibration curve of SSa by ELISA with MAb-3G10. Various concentrations of SSa were incubated with MAb-3G10 in the microtiter plate adsorbed with SSa-HSA (1 µg/ml). After washing with TPBS, the wells were again incubated with peroxidase-labeled anti-mouse IgG. Absorbance was measured at 405 nm

Fig. 5 indicates the calibration curve of SSa using MAb-1G6 by ELISA, showing that the full measuring range of the assay extended from 26 ng /ml to 1.5 µg/ml. Since the available measuring range of the HPLC method performed in our laboratory was 25 µg/ml to 400 µg/ml, it becomes evident that the ELISA is about 1000 times more sensitive than that of the HPLC method.

Fig. 6 indicates the calibration curve of SSa using MAb-3G10 by ELISA, showing that the full measuring range of the assay covers from 0.6 µg /ml to 2.3 µg/ml. Since the available measuring range of the HPLC method performed in our laboratory was 25 µg/ml to 400 µg/ml, it becomes evident that the ELISA is about 50 times more sensitive than that of the HPLC method.

3. New eastern blotting for saikosaponins

3.1 Extraction of crude drugs and Kampo medicines

Dried powders of various Bupleuri radix (20 mg) and Kampo medicine (50 mg) were extracted five times with 0.5 ml methanol with sonication and filtered using a Cosmonice filter W (0.45 µm filter unit, Nacalai Tesque, Kyoto, Japan). The combined extracts were diluted with methanol for ELISA and new eastern blotting analyses.

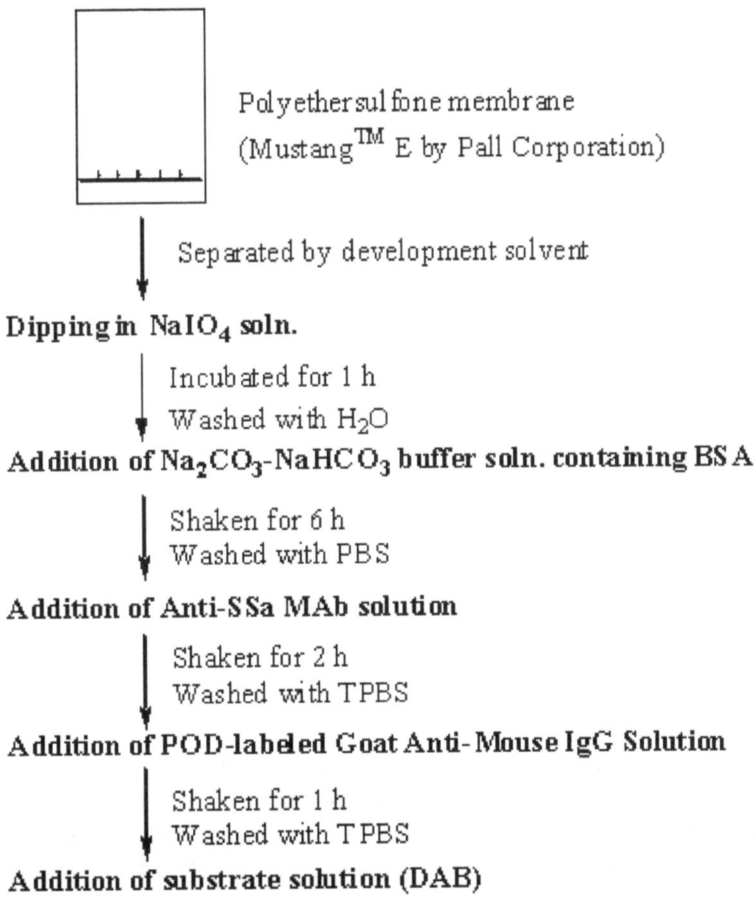

Fig. 7. New eastern blotting protocol

3.2 Visual detection of SSa, SSc, and SSd by new eastern blotting

New eastern blotting was performed except for separation by TLC plate and transfer to a PVDF membrane as reported previously (Tanaka et al., 1997) as following the protocol indicated in Fig. 7.

Saikosaponins and the extracts of Bupleuri radix and Kampo medicine were applied onto a positive-charged polyethersulfhone (PES) membrane (MustangTM E, Pall Corporation, East Hills, NY, USA). After drying, this membrane was hung in the tank and immersed and developed by acetonitrile-water (1:4, by volume). The developed PES membrane was dried and dipped into water containing $NaIO_4$ (10 mg/ml) for 1 h. After washing with water, 50 mM carbonate buffer solution (pH 9.6) containing BSA (1%) was added, and was stirred at room temperature for 3 h. After washing PES membrane with phosphate-buffered solution (PBS), the membrane was treated with PBS containing 5% skimmed milk (S-PBS) for 2 h to reduce nonspecific adsorption. The PES membrane was immersed in anti-SSa MAb (1G6) and stirred at room temperature for 2 h. After washing the PES membrane twice with PBS containing 0.05% Tween 20 (T-PBS) and water, a 1:1000 dilution of peroxidase-labeled goat anti-mouse IgG in PBS containing 0.02% gelatin was added, and the mixture was stirred at room temperature for 1 h. Then the PES membrane was washed twice with T-PBS and water and then exposed in Tris-HCl buffer (pH 7.5) containing 1 mg/ml 3,3′-diaminobenzidine tetrahydrochloride (DAB) and 0.02% H_2O_2 for 30 min at room temperature. The reaction was stopped by washing with water, and the immunostained PES membrane was allowed to dry.

3.3 Image analysis system and image acquisition

A graphic analysis system, which consisted of a Macintosh computer, a public domain program NIH Imaging 1.63 (developed at the U.S. National Institutes of Health and available on the internet at http://rsb.info.nih.gov/nih-image/), a desktop scanner and a scanning software Photoshop CS2 (Adobe Systems Inc., San Jose, CA, USA) was used.

Images were captured as 256 levels grayscale. The file size was 300 k bytes (200 dots per inch resolution). Digital output was transferred from the scanner to the computer and stored as a PICT file.

3.4 Image analysis using NIH Image

The immunostained PES membrane grayscale image was loaded and thresholded to make a binary image for the separation of objects and background. Then, we chose the analyze menu options and selected the area, ellipse major axis and ellipse minor axis commands to calculate the objects area as previously described (Masters et al., 1992; Root & Wang, 1993).

4. Establishment of new eastern blotting for immunodetection of saikosaponins

In a new approach, we demonstrated the immunodetection of saikosaponins on the positive-charged PES membrane. PES membrane is widely used for the ultrafiltration system (Duarte et al., 2003) and enzyme immobilization unit (Gomes et al., 2004). However, no success with immunodetection of small molecular compounds like saikosaponins using PES membrane has been reported yet. Fortunately, we found a new fact that the positive-charged PES membrane was suitable for the immunodetection of saikosaponins by dot blot analysis using anti-SSa MAb (1G6) (data not shown).

We also noticed its intrinsic hydrophilicity and strong physical property against organic solvents and believed it makes possible to separate saikosaponins chromatographically on this membrane. Although we tested various ratios of methanol-water as the solvent system, acceptable separation data was not obtained. However, fortunately we found its reverse phase property and tested various ratios of acetonitrile-water just following HPLC mobile phase for saikosaponins. All saikosaponin standards and Bupleuri radix (Mishima) extract were separated well with acetonitrile-water (1:4, by volume) as shown in Fig. 8.

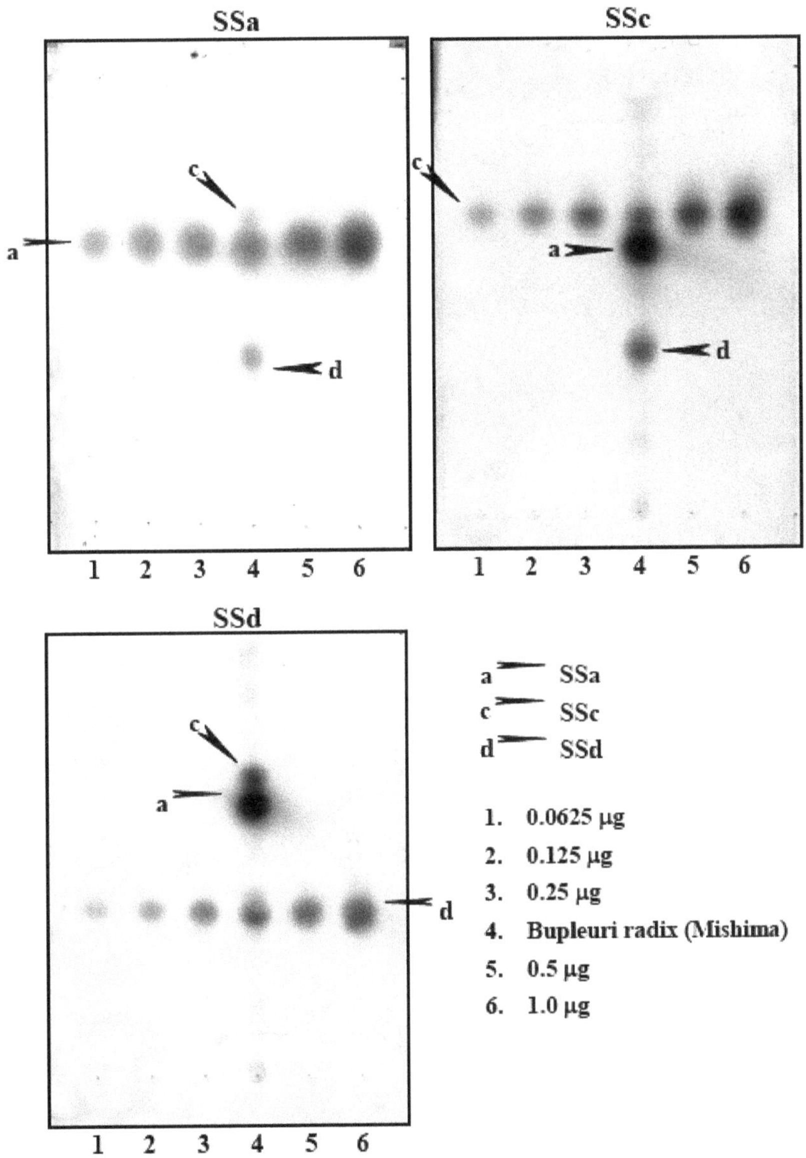

Fig. 8. Separation and immunodetection of saikosaponins by new eastern blotting using anti-SSa MAb (1G6)

The other important merit is the same as PVDF membrane depending on the increase of cross-reactivity as reported in the previous paper (Fukuda et al., 1999). The eastern blotting of SSa on a PES membrane using anti-SSa MAb (1G6) resulting in staining together with SSc and SSd. In this methodology, we separated the SSa molecule into two functional parts, the epitope part (mainly aglycone) and the sugar parts as commented above (See Fig. 2). The sugar parts in saikosaponins were oxidatively cleavaged to release aldehyde groups which were conjugated with protein to fix on a PES membrane. Because it was evident that a part of sugar moiety in SSa was immunized, the cleavage of sugar moiety by $NaIO_4$ expanded its cross-reactivity against other saikosaponins resulting in possibility of staining for SSc and SSd, though anti-SSa MAb (1G6) had weak cross-reactivity with SSc and SSd (2.65% and 3.76%, respectively).

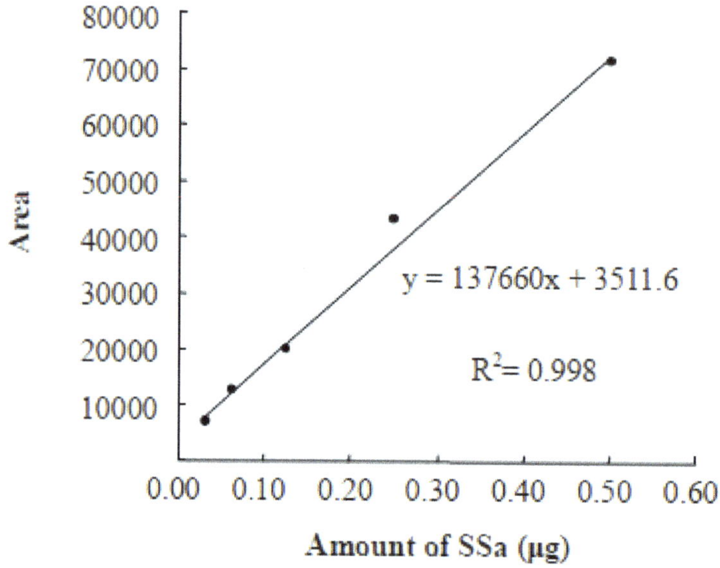

Fig. 9. Calibration curve of SSa obtained by new eastern blotting using anti-SSa MAb (1G6)

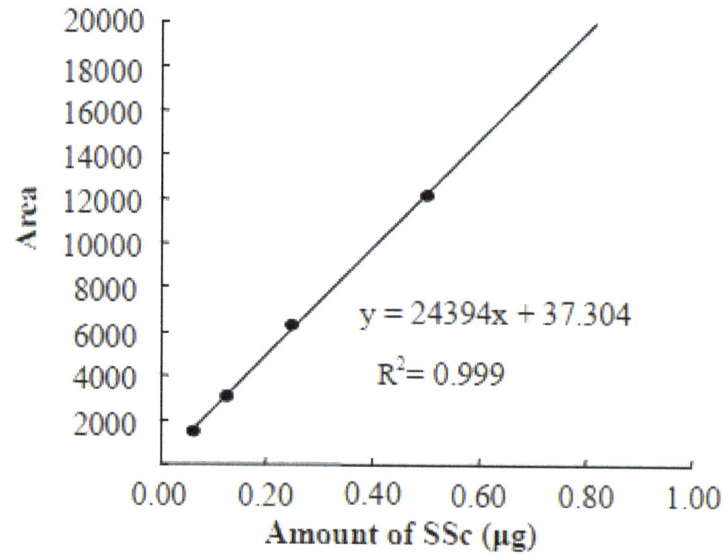

Fig. 10. Calibration curve of SSc obtained by new eastern blotting using anti-SSa MAb (1G6)

5. Application of new eastern blotting to quantitative immunoassay for saikosaponins

We applied the new eastern blotting to the quantitative immunoassay for saikosaponins using NIH Image because newly established method reflected direct sample amounts without transfer efficiency. For the calibration curves, each saikosaponin standard was spotted in five kinds concentration. By this method, the contents of saikosaponins can be determined individually. Calibration curve of each saikosaponin is indicated in Fig. 9 - 11.

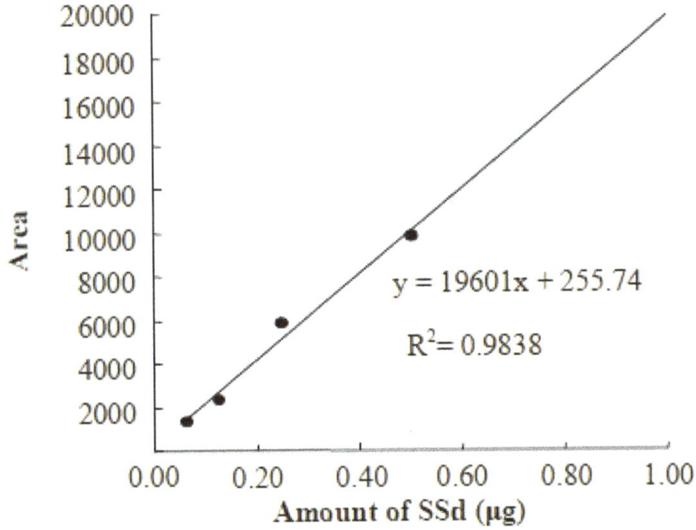

Fig. 11. Calibration curve of SSd obtained by new eastern blotting using anti-SSa MAb (1G6)

6. New eastern blotting as a tool for the quality control of Kampo medicines containing Bupleuri radix

New eastern blotting was also applied to the estimation of various Kampo medicines. Fig. 12 shows the new eastern blotting of Bupleuri radix and Kampo medicines prescribed with and without Bupleuri radix. Lane 10 shows Shoseiryuto prescription extract, which contains no Bupleuri radix resulting that no band was appeared by new eastern blotting. Compared to the result of Bupleuri radix, there was no SSd detected from Kampo medicines, because SSd will be converted into SSb_2 during the extraction processing.

On the other hand, the bands of SSa and SSc in Daisaikoto, Shosaikoto, Saikokyoyoto and Saikokaryukotsuboreito extracts (Fig. 12, lanes 6, 7, 8 and 9), which contain Bupleuri radix clearly appeared. These areas of the coloring spots on this membrane were calculated using graphic analysis by the NIH Image and the saikosaponins concentrations were determined as indicated in Table 2. These results were in a good agreement with those from the ELISA analysis (see Table 2).

In the case of SSb_2, only weak color development was observed in this method and no determination data was shown by using NIH Image analysis. It is suggested to be due to the quantitative determination limits of this NIH Image analysis system. However, this problem can be solved by using more sensitive anti-saikosaponin MAbs and/or color developing substrate and chemiluminescence system.

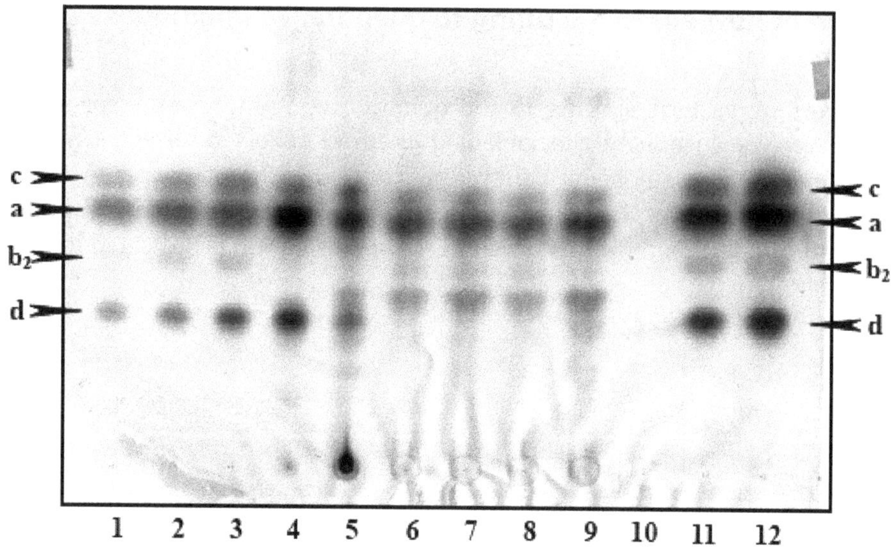

1. Saikosaponins standard (0.0625 μg)
2. Saikosaponins standard (0.125 μg)
3. Saikosaponins standard (0.25 μg)
4. Bupleuri radix (Mishima, Japanese species)
5. Bupleuri radix (Austria, Europe species)
6. Daisaikoto
7. Shosaikoto
8. Saikokyoyoto
9. Saikokaryukotsuboreito
10. Shoseiryuto (negative control)
11. Saikosaponins standard (0.5 μg)
12. Saikosaponins standard (1.0 μg)

Fig. 12. Immunodetection of saikosaponins in Bupleuri radix and various Kampo medicines by new eastern blotting using anti-SSa MAb (1G6)

	Concentration (μg/mg dry weight powder)						
	New Eastern Blotting					ELISA	
Sample	SSa	SSc	SSb_2	SSd	Total	SSa	Total
Bupleuri radix (Mishima)	8.38	1.39	ND	3.76	13.53	9.31	11.46
Bupleuri radix (Austria)	7.65	1.35	ND	1.55	10.55	7.90	8.94
Daisaikoto	0.63	0.19	(+)	ND	0.82	0.62	1.06
Shosaikoto	0.80	0.22	(+)	ND	1.02	0.76	1.19
Saikokyoyoto	0.69	0.13	(+)	ND	0.82	0.68	1.13
Saikokaryukotsuboreito	0.83	0.23	(+)	0.19	1.25	0.89	1.43
Shoseiryuto	ND	ND	ND	ND	ND	ND	ND

Table 2. Saikosaponins concentrations in Bupleuri radix and Kampo medicines determined by new eastern blotting using NIH Image. Data are the means of triplicate assays. ND= not detectable

7. Conclusion

Many analytical approaches have been used to identify saikosaponins in crude drugs and/or Kampo medicines. Among these methods, the use of HPLC in conjunction with mass spectrometry (MS) or photodiode array (PDA) is most frequently and widely used

(Ohtake et al., 2004; Li et al., 2005). The advantages of the new eastern blotting over the HPLC method are mainly its saving cost-performance (e.g., organic solvents and analytical equipments), speed, ease of use and more environmentally-soft determination method. Moreover, the new eastern blotting can analyze quantitatively and/or qualitatively at least three saikosaponins, SSa, SSc, and SSd by using a single MAb, anti-SSa MAb (1G6).

This is the first report of the separation and immunodetection of saikosaponins on positive-charged PES membrane and its application for quantitative immunoassay for saikosaponins. Although it has been believed difficult to determine the concentrations of small molecular compounds by western blotting technique, the methodology described here may open a wide field of comparable studies with other families of carbohydrates containing compounds of low molecular weight, such as glycosides, glucuronides, aminosugar conjugates and/or glycolipids and glycosphingolipids. It also should be conveniently used to survey for low concentrations of saikosaponins in plants and/or in experimental animals and humans.

8. Acknowledgement

This research was supported in part by Japan Science and Technology Agency, Grant-in-Aid from the Ministry of Education, Culture, Sports, Science and Technology of Japan, the research fund of Japan Society for the Promotion of Science (JSPS Asian Core Program) and Takeda Science Foundation.

9. References

Akahori, A. (1980). *Gendaitoyoigaku*, 1., 45-50.

Chabraoui, F.; Derrington, E. A.; Mallie-Didier, F.; Confavreux, C.; Quincy, C. & Caudie, C. (1993). Dot-blot immunodetection of antibodies against GM1 and other gangliosides on PVDF-P membranes. *J. Immunol. Methods*, 165., 225-230.

Duarte, R. M.; Santos, E. B. & Duarte, A. C. (2003). Spectroscopic characteristics of ultrafiltration fractions of fulvic and humic acids isolated from an eucalyptus bleached Kraft pulp mill effluent. *Water Res.*, 37., 4073-4080.

Fukuda, N.; Tanaka, H. & Shoyama, Y. (1999). Western blotting for ginseng saponins, ginsenosides using anti-ginsenoside Rb1 monoclonal antibody. *Biol. Pharm. Bull.*, 22., 219-220.

Fukuda, N.; Tanaka, H. & Shoyama, Y. (2000). Applications of ELISA, western blotting and immunoaffinity concentration for survey of ginsenosides in crude drugs of Panax species and traditional Chinese herbal medicines.*Analyst*, 125., 1425-1429.

Fukuda, N.; Tanaka, H. & Shoyama, Y. (2001). Double staining of ginsenosides by Western blotting using anti-ginsenoside Rb1 and Rg1 monoclonal antibodies. *Biol. Pharm. Bull.*, 24., 1157-1160.

Gomes, S. A.; Nogueira, J. M. & Rebelo, M. J. (2004). An amperometric biosensor for polyphenolic compounds in red wine. *Bios. Bioelec.*, 20., 1211-1216.

Granger, S. M.; Lloubes, R.; Murcia, G. & Schnarr, M. (1988). Specific protein-DNA complexes: immunodetection of the protein component after gel electrophoresis and Western blotting. *Anal. Biochem.*, 174., 235-238.

Ishiyama, M.; Shoyama, Y.; Murakami, H. & Shinohara, H. (1996). Production of monoclonal antibodies and development of an ELISA for solamargine. *Cytotechnology*, 18., 153-158.

Li, X. Q.; Gao, Q. T.; Chen, X. H. & Bi, K. S. (2005). High performance liquid chromatographic assay of saikosaponins from Radix Bupleuri in China, *Biol. Pharm. Bull.*, 28., 1736-1742.

Masters, D. B.; Griggs, C. T. & Berde, C. B. (1992). High sensitivity quantification of DNA from gels and autoradiograms with affordable optical scanning. *Biotechniques*, 12., 902-911.

Meisen, I.; Peter-Katalinic, J. & Muthing, J. (2004). Direct analysis of silica gel extracts from immunostained glycosphingolipids by nanoelectrospray ionization quadrupole time-of-flight mass spectrometry. *Anal. Chem.*, 76., 2248-2255.

Miyamoto, T.; Yamamoto, A.; Sakai, M.; Tanaka, H.; Shoyama, Y. & Higuchi, R. (2006). Immunochemical studies of starfish gangliosides: Production of monoclonal antibody against AG-2, the major ganglioside of starfish acanthaster plancei, and detecting its distribution in tissues by TLC immunostaining. *J. Marine Biosci. Biotech.*, 1., 298-304.

Morinaga, O.; Zhu, S.; Tanaka, H. & Shoyama, Y. (2006). Visual detection of saikosaponins by on-membrane immunoassay and estimation of traditional Chinese medicines containing Bupleuri radix. *Biochem. Biophys. Res. Commun.*, 346., 687-692.

Ohtake, N.; Nakai, Y.; Yamamoto, M.; Sakakibara, I.; Takeda, S.; Amagaya, S. & Aburada, M. (2004). Separation and isolation methods for analysis of the active principles of Sho-saiko-to (SST) oriental medicine. *J. Chromatogra. B.*, 812., 135-148.

Reig, J. A. & Klein, D. C. (1988). Submicrogram quantities of unstained proteins are visualized on polyvinylidene difluoride membranes by transillumination. *Appl. Theor. Electrophor.*, 1., 59-60.

Root, D. D. & Wang, K. (1993). Silver-enhanced copper staining of protein blots. *Anal. Biochem.*, 209., 15-19.

Shan, S.; Tanaka, H. & Shoyama, Y. (2001). Enzyme-linked immunosorbent assay for glycyrrhizin using anti-glycyrrhizin monoclonal antibody and an eastern blotting technique for glucuronides of glycyrrhetic acid. *Anal. Chem.*, 73., 5784-5790.

Suetake, K. & Yu, R. K. (2003). Thin-layer chromatography; immunostaining of glycolipid antigens; and interpretation of false-positive findings with acidic lipids. *Methods Enzymol.*, 363., 312-319.

Tanaka, H.; Putalun, W.; Tsuzaki, C. & Shoyama, Y. (1997). A simple determination of steroidal alkaloid glycosides by thin-layer chromatography immunostaining using monoclonal antibody against solamargine. *FEBS Lett.*, 404., 279-282.

Towbin, H.; Staehelin, T. & Gordon, J. (1979). Electrophoretic transfer of proteins from polyacrylamide gels to nitrocellulose sheets: Procedure and some applications. *Proc. Natl. Acad. Sci. USA*, 76., 4350-4354.

Towbin, H.; Schoenenberger, C.; Ball, R.; Braun, D. G. & Rosenfelder, G. (1984). Glycosphingolipid-blotting: an immunological detection procedure after separation by thin layer chromatography. *J. Immunol. Methods*, 72., 471-479.

Weiler, E. W. & Zenk, M. H. (1976). Radioimmunoassay for the determination of digoxin and related compounds in *Digitalis lanata*. *Phytochemistry*, 15., 1537-1545.

Zhu, S.; Shimokawa, S.; Tanaka, H. & Shoyama, Y. (2004). Development of an assay system for saikosaponin a using anti-saikosaponin a monoclonal antibodies. *Biol. Pharm. Bull.*, 27., 66-71.

Zhu, S.; Shimokawa, S.; Shoyama, Y. & Tanaka, H. (2006). A novel analytical ELISA-based methodology for pharmacologically active saikosaponins. *Fitoterapia*, 77., 100-108.

Zhu, S,; Morinaga, O,; Shimokawa, S,; Shon, T. K.; Lee, S. C.; Shoyama, Y. & Tanaka, H. (2007). Eastern blotting and use of anti-saikosaponin a monoclonal antibodies for detection of saikosaponins. *J. Nat. Med.*, 61., 178-183.

14

Stability Indicating Methods

Ana Paola Cione, Edivan Tonhi and Paulo Silva
Bioagri Laboratórios
Brazil

1. Introduction

1.1 How define a SIM?

According to FDA guideline (Guidance for Industry, Analytical Procedures and Methods Validation, FDA, 2000), a Stability Indicating Method (SIM) is defined as a validated analytical procedure that accurate and precisely measure active ingredients (drug substance or drug product) free from process impurities, excipients and degradation products. The FDA recommends that all assay procedures for stability should be stability indicating. The main objective of a stability indicating method is to monitor results during stability studies in order to guarantee safety, efficacy and quality. It represents also a powerful tool when investigating out-of-trend (OOT) (Swartz et al., 2004) or out-of-specification (OOS) results (CDER, 2006) in quality control processes.

1.2 How develop a SIM?

There are basically 3 steps necessary for developing a SIM:

1.2.1 Step 1: generation of degraded samples for testing selectivity of the method

Here lies one of the main concerns related to a development of a SIM, since the available guidance documents do not state the extent to which stress tests should be carried out - that is, how much stress should be applied or how much degradation should be aimed for.

In fact, there is not a "gold rule" that attends this issue and therefore, it is important to keep in mind that experimental conditions of stress tests, should be realistic and lead to "purposeful degradation" (Ngwa, G., 2010).

Stress tests should generate representative samples to assess drug substance and drug product stability, provide information about possible degradation pathway and demonstrate the stability indicating power of the analytical procedures applied.

1.2.1.1 Determination of Limit of Quantification (LoQ)

In close relation to the determination of the amount of degradation is the evaluation of Limit of Detection (LoD) and Limit of Quantification (LoQ) of the method. These limits should be closely related to the Reporting, Identification and Qualification of degradation products, as stated in ICH Q3B (R2) (EMEA, 2006). These thresholds are determined either as percentage of drug substance or total daily intake (TDI) of degradation product.

The analytical methods are usually expected to be validated for the ability to quantify potential degradation products and drug impurities with a LoD and LoQ at least as sensitive as the ICH threshold (see Figure 1).

Attachment 1: Thresholds for Degradation Products in New Drug Products

Reporting Thresholds

Maximum Daily Dose[1]	Threshold[2,3]
≤ 1 g	0.1%
> 1 g	0.05%

Identification Thresholds

Maximum Daily Dose[1]	Threshold[2,3]
< 1 mg	1.0% or 5 μg TDI, whichever is lower
1 mg - 10 mg	0.5% or 20 μg TDI, whichever is lower
>10 mg - 2 g	0.2% or 2 mg TDI, whichever is lower
> 2 g	0.10%

Qualification Thresholds

Maximum Daily Dose[1]	Threshold[2,3]
< 10 mg	1.0% or 50 μg TDI, whichever is lower
10 mg - 100 mg	0.5% or 200 μg TDI, whichever is lower
>100 mg - 2 g	0.2% or 3 mg TDI, whichever is lower
> 2 g	0.15%

Notes on Attachment 1

1 The amount of drug substance administered per day

2 Thresholds for degradation products are expressed either as a percentage of the drug substance or as total daily intake (TDI) of the degradation product. Lower thresholds can be appropriate if the degradation product is unusually toxic.

3 Higher thresholds should be scientifically justified.

Fig. 1. ICH thresholds for degradation products in New Drug Application (ICH Q3B)

The identification threshold (IT) varies from 0.1 to 1.0% of the labeled amount of active ingredient in the dosage form, or from 5 μg to 2 mg TDI, depending on the maximum daily dosage in the product´s professional labeling. The identification threshold may be lowered for degradation products that may be exceptionally toxic.

The Reporting Threshold (RT) is either 0.1% or 0.05% depending on the maxim daily dosage. For very low dose drug products, where this type of sensitivity is not attainable, even after exhaustive tentative, justification may be provided describing the failed reports.

Process-related drug substance impurities that are also degradation products should have the same limits as for ICH Q3B.

Ideally, the same analytical methodology should be used for Quality Control and Stability Studies. The determination of Out-of-Specification or Out-of-Trend results should be more reliable, when using a SIM, since LoD and LoQ used allows detection of impurities and/or degradation products adequately. In the situation in which a new peak arises during stability study and one may expect that it should not exist and hence it would constitute a type of OOT, the use of a well studied and well determined LoQ in a SIM, will help the applicator to decide if additional action are needed to investigate a new substance or a OOT. It should be mentioned that these thresholds are established for new drug products or New Drug Application (NDA). For Abbreviated New Drug Application (ANDA) or generic drugs, there are not specific regulations about this topic and even less, the companies dealing with these products, have background information as those obtained in the development of NDA. Such application is expected to contain a "full description of the drug substance including its physical and chemical characteristics and stability as well; such specifications and analytical methods are necessary to assure the identity, strength, quality, purity and bioavailability of drug product and stability data with proposed expiration date". As already cited, for ANDA, there are not specific regulations and the same ICH recommendation has been used. However, precisely because of the lack of information derived from the new drug development, the complexity and responsibility in developing/validating a SIM for an ANDA is high.

Information like aqueous solubility, pH versus solubility profile, excipients compatibility studies, etc, all information that enable fully assume the knowledge of the product ,will help to ensure that best (more appropriate) condition were chosen for developing a SIM, like those related to the forced degradation design.

1.2.1.2 Overstressing/Understressing

Care should be taken in order to avoid overstressing or understressing samples, with may lead to non representative or non-purposeful degradation. So, the use of a properly designed and executed forced degradation study will generate representative samples that will help to ensure that resulting method reflects adequately long-term stability (EMEA, 2003).

About the forced degradation (or stress test, both terms will be used in the text) design, it is recommended (Klick S., et al, 2005) to include alkaline and acidic hydrolysis, photolysis, oxidation, humidity and temperature stress. An compilation of data from literature (Klick S., et al, 2005; Alsante et al. 2007, Reynolds, et al. 2002, Reynolds, D.W, 2004; Kats M., 2005; Reynolds, D.W, 2002) is shown at Table 1 and compiles the more often used conditions to perform forced degradation studies.

These conditions can be used as a starting point in the development of a SIM. Changing conditions to harsher or softer levels, can be applied, when too little or too much degradation are obtained. For example, in cases in which too little degradation was obtained in the hydrolyses stress, it is recommended to increase concentrations to 1 Mol L^{-1} or higher; for oxidation stress, increase peroxide concentration to 10% or 20% (v/v) and/or time of reaction, as well as temperature. If co-solvents are necessary to increase solubility, it is recommended the use of acetonitrile that does not work as a sensitizer in photostability stress. Data needs to be evaluated as unusual degradants may form with co-solvents. If even not all conditions may cause degradation, document efforts and severity of conditions and should be include in final report.

By the other side, if too much degradation is detected, the severity of conditions may be decreased, by diluting acid/bases, neutralizing, reducing exposure time.

<table>
<tr><th colspan="4">Solid State</th></tr>
<tr><th colspan="2">Stress</th><th>Condition</th><th>Period of time</th></tr>
<tr><td colspan="2">Heat</td><td>60° C</td><td>Up to 1 month</td></tr>
<tr><td colspan="2">Humidity</td><td>75% RH</td><td>Up to 1 month</td></tr>
<tr><td colspan="2">Photostability</td><td>3 mm (powder)
Exposed and non-exposed samples ("control")</td><td>Follow ICH requirements (Q1B)</td></tr>
<tr><th colspan="4">Solution State</th></tr>
<tr><th colspan="2">Stress</th><th>Condition</th><th>Period of time</th></tr>
<tr><td rowspan="2">Hydrolys is</td><td>Acid</td><td>0.1 – 1 Mol L^{-1} HCl</td><td>Up to weeks and 60° C</td></tr>
<tr><td>alkaline</td><td>0.1 – 1 Mol L^{-1} NaOH</td><td>Up to weeks and 60° C</td></tr>
<tr><td colspan="2">Oxidation</td><td>H_2O_2 3% (v/v)</td><td>Up to 24 hours</td></tr>
<tr><td colspan="2">Photostability</td><td>Exposed and non-exposed samples ("control")</td><td>Follow ICH requirements (Q1B)</td></tr>
<tr><td colspan="2">Heat</td><td>60° C</td><td>Up to 1 month</td></tr>
</table>

Table 1. "More often" used conditions for forced degradation studies

Also, need to be clarified, that synthesis impurities when are not also degradation products do not need to be described in Stability Studies, but SIM may assure that these impurities do not interfere on degradation products determination.

1.2.1.3 Photostability studies

Photostability tests should follow ICH requirements (EMEA, 1998) , i.e., should be done in a sequential manner, starting with the fully exposed product and proceeding, if necessary to the immediate pack and then to the market pack, until studies demonstrate the drug product is adequately protected from exposure to light. Besides this, design of forced degradation test should consider the previous knowledge of the substance or product being tested, since photoreactivity is wavelength dependent and degradation pathways can be different for UV and visible ranges (case by case basis). It is recommended to use artificial sources of irradiation, like ID65 and specific filters to guarantee the exposure above 320 nm (indoor daylight standard). Also, forced degradation may be conducted on quartz glassware that does not filter radiation from the light sources and specific filters arrangement.

It can be found in literature (ICH Q1B) that exposition to an overall irradiation of not less than 1.2 million lux.hours and an integrated near ultraviolet energy of not less than 200 W h. m^{-2} may give reasonable degradation for photosensible active ingredients. Tests may only be valid when chemical actinometers are exposed simultaneously (preferably) to the samples and shows a pattern of degradation. Control samples (samples in the same condition of that exposed, except for the irradiation, i.e., protected from the light by aluminum foils for example) should also be analyzed, in order to guarantee that the degradation is really only due to the light and not to other factors like temperature (irradiation chamber should have rigorous temperature control) (Christensen, K. et. al 2000). In some cases, the ANDA holder justifies not performing photostability studies for the drug product based on the fact that the drug substance did not show photodegradation during forced degradation studies. However, this not must be acceptable, since in some cases, excipients or impurities may catalyze photodegradation of the main active in the drug product.

1.2.2 Step 2: method development (manipulating and evaluating selectivity/specificity)

Liquid chromatography is the most appropriate technique for developing/validating a SIM. The use of diode-array-detector and additionally mass spectrometers, gives best performances for people working with SIM development.

The goal is to manipulate selectivity by changing mobile phase composition, wavelength of detection and pH. Related to mobile phase pH, it can be said, that the advances in LC column technology have made possible the use of pH as a true selectivity tool for the separation of ionizable compounds (Neue, et. al, 1999; Cheng et. al, 2010). Columns mechanically strong, with high efficiency and that are operate over an extended pH range, should be preferred. Acidic compounds are more retained at low pH; while basic compounds are more retained at higher pH (neutral compounds are unaffected). At traditionally used pH values (pH 4 - 8), a slight change in pH would result in a significant shift in retention.

Type of chromatography used (e. g. HPLC or GC) and arrangements/detectors (GC/FID, GC/MS, LC/DAD or LC/MS) are certainly useful tools. For HPLC, different modes of chromatography can be used (normal or reversed phase, ion par or HILIC). Other powerful tool is the use of Light Scattering Detector (LSD) coupled to HPLC to monitor compounds without light absorption in uv/Vis region. Gas chromatography may only be used when no additional thermal degradation of the sample is produced (sample inlet works on high temperatures).

The use of HLPC coupled to diode-array detectors (DAD) in the achievement of peak purity usually give reasonable results, mainly related to reliable determination of the main active ingredient. It is possible to guarantee no co-elution with degradation peaks and other impurities. Indeed, the main feature of DAD detectors is that it is possible to collect spectra across a range of wavelengths at each data point collected across a peak, and through software manipulations involving multidimensional vector algebra, to compare each of the spectra to determine peak purity (Swartz & Krull, 2005; Gilliard & Ritter, 1997). In this manner, DAD detectors can distinguish spectral and chromatographic differences not readily observable by simple overlay comparisons (Gorenstein et al 1994; Young et al 1994, Warren et al 1995). DAD detectors can be limited on occasion the more similar the spectra, and the lower the relative absorbance, the more difficult it can be to distinguish co-eluted compounds. MS detection overcomes many of these limitations. MS can provide unequivocal peak purity information, exact mass, structural and quantitative information depending upon the type of instrument used. MS is also a very useful tool to track peaks to selectivity manipulations in method development. As disadvantage, MS detectors cannot handle non-volatile buffers, which are frequently used as mobile phase in drug analysis. The combination of both DAD and MS on a single instrument and software platform provides the type of valuable orthogonal information required when evaluating specificity on SIM development.

After determination of peak purity, in fact, the identification of degradation products and also mass balance determination usually are more complexes steps of analytical development, as in most of cases, commercial reference standards of degradation products are not available.

Calculations using area-percent-normalization (area %) are not precise, since it is necessary to take into consideration the response factors (area relative to amount). Degradation products may have not the same ultra-violet spectra of that of the parent drug and even if the UV spectra are similar, the absorptivity coefficient (Turro 2008) may have different values.

1.2.2.1 Case studies

Case study 1: Consider the analysis of a 100 mg tablet used in medical prescriptions as 3-dose per day and coming from a long term stability study (Figure 1).

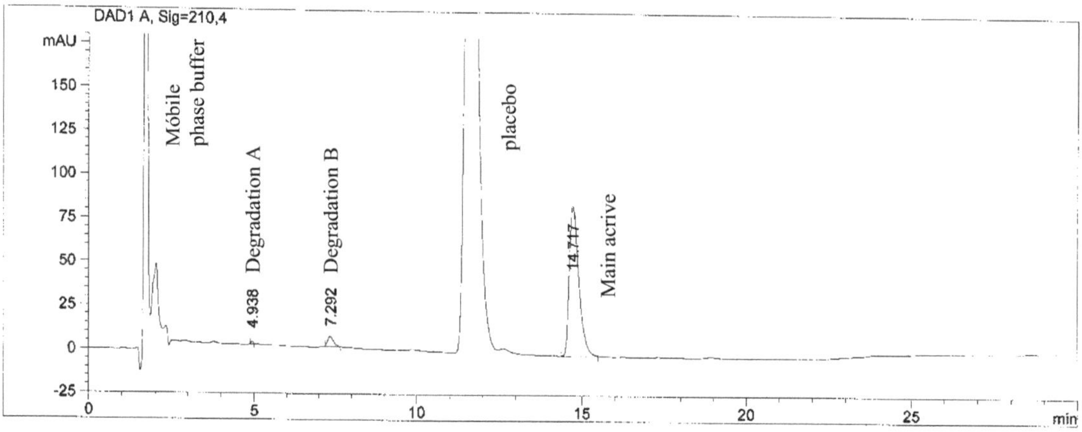

Fig. 1. Representative SIM chromatogram of long-term stability sample

The quantification of degradation product by %area results in 0.2% area for degradation A and 12% area for degradation B, related to the main active. It is confirmed that the degradation products are deriving from the main active, as a SIM was used. Information about UV spectra of both degradation products and main active are shown in Figure 2.

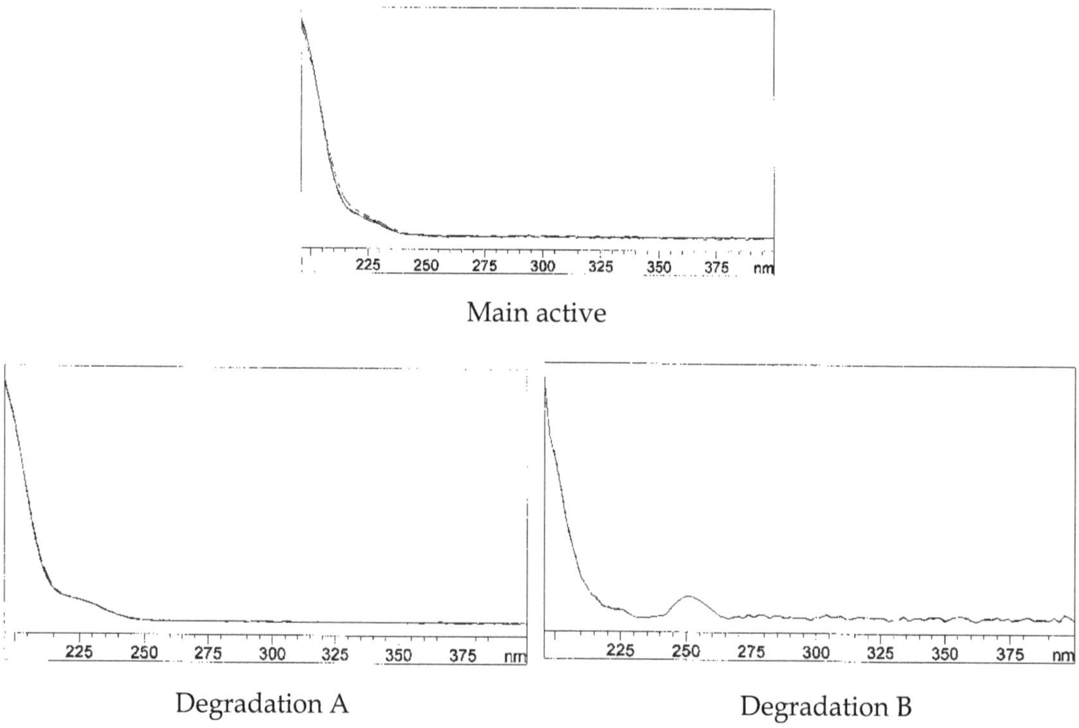

Fig. 2. Representative uv spectra of degradation products A and B

By simple comparison of spectra of main active and degradation A, it can be assumed that mass balance would be probably reached, due to high similarity between it; for degradation B mass balance may give unsatisfactory results, mainly if wavelength of detection and quantification is in the 250-275 nm region of the spectra. Other concern is related to the ICH threshold for the degradation products. In this case, the diary dose is 300 mg and degradation products A (0.2%) and B (12%) fall within the range of identification and qualification, which would means to define toxicity and mutagenicity potential of these two degradation products, and ultimately also redesign the drug product.

Case study 2:

In this second example (representative chromatogram showed on Figure 3), one may consider that when the sample is submitted to light stress the main active degrades to seven different products (see Table 2) and besides these seven common degradation more new two degradation can be detected in acidic stress (Table 3).

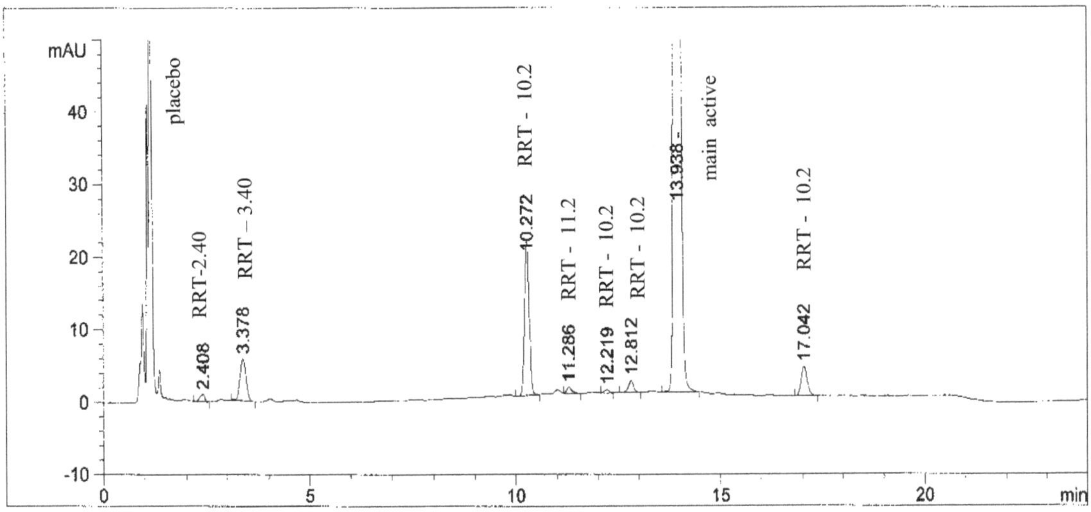

Fig. 3. SIM chromatogram of light stressed sample - 48 hours

Calculation of mass balance by considering % area of degradation product peaks, identified by Relative Retention Time (RRT) is also presented in tables 2 and 3.

% peak area												
RRT / λdetector	0.17	0.24	0.55	0.69	0.74	0.81	0.88	0.92	1.22	Sub-Total	Main Active* 74.1%	Total
210 nm	0.2	1.3	nd	nd	3.6	0.2	0.1	0.3	0.9	6.6		80.7
245 nm	0.3	2.4	nd	nd	0.5	0.15	<LoQ	<LoQ	1.0	4.75		78.9
360 nm	<LoQ	<LoQ	nd	nd	<LoQ	<LoQ	<LoQ	0.17	1.0	1.17		75.3

*this value represents % of main active on drug product, determined by external calibration with main active analytical standard; nd = non detected

Table 2. Peak % area degradation products after 48- hours of light stress

% peak area												
RRT / $\lambda_{detector}$	0.17	0.24	0.55	0.69	0.74	0.81	0.88	0.92	1.22	Sub-Total	Main Active*	Total
210 nm	0.3	0.2	0.2	0.2	2.3	1.85	<LQ	<LQ	<LQ	5.05	75.4%	80.45
245 nm	<LQ	<LQ	0.2	<LQ	0.3	1.4	<LQ	<LQ	<LQ	1.9		77.3
360 nm	<LQ	<LQ	<LQ	<LQ	<LQ	<LQ	<LQ	<LQ	<LQ	<LQ		<LQ

*this value represents % of main active on drug product, determined by external calibration with main active analytical standard.

Table 3. Peak % area degradation products after 120-hours of acidic stress

In the light stress (Table 2), the concentration of the main active after 48 hours is around 74.1%, and for an acceptable mass balance determination (values in % area or concentration around target concentration value), degradation products must account for 25.9% area. As can be seen at Figure 4, the UV spectra given from the DAD of these nine degradation products, there are significative differences in the profiles, i.e., different absorption intensities in different wavelength and this should be an indicative of difficulties on reaching satisfactory mass balance using % area.

When monitoring at 210 nm, mass balance reached 80.7%, since the sum of total % area of degradation products reached 6.6% area.

When doing the same calculation for 245 nm, mass balance was lower, reaching 78.9% and even lower at 360 nm, giving 75.3%. Degradation products identified at RRT-0.55 and RRT-0.69 were not detected at these three wavelengths, but were detected on acidic stress (Table 3) sample, when monitoring at 210 nm and 245 nm. Any degradation product was detected at 360 nm, in the acidic stress. Usually greater values are obtained in lower wavelengths.

Most frequently giving acceptable mass balance values, but not less complex, is the method in which chromatographic peaks of each degradation product is collected and identified (for example, by infrared spectroscopy, nuclear magnetic resonance as well as mass spectrometry analysis) and then used as analytical standards in a external calibration procedure. The method in which, response factor of each degradation product is achieved (also experimentally hard and complex), can give acceptable mass balance values. The determination of each degradation product is a critical work mainly when ICH thresholds are reached. This may trigger additional investigations about the drug product, so it is recommended to dedicate all analytical tools and expertise available in this step of method development.

1.2.3 Step 3: Method validation

Validation is not a efficient way to do method development so efforts should be dedicated in Specificity step of the method, working with the stressed samples. The validation routine may start with a protocol based on pharmacopeia and/or ICH guidelines (Q2B). For assay procedures, that are intended do measure the analyte present in a given sample, typical validation items should be considered: Accuracy, Precision (repeatability and intermediate precision), Specificity, Detection and Quantitation Limits, Robustness, Linearity and Range.

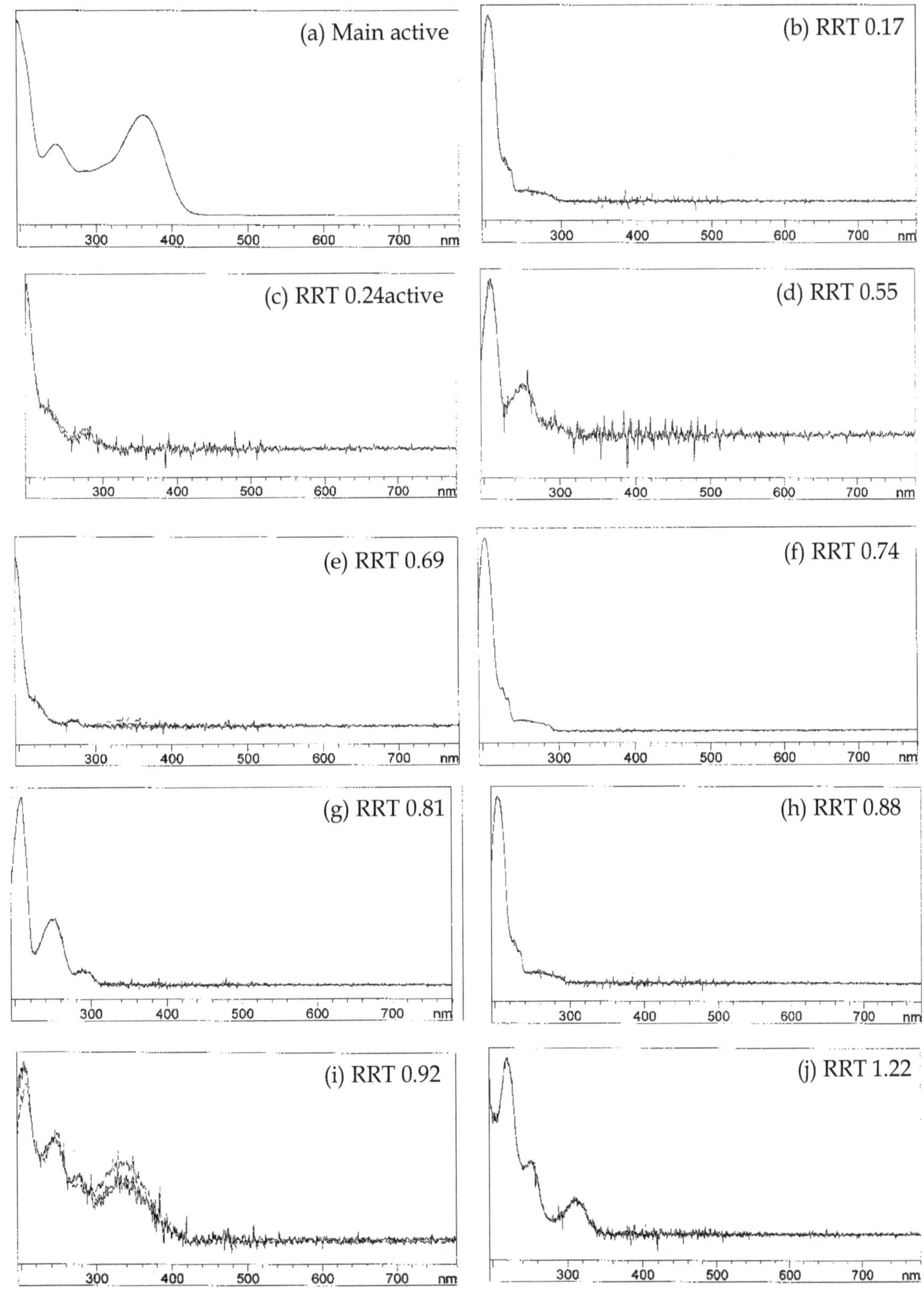

Fig. 4. UV-vis spectra of degradation products observed on light stressed samples (b, c, f to j) and acidic stressed samples (b to g).

2. Conclusion

Stress tests for developing a stability indicating method should always be designed and evaluated with common sense and chemical knowledge, keeping in mind the manufacturing process and the nature of the final drug product. The stability profile needs do be established for drug product to assure safety, efficacy and quality. The results coming from these studies can support formulation and packaging. The know-how coming from stress tests are useful to reduce time and money, related to the drug and final product development, giving the possibility of forecasting analytical problems.

A generic approach can be used as a starting point to set up a stress testing study, but a case-by-case approach for stress testing is essential to allow flexibility. This is also recognized by the regulatory agencies because very detailed instructions about how to perform stress testing are not given in the available guidance documents. In first instance, a SIM should be applied to quantification of the main active in a precise and accurately, even in the presence of interferences (degradation products, impurities, and placebo). In this manner, some evaluation of mass balance can be done, but the applicant must have in mind, the limitation about the obtained values, since %area is a useful but not precise/accurate tool to determine concentrations. If during long-term stability studies or quality control determinations, the main active concentration decreases, mass balance investigations may start, evaluating %peak, DAD spectra and in parallel, different/contributing analytical techniques.

3. References

Alsante K. M., Ando A., Brown R., Ensing J., Hatajik T. D., Wei K.& Tsuda, Y. (2007) The Role of Degradant Profiling in Active Pharmaceutical Ingredients and Drug Products. *Adv. Drug Delivery Rev.*, Vol. 59, No. 1, ISSN: 0169-409X.

Baertschi, S. W (Ed). (2005). Pharmaceutical Stress Testing: Predicting Drug Degradation. ISBN 0824740211.

Center for Drug Evaluation and Research (CDER). (2006). *Guidance for Industry Investigating Out-of-Specification (OOS) Test Results for Pharmaceutical Production.* Accessed on April, 2011. Available from: <http://www.fda.gov/downloads/Drugs/GuidanceComplianceRegulatoryInformation/Guidances/ucm070287.pdf>

Cheng, Y. -F, Walter, T. H., Lu, Z, Iraneta, P., Gendreau, C., Neue, V. D., Grassi, J. M., Carmody, J. L., O´Gara, J. E. & Fisk, R., P. (2000). Hybrid Organic-Inorganic Particle Technology: Breaking Through Traditional Barriers of HPLC Separations. *LCGC,* Vol. 18, No. 11, 1162 - 1172, ISSN: 1527-5949.

Christensen, K., Christensen, J. O., Frokjaer, S., Langballe, P., Hansen, L. L., Influence of temperature and storage time after light exposure on the quinine monohydrochloride actinometric system. (2000). *Eur. J. Pharm. Sci.*, Vol 9, No. 3, 317-321. ISSN: 0928-0987

European Medicines Agency ICH Topic Q1B. (1998). *Photostability Testing of New Active Substances and Medicinal Products.* Accessed on April, 2011. Available from: <http://www.ema.europa.eu/docs/en_GB/document_library/Scientific_guideline/2009/09/WC500002647.pdf>

European Medicines Agency. (1996). *Guidance for Industry Q2B Validation of Analytical Procedures: Methodology.* Accessed on April, 2011. Available from: <http://www.fda.gov/downloads/Regulator%20yInformation/Guidances/UCM128049.pdf>

European Medicines Agency. (2003). *ICH Topic Q 1 A (R2) - Stability Testing of new Drug Substances and Product.* Accessed on April, 2011. Available from: <http://www.ema.europa.eu/docs/en_GB/document_library/Scientific_guideline/2009/09/WC500002651.pdf>

European Medicines Agency. (2006). *ICH Topic Q 3 B (R2) Impurities in New Drug Products.* Accessed on April, 2011. Available from: <http://www.ema.europa.eu/docs/en_GB/document_library/Scientific_guideline/2009/09/WC500002676.pdf>

Gilliard, J. A., Ritter, C. Use of simulated chromatography-diode array detection data for the definition of a guide curve in purity assessment by spectral comparison. (1997). *J. Chrom. A.* Vol. 786, No. 1, 1-11. ISSN0021-9673.

Gorenstein, M. V., Li, J. B., Van Antwerp, J & Chapman, D. (1994). Detecting coeluted impurities by spectral comparison. *LCGC,* Vol.12, No. 10, 768-772, ISSN 0888-9090.

Kats, M. (2005). *Pharm International Forced Degradation Studies: Regulatory Considerations and Implementation.* Accessed on April, 2011. Available from: <http://biopharminternational.findpharma.com/biopharm/article/articleDetail.jsp?id=170505>

Klick S., Muijselaar P. G., Waterval. J., Eichinger T., Korn C., Gerding T. K. ; Debets A. J. ; Sanger-Van de Griend C., Van den Beld, C. ; Somsen G. W. ; De Jong G. J. (2005). Toward a Generic Approach for Stress Testing of Drug Substances and Drug Products. *Pharm. Technol.,* Vol. 29, No. 2, 48-57, ISSN: 1543-2521.

Neue, D, Walter, T. H., Alder, B. A., Jiang, Z., Fish, R. P., Cook, J. T., Glose, K. H., Carmody, J. L., Grassi, J. M., Cheng, Y. –F, Lu, Z & Crowley, R., J., (1999), Use of high performance LC packings from pH1 to pH 12. *Am. Lab,* 31-36. ISSN: 0044-7749.

Ngwa, G. (2010). Forced Degradation Studies. *Drug Delivery Technol.,* vol. 10 No. 3, June, ISSN 0976-1225.

Reynolds, D. W. (2004). Forced Degradation of Pharmaceuticals. *Am. Pharm. Rev,* May/June, 56-61, ISSN : 1099-8012.

Reynolds, D. W.; Facchine, K. L., Mullaney, F. F., Alsante, K. M., Hatajik, T., D. & Motto, M. (2002). Available Guidance and Best Practices for Conducting Forced Degradation Studies. *Pharm. Technol.,* Vol. 26, No. 2, 48-54, ISSN : 0147-8087.

Swartz, M., Krull, I., (2004). Investigating Out-Of-Specifications Results. *LCGC,* Vol. 22, No 2, 132-136, ISSN : 1527-5949.

Swartz, M., Krull, I., (2005). Developing and Validating Stability-Indicating Methods. *LCGC,* Vol. 23, No. 6, 586-593, ISSN : 1527-5949.

Turro, N. J., Ramamurthy, V., Scaiano, J. C. *Principles of Molecular Photochemistry: An Introduction.* University Science Book, 2008. ISBN 978-0849384066.

Warren, W., J., Stanick, M. V., Gorenstein, M. V. & Young, P. M.. (1995). HPLC analysis of synthetic oligonucleotides using spectral contrast techniques. *Biotechniques*, Vol 18, No. 2, 282-297, ISSN: 0736-6205.

Young, P. M., Gorenstein, M. V., (1994) Tryptic mapping by reversed-phase HPLC with photodiode-array detection incorporating the spectral-contrast technique. *LCGC*, Vol 12, No. 11, 832-838. ISSN: 0888-9090.

Permissions

All chapters in this book were first published in QCHMRA, by InTech Open; hereby published with permission under the Creative Commons Attribution License or equivalent. Every chapter published in this book has been scrutinized by our experts. Their significance has been extensively debated. The topics covered herein carry significant findings which will fuel the growth of the discipline. They may even be implemented as practical applications or may be referred to as a beginning point for another development.

The contributors of this book come from diverse backgrounds, making this book a truly international effort. This book will bring forth new frontiers with its revolutionizing research information and detailed analysis of the nascent developments around the world.

We would like to thank all the contributing authors for lending their expertise to make the book truly unique. They have played a crucial role in the development of this book. Without their invaluable contributions this book wouldn't have been possible. They have made vital efforts to compile up to date information on the varied aspects of this subject to make this book a valuable addition to the collection of many professionals and students.

This book was conceptualized with the vision of imparting up-to-date information and advanced data in this field. To ensure the same, a matchless editorial board was set up. Every individual on the board went through rigorous rounds of assessment to prove their worth. After which they invested a large part of their time researching and compiling the most relevant data for our readers.

The editorial board has been involved in producing this book since its inception. They have spent rigorous hours researching and exploring the diverse topics which have resulted in the successful publishing of this book. They have passed on their knowledge of decades through this book. To expedite this challenging task, the publisher supported the team at every step. A small team of assistant editors was also appointed to further simplify the editing procedure and attain best results for the readers.

Apart from the editorial board, the designing team has also invested a significant amount of their time in understanding the subject and creating the most relevant covers. They scrutinized every image to scout for the most suitable representation of the subject and create an appropriate cover for the book.

The publishing team has been an ardent support to the editorial, designing and production team. Their endless efforts to recruit the best for this project, has resulted in the accomplishment of this book. They are a veteran in the field of academics and their pool of knowledge is as vast as their experience in printing. Their expertise and guidance has proved useful at every step. Their uncompromising quality standards have made this book an exceptional effort. Their encouragement from time to time has been an inspiration for everyone.

The publisher and the editorial board hope that this book will prove to be a valuable piece of knowledge for researchers, students, practitioners and scholars across the globe.

List of Contributors

Takuhiro Uto and Nguyen Huu Tung
Nagasaki International University Japan

Nancy Ornelas-Soto and Oracio Barbosa-García
Centro de Investigaciones en Óptica, León, Gto.

Pedro L. Lopez-de-Alba
Departamento de Química. Universidad de Guanajuato. Gto. México

Hiroyuki Tanaka
Faculty of Pharmaceutical Sciences, Kyushu University Japan

Sigrid Mennickent, Marta de Diego, Mario Vega and Carmen Gloria Godoy
Faculty of Pharmacy, University of Concepción, Concepción Chile

Zhang Zhen
Center for Drug Evaluation, State Food and Drug Administration, Beijing
Shenyang Pharmaceutical University, Shenyang, Liaoning, China

Bi Kaishun
Shenyang Pharmaceutical University, Shenyang, Liaoning, China

Chih-Sheng Chen, Ruey-Shyang Hseu and Ching-Tsan Huang
National Taiwan University, Taipei Taiwan, Republic of China

Kapil Kalra
Dev Bhoomi Institute of Pharmacy and Research, Dehradun, Uttarakhand, India

Zhang Yongyu, Sun Shujun, Dai Jianye, Wang Wenyu, Cao Huijuan, Wu Jianbing and Gou Xiaojun
Shanghai University of Traditional Chinese Medicine P.R. China

Ahmed Badr Eldin
Sigma Pharmaceutical Corp., Egypt

A. Coşkun Dalgiç and K. Bülent Belibağli
Department of Food Engineering, University of Gaziantep, Gaziantep

Hasan Vardin
Department of Food Engineering, University of Harran, Şanlıurfa, Turkey

José Otávio Carréra Silva Júnior, Roseane Maria Ribeiro Costa, Francisco Martins Teixeira and Wagner Luiz Ramos Barbosa
Universidade Federal do Pará, Instituto de Ciências da Saúde, Faculdade de Farmácia Rua Augusto Corrêa n. 1, Cidade Universitária Professor José da Silveira Neto, CEP: 66.075-110, Belém-Pa, Brazil

Samuele E. Burastero
San Raffaele Scientific Institute, via Olgettina, 58, Milan Italy

Osamu Morinaga
Faculty of Pharmaceutical Sciences, Nagasaki International University, Japan

Xiao-Wei Li
School of Pharmaceutical Sciences, Peking University, China

Shunsuke Fujii
Graduate School of Health Management, Nagasaki International University, Japan

Ana Paola Cione, Edivan Tonhi and Paulo Silva
Bioagri Laboratórios Brazil

Index

www.ingramcontent.com/pod-product-compliance
Lightning Source LLC
LaVergne TN
LVHW080639210926
848485LV00003B/297
* 9 7 8 1 6 3 9 8 9 1 3 6 8 *